Parkinson's Disease

METHODS IN MOLECULAR MEDICINE™

John M. Walker, Series Editor

68. **Molecular Analysis of Cancer,** edited by *Jacqueline Boultwood and Carrie Fidler,* 2002
67. **Meningococcal Disease:** *Methods and Protocols,* edited by *Andrew J. Pollard and Martin C. J. Maiden,* 2001
66. **Meningococcal Vaccines:** *Methods and Protocols,* edited by *Andrew J. Pollard and Martin C. J. Maiden,* 2001
65. **Nonviral Vectors for Gene Therapy:** *Methods and Protocols,* edited by *Mark A, Findeis,* 2001
64. **Dendritic Cell Protocols,** edited by *Stephen P. Robinson and Andrew J. Stagg,* 2001
63. **Hematopoietic Stem Cell Protocols,** edited by *Christopher A. Klug and Craig T. Jordan,* 2001
62. **Parkinson's Disease: *Methods and Protocols,*** edited by *M. Maral Mouradian,* 2001
61. **Melanoma Techniques and Protocols: *Molecular Diagnosis, treatment, and Monitoring,*** edited by *Brian J. Nickoloff,* 2001
60. **Interleukin Protocols,** edited by *Luke A. J. O'Neill and Andrew Bowie,* 2001
59. **Molecular Pathology of the Prions,** edited by *Harry F. Baker,* 2001
58. **Metastasis Research Protocols: *Volume 2, Cell Behavior In Vitro and In Vivo,*** edited by *Susan A. Brooks and Udo Schumacher,* 2001
57. **Metastasis Research Protocols: *Volume 1, Analysis of Cells and Tissues,*** edited by *Susan A. Brooks and Udo Schumacher,* 2001
56. **Human Airway Inflammation:** *Sampling Techniques and Analytical Protocols,* edited by *Duncan F. Rogers and Louise E. Donnelly,* 2001
55. **Hematologic Malignancies:** *Methods and Protocols,* edited by *Guy B. Faguet,* 2001
54. ***Mycobacterium tuberculosis* Protocols,** edited by *Tanya Parish and Neil G. Stoker,* 2001
53. **Renal Cancer:** *Methods and Protocols,* edited by *Jack H. Mydlo,* 2001
52. **Atherosclerosis: *Experimental Methods and Protocols,*** edited by *Angela F. Drew,* 2001
51. **Angiotensin Protocols,** edited by *Donna H. Wang,* 2001
50. **Colorectal Cancer: *Methods and Protocols*,** edited by *Steven M. Powell,* 2001
49. **Molecular Pathology Protocols,** edited by *Anthony A. Killeen,* 2001
48. **Antibiotic Resistance Methods and Protocols,** edited by *Stephen H. Gillespie,* 2001
47. **Vision Research Protocols,** edited by *P. Elizabeth Rakoczy,* 2001
46. **Angiogenesis Protocols,** edited by *J. Clifford Murray,* 2001
45. **Hepatocellular Carcinoma: *Methods and Protocols*, edited by** *Nagy A. Habib,* 2000
44. **Asthma: *Mechanisms and Protocols*, edited by** *K. Fan Chung and Ian Adcock,* 2001
43. **Muscular Dystrophy: *Methods and Protocols,* edited by** *Katherine B. Bushby and Louise Anderson,* 2001
42. **Vaccine Adjuvants: *Preparation Methods and Research Protocols*,** edited by *Derek T. O'Hagan,* 2000
41. **Celiac Disease: *Methods and Protocols*,** edited by *Michael N. Marsh,* 2000
40. **Diagnostic and Therapeutic Antibodies,** edited by *Andrew J. T. George and Catherine E. Urch,* 2000
39. **Ovarian Cancer: *Methods and Protocols*,** edited by *John M. S. Bartlett,* 2000
38. **Aging Methods and Protocols,** edited by *Yvonne A. Barnett and Christopher R. Barnett,* 2000
37. **Electrochemotherapy, Electrogenetherapy, and Transdermal Drug Delivery:** *Electrically Mediated Delivery of Molecules to Cells*, edited by *Mark J. Jaroszeski, Richard Heller, and Richard Gilbert,* 2000
36. **Septic Shock Methods and Protocols,** edited by *Thomas J. Evans,* 2000
35. **Gene Therapy of Cancer: *Methods and Protocols*,** edited by *Wolfgang Walther and Ulrike Stein,* 2000

METHODS IN MOLECULAR MEDICINE™

Parkinson's Disease

Methods and Protocols

Edited by

M. Maral Mouradian, MD

National Institute of Neurological Disorders and Stroke
National Institutes of Health, Bethesda, MD

Humana Press Totowa, New Jersey

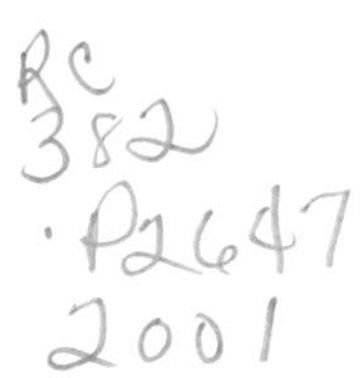

999 Riverview Drive, Suite 208
Totowa, New Jersey 07512

This publication is printed on acid-free paper. ∞

ANSI Z39.48-1984 (American Standards Institute) Permanence of Paper for Printed Library Materials.

Cover design by Patricia F. Cleary.

Cover illustration: Immunolabeling of synthetic α-synuclein filaments and filaments extracted from dementia with Lewy bodies and multiple system atrophy brains (*see* full caption for Fig. 10 on page 47).

For additional copies, pricing for bulk purchases, and/or information about other Humana titles, contact Humana at the above address or at any of the following numbers: Tel: 973-256-1699; Fax: 973-256-8341; E-mail: humana@humanapr.com, or visit our Website at www.humanapress.com

Printed in the United States of America. 10 9 8 7 6 5 4 3 2 1

Library of Congress Cataloging-in-Publication Data

Parkinson's disease: methods and protocols/edited by Maral Mouradian.
p. cm.--(Methods in molecular medicine; v. 62)
Includes bibliographical references and index.
ISBN 0-89603-761-4 (alk. paper)
1. Parkinson's Disease--Laboratory manuals. 2. Pathology, Molecular--Laboratory manuals. I. Mouradian, Maral M. II. Methods in molecular medicine (Totowa, N.J.); v. 62.
RC382.P2647 2001
616.8'33--dc21

00-047142

Preface

Parkinson's disease is a progressive neurodegenerative disorder characterized clinically by tremor, rigidity, slow movements, and postural instability. Pathologically, dopaminergic neurons of the substantia nigra bear the brunt of the degeneration, though other neuronal groups can be affected as well. Although Parkinson's disease is the only neurodegenerative disorder for which effective therapies are available, these treatment options are only symptomatic, do not influence the underlying degenerative process, and are associated with a high incidence of complications, particularly with their long-term use. The progressive nature of the disease and the limitations of its palliative therapies result in significant functional impairment. The chronic disability and the increased prevalence of the disease with the prolongation of life expectancy in developed countries make the social and economic impact of this disease quite high. Fortunately, systematic basic and clinical research in this disease has yielded major new advances that render patients' hopes for a cure considerably closer to reality.

The application of molecular biologic methodologies in the study of Parkinson's disease has begun to have a major impact only in recent years. Consequently, the utility of these technologies is largely in the research arena, although their clinical applications are now being realized. Therefore, the goal of *Parkinson's Disease: Methods and Protocols* is to introduce scientists and clinicians interested in Parkinson's disease, in particular, and neurodegenerative diseases, in general, to the progress and potential of molecular biology and genetics in unraveling the mysteries of these disorders and in devising innovative therapeutic strategies. The timeliness of this subject stems from the recent explosion of information about the genetic etiologies of Parkinson's disease. Naturally, these findings have sparked tremendous research interest and multiplied opportunities to elucidate the molecular pathogenesis of this disease. In addition, advances in cellular and molecular biology have fueled the need to develop new and improved therapeutic modalities for this disorder.

Genetic discoveries in pedigrees with familial Parkinson's disease have revolutionized our concept of this disorder. These findings have now made it clear that Parkinson's disease is not a single disorder. Rather it represents multiple underlying defects with similar clinical phenotypes. This etiologic disparity, in fact, demands the pursuit of many different research hypotheses about the molecular pathogenesis of the disease and requires the use of varied experimental tools.

In short, these genetic discoveries constitute the ground work for the next set of important questions in this field, namely, how these genetic defects result in the death of dopaminergic neurons and how to prevent or slow this process.

Parkinson's Disease: Methods and Protocols covers the main basic research disciplines and molecular methodologies that are actively being pursued in studies of Parkinson's disease. It compiles state-of-the-art molecular methods that are currently being used to advance our understanding of the etiologies and pathogenesis of the neurodegeneration in this disorder. This book also provides a concise and comprehensive review of the background and significance of each protocol described in order to give the reader a fundamental understanding of the subject matter and its implications.

Four broad fields relevant to Parkinson's disease are covered in this book. Part I, Genetics, describes the two established gene defects known to cause this disease, namely, missense mutations in the α-synuclein gene, which result in autosomal dominant disease, and deletions or point mutations in the parkin gene, which lead to autosomal recessive disease. Part II, Molecular Pathogenetic Studies, describes several recent biochemical hypotheses and findings thought to be important in the death of nigral dopaminergic neurons. These include experiments to elucidate biochemical and structural changes that result from α-synuclein mutations, characterization of apoptotic dopaminergic neurons, and investigating the role of nitric oxide and oxidative stress in the death of these neurons. Part III, Molecular Aspects of Basal Ganglia Function, describes methods used to study various aspects of the nigrostriatal neural circuitry, including quantification of tyrosine hydroxylase mRNA, immunochemical studies of dopamine transporters, transcription control mechanisms for dopamine receptor genes, in situ hybridization for genes expressed in the basal ganglia, and the functional regulation of NMDA receptors in striatal medium spiny neurons in experimental parkinsonism. Lastly, Part IV, Molecular Therapies, describes novel experimental treatment approaches that have been tested recently in animal models of Parkinson's disease, including intracerebral delivery of trophic factors, grafting genetically engineered cells into the striatum using either naked cells or encapsulated implants, and the use of neural stem cells.

We hope that *Parkinson's Disease: Methods and Protocols* will enhance the awareness of the scientific and medical communities about recent landmark discoveries in Parkinson's disease. This book makes currently employed research protocols readily available under one cover for scientists who plan to enter this field. We trust this will attract new investigators to study Parkinson's disease and, therefore, accelerate the progress toward a cure.

***M. Maral Mouradian,** MD*

Contents

Contributors

PATRICK AEBISCHER • *Division of Surgical Research and Gene Therapy Center, Lausanne University Medical School, Lausanne, Switzerland*

RICHARD J. E. ARMSTRONG • *Cambridge Centre for Brain Repair, Cambridge, United Kingdom*

KRYS S. BANKIEWICZ • *Molecular Therapeutics Section, Laboratory of Molecular Medicine and Neuroscience, National Institute of Neurological Disorders and Stroke, National Institutes of Health, Bethesda, MD*

ROGER A. BARKER • *Cambridge Centre for Brain Repair and Department of Neurology, University of Cambridge, Cambridge, United Kingdom*

ARI BARZILAI • *Department of Neurochemistry, The George Wise Faculty of Life Sciences, Tel-Aviv University, Tel-Aviv, Israel*

ROBERT E. BURKE • *Departments of Neurology and Pathology, Columbia University, The College of Physicians and Surgeons, New York, NY*

MARC G. CARON • *Departments of Cell Biology and Medicine, Howard Hughes Medical Institute, Duke University Medical Center, Durham, NC*

R. ANTHONY CROWTHER • *Medical Research Council, Laboratory of Molecular Biology, Cambridge, United Kingdom*

TED M. DAWSON • *Departments of Neurology and Neuroscience, Johns Hopkins University School of Medicine, Baltimore, MD*

NOAM DRIGUES • *Faculty of Medicine and Department of Pharmacology, Technion, Haifa, Israel*

STEPHEN B. DUNNETT • *Cambridge Centre for Brain Repair, Forvie Site, Cambridge; School of Biosciences, Cardiff University, Cardiff, United Kingdom*

DENNIS D. ELSBERRY • *Medtronic Neurological, Minneapolis, MN*

RAUL R. GAINETDINOV • *Departments of Cell Biology and Medicine, Howard Hughes Medical Institute, Duke University Medical Center, Durham, NC*

DON M. GASH • *Department of Anatomy and Neurobiology, University of Kentucky Medical Center, Lexington, KY*

GREG A. GERHARDT • *Department of Psychiatry and Pharmacology, University of Colorado Health Sciences Center, Denver, CO*

MICHEL GOEDERT • *Medical Research Council, Laboratory of Molecular Biology, Cambridge, United Kingdom*

RICHARD GRONDIN • *Department of Anatomy and Neurobiology, University of Kentucky Medical Center, Lexington, KY*

YOSHINOBU HARA • *Laboratory of Molecular Neurobiology, Human Gene Sciences Center, Tokyo Medical and Dental University, Bunkyo-ku, Tokyo, Japan*

NOBUTAKA HATTORI • *Department of Neurology, Juntendo University School of Medicine, Bunkyo, Tokyo, Japan*

HIROSHI ICHINOSE • *Institute for Comprehensive Medical Science, Graduate School of Medicine, Fujita Health University, Tokoake, Aichi, Japan*

HIDEHITO INAGAKI • *Institute for Comprehensive Medical Science, Graduate School of Medicine, Fujita Health University, Tokoake, Aichi, Japan*

ROSS JAKES • *Medical Research Council, Laboratory of Molecular Biology, Cambridge, United Kingdom*

POUL HENNING JENSEN • *Department of Medical Biochemistry, University of Aarhus, Denmark*

CLAAS-HINRICH LAMMERS • *Department of Psychiatry and Psychotherapy, University of Luebeck, Luebeck, Germany*

SANG-HYEON LEE • *Department of Bioscience and Biotechnology, Silla University, Sasang-gu, Pusan, Korea*

ALLAN I. LEVEY • *Department of Neurology, Emory University School of Medicine, Atlanta, GA*

EUGENE O. MAJOR • *Molecular Therapeutics Section, Laboratory of Molecular Medicine and Neuroscience, National Institute of Neurological Disorders and Stroke, National Institutes of Health, Bethesda, MD*

SILVIA MANDEL • *Faculty of Medicine and Department of Pharmacology, Technion, Haifa, Israel*

HIROTO MATSUMINE • *Department of Neurology, Juntendo University School of Medicine, Bunkyo-ku, Tokyo, Japan*

ELDAD MELAMED • *Department of Neurology, Tel Aviv University, Rabin Medical Center, Campus Beilinson, Petah-Tiqva, Israel*

GARY W. MILLER • *Division of Pharmacology and Toxicology, College of Pharmacy, University of Texas at Austin, Austin, TX*

YOSHIKUNI MIZUNO • *Department of Neurology, Juntendo University School of Medicine, Bunkyo-ku, Tokyo, Japan*

M. MARAL MOURADIAN • *Genetic Pharmacology Unit, Experimental Therapeutics Branch, National Institute of Neurological Disorders and Stroke, National Institutes of Health, Bethesda, MD*

TOSHIHARU NAGATSU • *Institute for Comprehensive Medical Science, Graduate School of Medicine, Fujita Health University, Tokoake, Aichi, Japan*

Daniel Offen • *Department of Neurology, Rabin Medical Center, Petah-Tiqva, Israel*

Justin D. Oh • *Experimental Therapeutics Branch, National Institute of Neurological Disorders and Stroke, National Institutes of Health, Bethesda, MD*

Tamae Ohye • *Institute for Comprehensive Medical Science, Graduate School of Medicine, Fujita Health University, Tokoake, Aichi, Japan*

Tinmarla F. Oo • *Department of Pathology, Columbia University, The College of Physicians and Surgeons, New York, NY*

Abbas Parsian • *Department of Molecular and Cellular Biology, University of Louisville Health Sciences Center, Louisville, KY*

Joel S. Perlmutter • *Department of Neurology, Washington University School of Medicine, St. Louis, MO*

Phillip Pivirotto • *Molecular Therapeutics Section, Laboratory of Molecular Medicine and Neuroscience, National Institute of Neurological Disorders and Stroke, National Institutes of Health, Bethesda, MD*

Serge Przedborski • *Departments of Neurology and Pathology, Columbia University, New York, NY*

Anne E. Rosser • *Cambridge Centre for Brain Repair and Department of Neurology, University of Cambridge, Cambridge, United Kingdom*

Rosario Sanchez-Pernaute • *Molecular Therapeutics Section, Laboratory of Molecular Medicine and Neuroscience, National Institute of Neurological Disorders and Stroke, National Institutes of Health, Bethesda, MD*

Anat Shirvan • *Department of Neurology, Rabin Medical Center, Petah-Tiqva, Israel*

Maria Grazia Spillantini • *Cambridge Centre for Brain Repair; Department of Neurology, University of Cambridge, Cambridge, United Kingdom*

Takahiro Suzuki • *Institute for Comprehensive Medical Science, Graduate School of Medicine, Fujita Health University, Tokoake, Aichi, Japan*

Jack L. Tseng • *Division of Surgical Research and Gene Therapy Center, Lausanne University Medical School, Lausanne, Switzerland*

Yan-Min Wang • *Departments of Cell Biology and Medicine, Howard Hughes Medical Institute, Duke University Medical Center, Durham, NC*

Moussa B. H. Youdim • *Faculty of Medicine and Department of Pharmacology, Technion, Haifa, Israel*

Zhiming Zhang • *Department of Anatomy and Neurobiology, University of Kentucky Medical Center, Lexington, KY*

Ilan Ziv • *Department of Neurology, Rabin Medical Center, Petah-Tiqva, Israel*

I

Genetics

1

Point Mutations in the α-*Synuclein* Gene

Abbas Parsian and Joel S. Perlmutter

1. Introduction

Idiopathic Parkinson's disease (PD) is an age-dependent, neurodegenerative disorder and is predominantly sporadic. Only 20–30% of patients have a positive family history for PD with a complex mode of inheritance. In a few extended families, the disease is inherited as an autosomal dominant trait. Linkage to chromosome 4 was reported in a large Italian kindred multiply affected by an early-onset form of PD *(1)*. However, this finding was not replicated in a sample of 94 Caucasian families by Scott et al. *(2)*, or in 13 multigenerational families by Gasser et al. *(3)*. It has recently been demonstrated that a mutation within the *a-synuclein* gene on chromosome 4 segregates with disease in the Italian family *(4)*. It was further demonstrated that the same missense mutation was also present in three Greek families with early onset PD. Sequence analysis of exon 4 of the gene revealed a single base pair change at position 209 from G to A (G209A). This mutation results in an Ala to Thr substitution at position 53 of the protein (Ala53Thr) and creates a Tsp45I restriction site *(4)*. This is the first report of a mutation causing clinically and pathologically defined idiopathic PD associated with the critical pathologic finding, the intraneuronal inclusions called Lewy bodies in brainstem nuclei including the substantia nigra. However, Krüger et al. *(5)* reported a G→C transversion at position 88 of the coding sequence in two sibs and the deceased mother in a German family. It was concluded that this mutation is the cause of PD in this family.

More recently, Papadimitriou et al. *(6)* reported two additional Greek families with autosomal dominant PD associated with the G209A mutation in the α-*synuclein* gene. These families are clinically similar to other PD families with the mutation in the α-*synuclein* gene since they also have early onset, infrequent resting tremor, relatively rapid progression, and excellent response

From: *Methods in Molecular Medicine, vol. 62: Parkinson's Disease: Methods and Protocols*
Edited by: M. M. Mouradian © Humana Press Inc., Totowa, NJ

to levodopa. Asymptomatic carriers older than the expected age of onset were identified in both families. Therefore, it was concluded that the issue of incomplete penetrance or the early age of onset needs to be reevaluated.

To determine the involvement of the α-*synuclein* gene in the etiology of PD in our sample, 83 PD subjects with a positive family history were screened for the G→A mutation at position 209 in exon 4 by polymerase chain reaction (PCR) assay *(7)*. None of our subjects carried this mutation. The exons of the α-*synuclein* gene were sequenced from 20 patients with a positive family history for PD to determine whether there were other mutations in the gene that might cosegregate in our families. No mutation was found in any exons of the gene in these subjects, confirming our mutation analysis for exon 4. However, we did detect an A→G neutral polymorphism in intron 5 of the gene. The polymorphism creates a *Mnl*I site (G). The frequency of this polymorphism is 0.56 (G) and 0.44 (A) based on 24 individuals. The direct PCR sequencing protocol used in this study included several major steps, namely, PCR amplification of the candidate region (exons); cycle sequencing using D-rhodamine terminator (PE Applied Biosystems), and capillary electrophoresis using an ABI Sequencer 310 (PE Applied Biosystems). These steps are described in detail in the Methods section.

2. Materials

The materials used in the following methods are divided into three categories based on the requirements of the different methods. Some of the required reagents overlap among the different methods.

2.1. PCR Reagents

These reagents are needed to amplify genomic DNA for sequencing or mutation screening.

1. PCR buffer: 5X PCR buffer consists of 250 m*M* KCl, 50 m*M* Tris-HCl, pH 8.3, and 7.5 m*M* $MgCl_2$ (all from Sigma). To make 100 mL of the buffer, mix: 12.5 mL 2 *M* KCl, 5.0 mL 1 *M* Tris-HCl, pH 8.3, 0.75 mL 1 *M* $MgCl_2$. Stir well and store in –20°C freezer in 10-mL centrifuge tubes.
2. DNTPs (nucleotide triphosphate mix of A, T, C, G) from Boehringer Mannheim.
3. DNA Taq polymerase (Promega).
4. Dimethylsulfoxide (DMSO; Sigma).
5. Ethidium bromide (Sigma).
6. TBE buffer: This buffer is made as 20X 3:1 which consists of 324.6 g Tris Base (Sigma), 55.0 g boric acid (Sigma), 5.0 mL 0.5 *M* EDTA (Sigma), and 995 mL ddH2O. Stir until completely dissolved and store at room temperature. When ready to use, make 1X dilution with ddH2O.
7. Agarose (Sigma).

2.2. Sequencing Reagents

These reagents are specific for direct sequencing of PCR products using an ABI Genetic Analyzer. Other sequencing kits available may require optimization.

1. Low melting temperature agarose (Gibco-BRL).
2. Qiaquick PCR Purification Kit (Qiagen).
3. Wizard PCR Prep DNA Purification Kit (Promega).
4. ABI Cycle Sequencing Kit (PE Applied Biosystems).
5. ABI POP-6 polymer (PE Applied Biosystems).
6. Deionized formamide (PE Applied Biosystems).
7. Ficoll loading dye: 0.25% bromophenol blue, 0.25% xylene cyanol, 15% Ficoll Type 400, and 100 m*M* EDTA.
8. 3-mL Syringe (Fisher).

2.3. Mutation Screening Reagents

These reagents are required for mutation screening of the α-*synuclein* gene (G209A). All except the restriction enzyme could be used for other mutations in the gene.

1. Restriction enzyme Tsp45I (New England Biolabs).
2. Ethidium bromide.
3. TBE buffer: Described in **Subheading 2.1, item 6.**
4. Polyacrylamide gel (Sequagel, National Diagnostics).

3. Methods

The methods used in screening for new mutations in candidate genes are cycle sequencing and PCR assay following a digestion with restriction enzyme. The major steps are described below.

3.1. Designing Primers

Primers are short oligonucleotides (20–25 base pairs) that initiate DNA amplification. The first step in amplification of any genomic region is to design the primers to produce PCR products that are maximally specific for the desired stretch of DNA. Since DNA amplification is sensitive to the conditions of the PCR, it is important to identify optimal conditions for the reaction. We have been successful in designing primers for sequencing exons of genes using the 'PRIMER' computer program developed by Eric Lander (personal communication). The major steps in designing primers are as follows:

1. The sequence of the DNA template needs to be provided as a file.
2. The program then designs more than 100 forward and reverse primers and selects the best pair based on preselected criteria. Forward primers duplicate DNA from the 5' to the 3' end of the strand, and reverse primers duplicate the strand in the opposite direction. Forward and corresponding reverse primer pairs are used together to limit the length of the amplified segment.

3. The program also provides the optimal temperature conditions for the PCR, thereby substantially reducing the time for reaction optimization.
4. Based on our experience, sequencing PCR products in the range of 200–350 bp is more accurate, efficient, and cost effective than longer PCR products in screening subjects for new mutations.
5. The sequence of most cloned genes is available on the GeneBank database at the National Center for Biotechnology Information (NCBI) and can easily be obtained through the Web site http://www.ncbi.nlm.nih.gov.
6. To sequence the entire exon efficiently, the target template should cover at least 50 bp of intronic sequence on each side of the exon.

3.2. Sequencing of Exons

The direct sequencing protocol routinely used in our laboratory includes several major steps *(8)*, namely, PCR amplification of the candidate exons; cycle sequencing using D-rhodamine terminator (PE Applied Biosystems); and capillary electrophoresis using an ABI 310 Genetic Analyzer (PE Applied Biosystems).

3.2.1. PCR Amplification of Candidate Regions

1. Genomic DNA from subjects is amplified with primers corresponding to intronic sequences flanking each exon.
2. The PCR reactions usually include 250 ng genomic DNA, 1X PCR buffer, 250 μ*M* of each dNTP, 2.5 U Taq DNA polymerase, and 10 μ*M* of each primer in a total volume of 100 μL.
3. The reaction mix is denatured at 94°C for 5 min in a Perkin-Elmer-Cetus 9600 thermal cycler (Norwalk, CT). This will be followed by 30 cycles of denaturation at 94°C for 1 min, annealing at 55°C for 45 s, and extension at 72°C for 45 s with a final extension of 10 min at 72°C.
4. To check the quality of the PCR product, 5 μL of the reaction is loaded on a 1.5% agarose gel, electrophoresed for 1 h, stained with ethidium bromide, and visualized with UV transillumination.

3.2.2. Purification of PCR Products

Based on the quality and specificity of the PCR product on the gel (as described above), two approaches could be used to purify the product. If the PCR product is highly specific with few or no nonspecific bands, a Qiaquick PCR purification kit could be used. However, if there are nonspecific bands, then gel purification followed by column purification is needed. This is a critical step since the nonspecific products will degrade the quality of DNA sequencing due to their addition in the reaction mixture and their potential hybridization with the sequencing primers.

3.2.2.1. Gel Purification of PCR Products

1. Prepare 1% low melting temperature agarose gel (Gibco-BRL) in 1X TBE buffer with large wells (8 X 1.0 mm) that would hold 50 μL of the PCR product.
2. Mix the PCR product with 8 μL of 9X loading Ficoll dye and load the entire sample onto the gel. The electrophoresis voltage should not exceed 65 V since it would melt the gel.
3. Stain the gel with ethidium bromide. Under long-wavelength ultraviolet (UV; 365 nm; *see* **Note 1**) transillumination, excise each band and place it in a 1.5-mL microfuge tube.
4. Incubate the samples at 70°C until the agarose is completely melted. Then, add 1 mL of resin to the melted agarose and mix thoroughly by hand (do not vortex; *see* **Note 2**).
5. For each PCR sample, prepare one Wizard Minicolumn (Promega), remove and set aside the plunger from a 3-mL disposable syringe, and attach the syringe barrel provided to the extension of each Minicolumn.
6. Pipet the resin/DNA mix into the syringe barrel, insert the syringe plunger slowly, and gently push the slurry into the Minicolumn with the syringe plunger.
7. Detach the syringe from the Minicolumn, remove the plunger, and reattach the syringe barrel to the Minicolumn.
8. Pipet 2 mL of 80% isopropanol into the syringe to wash the column, insert the plunger into the syringe, and gently push the isopropanol through the Minicolumn.
9. Remove the syringe and transfer the Minicolumn to a 1.5-mL microcentrifuge tube and centrifuge for 20 s at 12,000*g* to dry the resin.
10. Transfer the Minicolumn to a new microcentrifuge tube, apply 50 μL water or TE buffer to the Minicolumn, and wait 1 min. Then, centrifuge the Minicolumn for 20 s at 12,000*g* to elute the bound DNA fragment.
11. Remove and discard the Minicolumn. The purified DNA may be stored in the microcentrifuge tube at 4°C or –20°C.

3.2.2.2. Column Purification of PCR Product

As mentioned above, if the PCR products are very specific, they could be purified using a Qiaquick PCR purification kit (Qiagen) without the gel purification step. The reagents and protocol are included in the kit. Briefly,

1. Add buffer PB to your PCR product in the microcentrifuge tube at a 5:1 ratio. Place a Qiaquick spin column in the 2-mL collection tube provided and add your sample to the column.
2. Centrifuge at 8500*g* (13,000 rpm) for 1 min. During this process the DNA binds to the column. Discard the flow-through buffer and place the column back into the same tube.
3. Add 0.75 mL buffer PE to the column and centrifuge as above for 1 min to wash the DNA. Discard the flow-through buffer and put the column back in the same tube.

4. Centrifuge the column at 14,000 rpm speed for an additional minute. Place the column in a clean 1.5-mL microfuge tube.
5. Add 50 µL buffer EB (10 m*M* Tris-HCl, pH 8.5) or water to the center of the column and centrifuge as above for 1 min to elute the DNA from the column. To increase the DNA concentration, add less buffer EB to the column and let stand for 1 min before centrifugation.

3.2.3. Cycle Sequencing

The second step is the cycle sequencing reaction, which includes 8 µL D-rhodamine dye terminator premix (PE Applied Biosystems), 5 pmole forward primer, and DNA template (PCR products, 50–100 ng) in a total volume of 20 µL.

1. Denature the mixture at 96°C for 1 min, and is followed by 20–30 cycles of 96°C for 30 s, 45°C for 15 sec, and 60°C for 4 min in a Perkin-Elmer-Cetus 9600 thermal cycler.
2. Then stop the sequencing reactions by precipitation with 2 m*M* $MgCl_2$ and 95% cold (–20°C) ethanol for 15 min on ice (*see* **Note 3**).
3. Centrifuge the precipitates, dry the pellets, and add 25 µL of template suppression reagent (TSR) to each reaction.
4. Mix the reactions thoroughly and heat at 95°C for 2 min. Chill them on ice and keep on ice until loaded on an ABI 310 Genetic Analyzer.

3.2.4. Installing the Syringe and the Capillary

Since every capillary electrophoresis system has different features and since manufacturers provide detailed step-by-step instructions for preparation of gels and samples, we only briefly describe the major steps for the ABI 310 Genetic Analyzer used in our *α-synuclein* sequencing project.

1. Equilibrate the POP-6 polymer (PE Applied Biosystems) at room temperature, fill the syringe manually (1 mL), and remove the air bubbles (*see* **Note 4**). Clean the syringe and place in the instrument.
2. Install the capillary system and secure to the heat plate with a piece of tape. The autosampler must be calibrated every time the capillary is changed.
3. Samples are prepared by mixing 1 µL of sequencing products with 12 µL of deionized formamide and 0.5 µL of size standards in sample tubes for 48- or 96-well trays.
4. Seal the sample tubes, denature at 95°C for 3 min, and cool quickly in an ice-water bath.

3.2.5. Sequence Analysis

The sequence analysis procedure described here is for the ABI 310 Genetic Analyzer. This process is usually performed in two steps. The first step is base calling or reading to determine the sequence of the samples using the sequencing software installed on the ABI sequencer. The second step is sequence alignment with published sequences using the BLAST software programs.

The first step includes the following:

1. Start by using the FACTURA program and specify the gel matrix, then add sequences to the batch worksheet, submit the batch worksheet, save the results, print, and save the batch report.
2. This software is also used to enter multiple sample files from the same run or different runs into a batch worksheet and process all samples in the batch worksheet at one time.
3. The important variables that must be considered in this step are the signal-to-noise ratio, variation in peak heights, and irregular migration of the sample on the gel.

The next step is sequence analysis using the NAVIGATOR software. This software can align multiple sequences using a Clustal alignment algorithm. The process involves several steps that include the following:

1. Opening a layout and importing a batch worksheet, producing reverse/complimentary sequences, aligning multiple sequences, displaying electropherograms for ambiguous bases, creating a consensus sequence, saving the layout, saving the changes to individual sequence files, and printing the layout.
2. These steps are detailed in the manuals of every sequencer and are specific for a particular instrument. After the sequence of a sample is determined, it is matched with known sequences deposited in GeneBank.

3.3. Mutation Analysis of α-Synuclein

In general, mutations in a gene are identified by sequence analysis. However, if the sequence variant creates or destroys a restriction enzyme site, then PCR followed by digestion can be used to screen larger samples of patients and controls. In this case, primer pairs that are designed for amplification of exons in the sequencing phase will be used. If no restriction enzyme site is altered, a mismatch primer can be created so that PCR and a restriction digestion can be used for screening. In the latter approach, one of the previously designed primers and a mismatched primer will be used for any particular exon with a mutation.

1. The G→A mutation at bp 209 described in the Italian PD kindred creates a *Tsp*45I restriction site, which is used to detect the variant. The primers published by Polymeropoulos et al. *(4)* are used to amplify exon 4 of the *α-synuclein* gene, and the product is genotyped by restriction enzyme *Tsp*45I digestion following PCR.
2. The PCR reaction includes 5% DMSO, 250 μ*M* dNTP, 10 pmol of each primer, 50 ng genomic DNA, and 0.5 U Taq polymerase (Promega) in PCR buffer.
3. The PCR reactions are denatured for 5 min at 94°C followed by 30 cycles of 94°C for 1 min, 56°C for 45 s, and 72°C for 45 s with a final extension at 72°C for 5 min. PCR cycling is performed with a Perkin-Elmer-Cetus 9600 thermocycler (any other thermal cycler could be used instead).
4. The PCR products are digested with *Tsp*45I at 65°C for several hours.

5. The products are electrophoresed on 8% nondenaturing polyacrylamide gel (*see* **Note 5**), stained with ethidium bromide, visualized under UV light, and photographed by the UVP Image-Store 7500 system.

4. Notes

1. It is very important to use either long-wavelength UV or a fluorescent transilluminator so that the DNA is not damaged.
2. Work quickly because repolymerization of the agarose gel/resin mix will decrease the yield.
3. Cleaning the sequencing reaction product by ethanol precipitation will result in loss of the first 50 bases immediately following the sequencing primer. Cleaning with spin column purification will provide sequence data within 5 bases of the sequencing primer.
4. Do not use the polymer that has been on the instrument for more than 3 d.
5. Based on the fragment size of the digested PCR product, a 2–3% agarose gel could also be used to separate the fragments. The advantage of agarose is its nontoxic nature.

Acknowledgments

This work was supported by NIH grants AA09515, MH31302, and NS-31001, the Greater St. Louis Chapter of the American Parkinson's Disease Association, the Robert & Mary Bronstein Foundation, the Clinical Hypotheses Research Section of the Charles A. Dana Foundation, and the McDonnell Center for Higher Brain Function.

References

1. Polymeropoulos, M. H., Higgins, J. J., Golbe, L. J., Johnson, W. G., Ide, S. E., Di Iorio, G., et al. (1996) Mapping of a gene for Parkinson's Disease to chromosome 4q21-q23. *Science* **274,** 1197–1199.
2. Scott, Wk, Stajich, J. M., Yamaoka, L. H., Spur, M. C., Vance, J. M., Roses, A. D., et al. (1997) Genetic complexity and Parkinson's disease. *Science* **277,** 387.
3. Gasser, T., Muller-Myhsok, B., Wszolek, Z. K., Dhrr, A., and Vaughan, J. R. (1997) Genetic complexity and Parkinson's disease. *Science* **277,** 388-390.
4. Polymeropoulos, M. H., Lavedan, C., Leroy, E., Ide, S. E., et al., (1997) Mutation in the α-synuclein gene identified in families with Parkinson's disease. *Science* **276,** 2045–2047.
5. Kruger, R., Kuhn, W., Muller, T., Woitalla, D., Graeber, M., Kosel, S., et al. (1998) Ala30 Pro mutation in the gene encoding α-synuclein in Parkinson's Disease. *Nature Genet.* **18,** 106–108.
6. Papadimitriou, A., Veletza, V., Hadjigeorgiou, G. M., Partikiou, A., Hirano, M., and Anastasopoulos, I. (1999) Mutated α-synuclein gene in two Greek kindreds with familial PD: Incomplete penetrance? *Neurology* **52,** 651–654.

7. Parsian, A., Racette, B., Zhang, Z. H., Chakraverty, S., Rundle, M., Goate, A., et al. (1998) Mutation, sequence analysis, and association studies of α-synuclein in Parkinson's disease. *Neurology* **51,** 1757–1759.
8. Parsian, A. (1999) Sequence analysis of exon eight of MAOA gene in alcoholics with antisocial personality and normal controls. *Genomics* **55,** 290–295.

2

Autosomal Recessive Juvenile Parkinsonism (AR-JP): Genetic Diagnosis

Hiroto Matsumine, Nobutaka Hattori, and Yoshikuni Mizuno

1. Introduction

Autosomal recessive juvenile parkinsonism (AR-JP) is a familial levodopa-responsive parkinsonism resulting from Lewy body negative degeneration of nigral neurons in the zona compacta of the substantia nigra *(1–4)*. The first proposal for a distinct clinical entity with recessively inherited parkinsonism was made in Japan and was termed "paralysis agitans with marked diurnal fluctuations of symptoms" *(1)*. This syndrome was later designated as autosomal recessive form of juvenile parkinsonism *(2)*. It was subsequently found to be linked to the 17-cM region on chromosome 6q25.2-27, and the locus was recently designated Park2 *(3,5)*. Through the study of a patient who had homozygous microdeletion of the marker D6S305 *(5)*, the responsible gene was identified by positional cloning and was designated *parkin (6)*. Linkage and mutation analysis to date have shown that founders of mutations in this gene are multiple and widely distributed in the world *(7–13)*. Abnormalities in this gene, which are specific for AR-JP, include homozygous exonic deletions, small deletions, and point mutations. The presence of homozygous exonic deletions strengthens the notion that nigral neurodegeneration in AR-JP is caused by loss of function of the parkin protein.

1.1. Assessment of the AR-JP Phenotype

1.1.1. Clinical and Pathologic Manifestations of AR-JP

The cardinal features of AR-JP are early-onset parkinsonism with a benign course and remarkable response to levodopa. The following clinical features are also important to support the diagnosis of AR-JP (**Table 1**):

From: *Methods in Molecular Medicine, vol. 62: Parkinson's Disease: Methods and Protocols*
Edited by: M. M. Mouradian © Humana Press Inc., Totowa, NJ

Table 1
Major and Minor Manifestations Useful for the Clinicopathologic Diagnosis of AR-JP

Type of finding	Feature
Major clinical features	Early-onset parkinsonism (mean age 27.0 ± 9.0 years; range: 8–58 yr)
	A clear levodopa-response
	Frequent and early dopa induced dyskinesias and wearing-off phenomenon
	No dementia and rare autonomic dysfunction
	Extremely slow progression (Hoehn-Yahr stage 2.6 ± 0.7, after 20–30 yr from onset
Minor clinical features	Sleep benefit (improvement of symptoms after sleep lasting 30–120 min)
	Mild foot dystonia (dorsiflexion of big toe or pes equinovarus)
	Fine postural tremor
	Hyperreflexia with negative Babinski sign
Pathological findings	Lewy body-negative neuron loss with severe gliosis in the substantia nigra pars compacta
	Mild neuron loss in the locus ceruleus

Data from **ref. *4***.

1. Mild focal dystonia, which often manifests as unilateral foot dystonia-dorsiflexion of the big toe or pes equinovarus deformity. Dorsiflexion of the big toe can be easily observed when the patient sits on a high chair or walks with bare feet. In some cases, truncal dystonia is the first symptom.
2. Sleep benefit, which can be identified by asking patients whether their parkinsonian symptoms improve after naps, or whether their symptoms are much milder upon awakening in the morning compared with the evening.
3. Extremely slow progression of the disease and absence of dementia even in the terminal stages of the disease.
4. Rare occurrence of autonomic dysfunction such as constipation or neurogenic bladder.
5. Fine postural finger tremor.
6. Hyperactive deep tendon reflexes with a negative Babinski sign.
7. Dopa-induced dyskinesia, which soon follows the dramatic dopa responsiveness.
8. Wearing-off phenomenon, which is frequently encountered in a relatively early phase of the disease.

1.1.2. Family Interview

Family interviews typically reveal multiple affected individuals in one generation with no appearance of the disease in previous generations or offspring of pateints. Thus, if the patient has no siblings, AR-JP can manifest as a sporadic early-onset parkinsonism. Although 51% of AR-JP families (9/17) have consanguineous marriages ***(4)***, a sufficiently large proportion (49%) have no history of consanguinity despite exhaustive family interviews ***(4)***. Nevertheless, patients from these non-consanguineous families frequently have homozygous haplotypes (63%; *see* **Subheading 1.2.4.**), which indicates the presence of an ancient consanguineous loop. In such cases, the parents' families frequently originated from the same geographic area.

1.2. Analysis of Mutations in the parkin *Gene*

1.2.1. Structure and Expression of the parkin *Gene*

The *parkin* gene consists of 12 exons encoding 465 amino acids, with a molecular weight of 51,652 D (**Fig. 1**). The full-length cDNA, which has been isolated from human skeletal muscle and fetal brain cDNA libraries consists of 2860 bp with an open reading frame of 1395 bp. The N-terminal 76 amino acid residues show homology to ubiquitin (65% positive, 33% identical). The characteristic cysteine-rich motif (Cys-X2-Cys-X9-Cys-X1-His-X2-Cys-X4—Cys-X4-Cys-X2-Cys) is also found at the C-terminus of parkin. The *parkin* gene is ubiquitously transcribed. Northern blot analysis using full-length *parkin* cDNA as probe revealed a 4.5 kb mRNA in almost all tissues (6). In the brain, *parkin* mRNA is present in several regions, including cerebellum, substantia nigra, cerebral cortex, brainstem, putamen, caudate, hippocampus, amygdala, and thalamus. Reverse transcriptase polymerase chain reaction (RT-PCR) analysis using leukocyte RNA revealed no full-length mRNA but a shorter transcript in which exons 3, 4, and 5 are spliced out. In the brain, the full-length transcript, as well as a small amount of mRNA with a spliced-out exon 5, has been detected by RT-PCR ***(14)***.

1.2.2. Analysis of Exon Deletions by Genomic PCR

A wide variety of deletion mutations in the *parkin* gene have been reported so far (**Table 2**). If the patient is homozygous for the deletion, it is detectable by lack of a genomic PCR product using intron primers encompassing the deleted exons. However, if a patient is heterozygous for the deletions (compound heterozygote: *see* **Note 1**), only the exon whose deletion is shared by both chromosomes fails to be amplified. If no part of the deletion is shared between the two chromosomes, exon PCR cannot detect any deletion. For example, if an individual receives exon 3 deletion from the father and exon 4 deletion from the mother, exon PCR cannot detect any deletion. Southern blot analysis is not dependable for evaluation of such small changes in gene dosage. Accordingly, when the patient shows a heterozygous haplotype for mark-

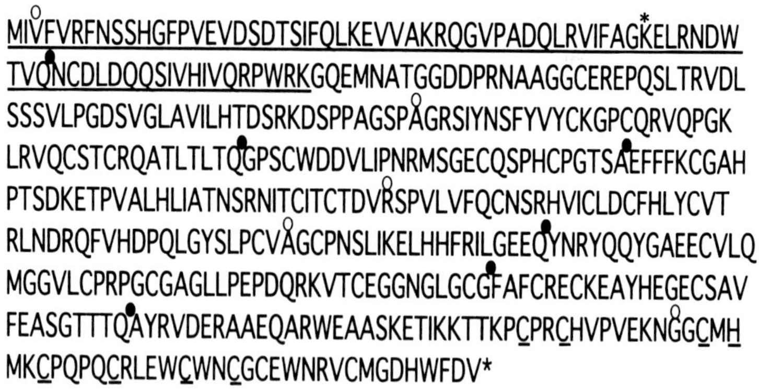

MIVFVRFNSSHGFPVEVDSDTSIFQLKEVVAKRQGVPADQLRVIFAGKELRNDW
TVQNCDLDQQSIVHIVQRPWRKGQEMNATGGDDPRNAAGGCEREPQSLTRVDL
SSSVLPGDSVGLAVILHTDSRKDSPPAGSPAGRSIYNSFYVYCKGPCQRVQPGK
LRVQCSTCRQATLTLTQGPSCWDDVLIPNRMSGECQSPHCPGTSAEFFFKCGAH
PTSDKETPVALHLIATNSRNITCITCTDVRSPVLVFQCNSRHVICLDCFHLYCVT
RLNDRQFVHDPQLGYSLPCVAGCPNSLIKELHHFRILGEEQYNRYQQYGAEECVLQ
MGGVLCPRPGCGAGLLPEPDQRKVTCEGGNGLGCGFAFCRECKEAYHEGECSAV
FEASGTTTQAYRVDERAAEQARWEAASKETIKKTTKPCPRCHVPVEKNGGCMH
MKCPQPQCRLEWCWNCGCEWNRVCMGDHWFDV*

Fig. 1. Exon boundaries in the parkin protein. Open circles, exon boundary breaks three nucleotide amino acid codes; closed circles, exon boundary does not break the amino acid code. Ubiquitin-like sequences in the N-terminal portion of parkin protein are underlined. The conserved site of polyubiquitination (Lys at 48) is shown by asterisks. A ring finger-like cysteine-rich motif at the C-terminal portion is indicated by underlined cysteine (C) and histidine (H) residues within this motif.

ers on the AR-JP locus, negative results from exon PCR do not necessarily mean that the patient has no deletion in the AR-JP gene.

To date, exon PCR has been effective for the detection of deletions in 57% of chromosome 6q-linked recessive juvenile parkinsonism (12 of 21 families) in Japan and in 25% (3 of 12 families) in Europe and North Africa ***(11)***. Thus, 25–57% of clinical AR-JP can be detected by exon PCR.

1.2.3. Exon Sequencing

When exon PCR shows no deletion, the next step is to sequence each exon and its boundaries. A wide variety of point mutations in the *parkin* gene have been reported so far (**Table 2**).

Homozygous one-point mutations, small insertions or deletions at the same nucleotide site on both chromosomes could be detected. Alternatively, if the patient is a compound heterozygote (*see* **Note 1**), one-point heterozygous mutation at the same nucleotide position might also be detected. When a heterozygous point mutation is observed, the presence of a compound heterozygote with a deletion in the other chromosome is possible. When two-point mutations are observed at different sites, it is necessary to exclude the possible presence of two mutations residing on the same chromosome. This can be done by sequencing a carrier who has only one disease chromosome, which can be detected by haplotype analysis. If only one of these two-point mutations is

Table 2
Mutations in the *parkin* Gene

Exonic deletions detected by exon PCR
Exon 3
Exons 3, 4
Exons 3, 4, 5, 6, 7
Exon 4
Exons 4, 5, 6
Exon 5
Exons 5, 6, 7
Exons 8, 9
Point mutations
Lys161Asn (exon 4)
Thr240Arg (exon 6)
Arg256Cys (exon 7)
Arg275Trp (exon 7)
Thr415Asn (exon 11)
Gln311Stop (exon 8)
Trp453Stop (exon 12)
Small deletions or insertions
202-3del (exon 2)
255del (exon 3)
321-2ins (exon 3)
535del (exon 5)
Polymorphic mutations
Ser167Asn (exon 4)
Arg366Trp (exon 10)
Val380Leu (exon 10)
Asp394Asn (exon 11)

Data from **refs.** ***9–12***, ***14***, ***15***, and ***19***.

observed in the carrier, the patient is a compound heterozygote. If both of the two-point mutations are present in the carrier, the patient may have two point mutations in one chromosome. In the latter case, it is still possible that the patient is a compound heterozygote with a deletion in one chromosome and two-point mutations in the other. When a new homozygous one-point mutation is identified, the possibility of polymorphic mutation should be assessed. Several polymorphic mutations in the *parkin* gene have been reported (**Table 2**) ***(13,15)***.

1.2.4. Haplotype Analysis

As mentioned above, haplotype analysis is mandatory to interpret correctly the results of exon deletions and point mutations (*see* **Note 2**). If an affected patient has a heterozygous haplotype for the *parkin* gene, he/she is expected to be a compound heterozygote, receiving different mutations from each parent. In AR-JP derived from a consanguineous marriage, the patient usually receives the identical mutation from both parents, and thus should be homozygous for polymorphic marker alleles located in and around the *parkin* gene. However, in AR-JP, mutations in the *parkin* gene are variable and widely distributed in the world. This multiple-founder effect increases the likelihood of the occurrence of the disease from nonconsanguineous marriages, resulting in compound heterozygotes.

It should be noted that although the normal carrier state (heterozygote) of a deletion cannot be detected by conventional exon PCR, it can be detected by haplotype analysis if the individual belongs to the same family as the affected proband and the parents have heterozygous haplotypes (**Figs. 2–4**). When only patients' samples are available, it is desirable to calculate allele frequencies of the markers in the general population from which affected families originate. If the frequencies of the marker alleles are rare, haplotype homozygosity alone is sufficient to indicate the true linkage of the haplotype to the disease (*see* **Note 3**).

1.2.5. Analysis of parkin mRNA and Protein

Absence or truncation of *parkin* transcripts can be detected by RT-PCR using tissue RNA samples. The presence of tissue-specific splicing of *parkin* transcripts should be taken into consideration. For example, full-length *parkin* transcript is absent in peripheral leukocytes ***(14)***. When a specific antibody is available, Western blot analysis using tissue samples can detect abnormalities of parkin translated products. Analysis of the *parkin* mRNA and protein has just begun, and further studies should become available in the near future. Such analyses would be helpful in the diagnosis of AR-JP when genomic studies are not informative.

1.2.6. Perspectives

Even when PCR-based studies of homozygous exonic deletions and point mutations are negative in a particular patient, the diagnosis of AR-JP cannot be excluded if haplotype analysis shows a heterozygous haplotype. Individual patients might be compound heterozygotes having two different exonic deletions that do not share a common segment. When a hetrozygous point mutation is present in a patient, a compound state with one deletion and one point mutation should be evaluated. Thus, without a sensitive method to detect small changes in gene dosage such as heterozygous deletions, the diagnosis of AR-JP should depend on the efforts to put together the results of PCR-based analysis of the mutation and haplotype studies of the pedigree.

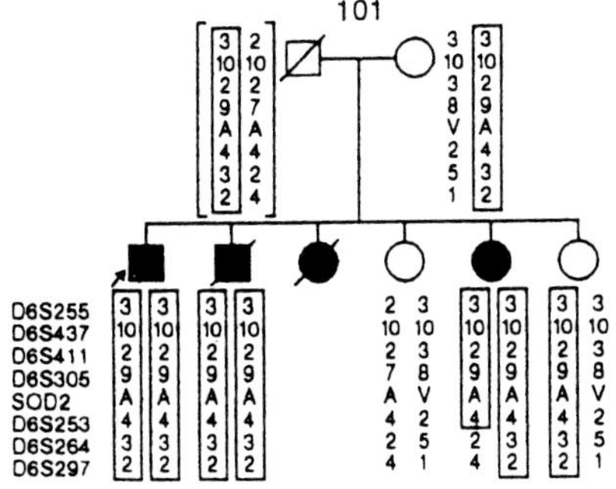

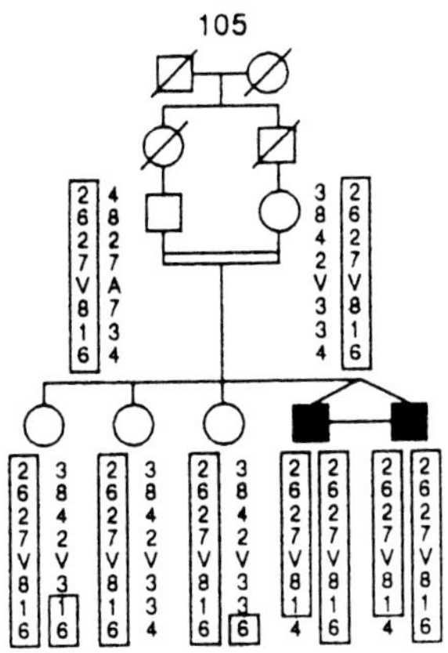

Fig. 2. Haplotype analysis and carrier detection in AR-JP pedigrees *(3)*. Homozygous segregation of haplotypes and diagnosis of carrier state are possible in these two AR-JP families. The haplotype of the disease chromosome is enclosed by the rectangle. Markers used are D6S441, D6S255, D6S437, D6S305, alanine (A)/valine (V) dipolymorphism of MnSOD, D6S253, D6S264, and D6S297. As seen in pedigree 101, multiple affected siblings and homozygous segregation are frequently seen with no apparent consanguinity. In this family, the second daughter is not a carrier of the disease chromosome. However, both parents and the fourth daughter are carriers (heterozygote), with one disease chromosome whose haplotype is 3-10-2-9-A-4-3-2. All affected individuals are homozygous for the haplotype 3-10-2-9-A-4-3-2. Recombination is observed between markers D6S253 and D6S264 on the paternal chromosome of the third affected daughter. This family has exon 4 deletion. Note the first-degree cousin marriage in family 105. Only the patients (monozygotic twins) show homozygosity of the disease chromosome with the haplotype 2-6-2-7-V-8-1. All other siblings and their parents are carriers of the disease chromosome. Several recombinations are observed in members of this family except in the second unaffected daughter. This family has exon 5 deletion.

The existence of multiple founder mutations in the *parkin* gene and the high proportion of nonconsanguinity in AR-JP pedigrees (49%) indicate a high frequency of compound heterozygotes and asymptomatic carriers of *parkin* mutations in the normal population, resulting in a potentially high prevalence of sporadic cases of AR-JP *(4)*. The major obstacle for assessing the latter possibility is the difficulty in detecting deletion heterozygotes.

Recently, real-time PCR monitoring by fluorescent-energy transfer techniques such as TaqMan or LightCycler system have been introduced to detect such small differences in gene dosage *(16)*. These technical improvements could enable the detection of deletion heterozygotes in the *parkin* gene. At the

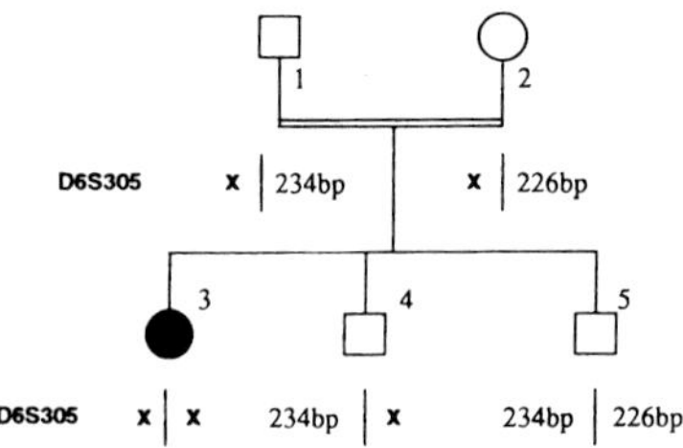

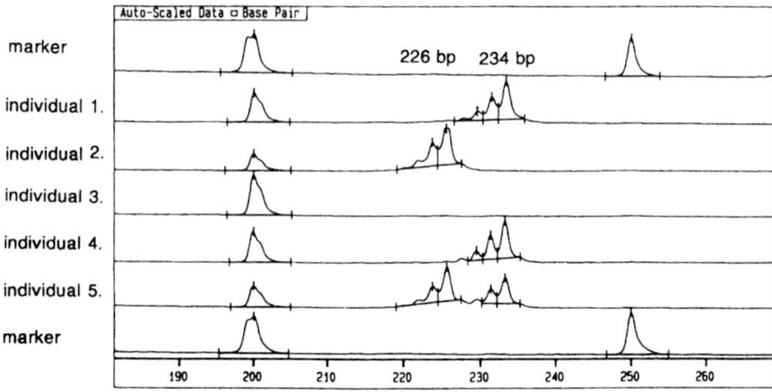

Fig. 3. Allotype analysis of the microsatellite marker D6S305 in the family of an AR-JP patient using the Pharmacia ALF2 Fragment manager *(5)*. Data are obtained by the Pharmacia ALF2 sequencer and analyzed by Fragment manager software. FITC-labeled PCR products of the microsatellite marker D6S305 were electrophoresed. In each of these lanes, size markers (200 and 300 bp) were also run. This zoomed-in figure does not show the peak at 300 bp. In lanes designated as markers, a 50-bp size ladder was run. Note the 200- and 250-bp peaks in each marker lane. The ordinate represents nucleotide length (bp). PCR products generate a complex of peaks, with several smaller peaks are located left of the highest peak, which represents shorter products generated by the skipping phenomenon of amplification. This phenomenon is often observed in amplification of short nucleotide repeats. The length difference between each of these skipping peaks is 2 bp, because D6S305 is a dinucleotide repeat polymorphic marker. Two alleles (226 and 234 bp) are seen in this family. Individuals 1 and 2 are parents who are first cousins. Individual 1 shows a single allele (234 bp). Individual 2 shows a single allele, which is different in size from that of individual 1 (226 bp). If individuals 1 and 2 are homozygotes, all offspring should show a heterozygous allotype (226/234 bp). However, individual 4 shows a single allele (234 bp), indicating that this person received a null (deleted) allele (shown as X in the family pedigree) from individual 2. This in turn suggests that individual 2 has heterozygous deletion of this marker (X/226 bp). On the other hand, individual 3, who has clinical AR-JP, shows no PCR product, indicating that she received two deleted alleles, one from each parent (X/X). The latter observation means that individual 1 also has a heterozygous deletion of the marker (X/234 bp). Individual 5 shows a heterozygous allotype (226/234 bp), indicating that he received no deleted allele from either parent. These findings taken together indicate that the responsible gene for AR-JP resides in close proximity to D6S305.

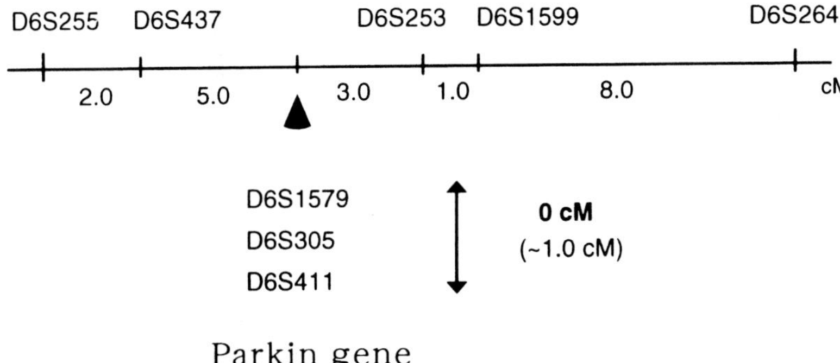

Fig. 4. Genetic map of polymorphic microsatellite markers in and around the *parkin* gene on chromosome 6q25.2-27 ***(3–5)***. The microsatellite marker D6S305 is located within the *parkin* gene ***(5,6)***.

same time, the full sequencing of the genomic region in and around the *parkin* gene is in progress, which will enable the detection of mutations in the noncoding region of this gene as well.

α-Synuclein aggregation is considered a major cause of Lewy body formation. Nonetheless, the cell death pathway triggered by α-synuclein aggregation is not clear. The unique feature of neuronal death in AR-JP, namely, absence of Lewy body formation, suggests the possibility that the downstream event in the cell death cascade triggered by α-synuclein aggregation might share the same biochemical pathway involving *parkin* ***(17)***. Genetic analysis of mutations in the *parkin* gene in AR-JP patients will eventually contribute to the elucidation of the functional role of parkin in the pathogenesis of Parkinson's disease.

2. MATERIALS

2.1. Exon Deletions

1. Chimeric primers with M13 universal and reverse primer sequences at their 5' ends are used for exon PCR as well as for exon sequencing (**Table 3**, *see* **Note 4**).
2. Ampli Taq Gold DNA polymerase (Perkin-Elmer, Applied Biosystems Division, Foster City, CA).
3. 10X PCR buffer: 500 m*M* KCl, 100 m*M* $MgCl_2$, 0.1% gelatin.
4. 10 m*M* dNTPs.
5. PCR thermal cycler.

2.2. Exon Sequencing

1. The PCR product obtained by exon PCR (*see* **Subheading 3.1.**).
2. Ultrafree-MC centrifugal filter (Millipore, Tokyo, Japan).

Table 3
PCR Primer Sequences for Exon PCR[a]

Exon number	Primer sequences	Product length (bp)
1	Forward: 5'-caggaaacagctatgaccgcgcggctggcgccgctgcgcgca-3'	147
	Reverse: 5'-tgtaaaacgacggccagtgcggcgcagagaggctgtac-3'	
2	Forward: 5'-caggaaacagctatgaccatgttgctatcaccatttaaggg -3'	343
	Reverse: 5'-tgtaaaacgacggccagtagattggcagcgcaggcggcatg-3'	
3	Forward: 5'-caggaaacagctatgaccacatgtcacttttgcttccct-3'	462
	Reverse: 5'-tgtaaaacgacggccagtaggccatgctccatgcagactgc-3'	
4	Forward: 5'-caggaaacagctatgaccacaagcttttaaagagtttcttgt-3'	296
	Reverse: 5'-tgtaaaacgacggccagtaggcaatgtgttagtacaca-3'	
5	Forward: 5'-caggaaacagctatgaccacatgtcttaaggagtacattt-3'	262
	Reverse: 5'-tgtaaaacgacggccagttctctaatttcctggcaaacagtg-3'	
6	Forward: 5'-caggaaacagctatgaccagagattgtttactgtggaaaca-3'	303
	Reverse: 5'-tgtaaaacgacggccagtgagtgatgctatttttagatcct-3'	
7	Forward: 5'-caggaaacagctatgacctgcctttccacactgacaggtact-3'	274
	Reverse: 5'-tgtaaaacgacggccagttctgttcttcattagcattagaga-3'	
8	Forward: 5'-caggaaacagctatgacctgatagtcataactgtgtgtaag-3'	241
	Reverse: 5'-tgtaaaacgacggccagtactgtctcattagcgtctatctt-3'	
9	Forward: 5'-caggaaacagctatgaccgggtgaaatttgcagtcagt-3'	313
	Reverse: 5'-tgtaaaacgacggccagtaatataatcccagcccatgtgca-3	
10	Forward: 5'-caggaaacagctatgaccattgccaaatgcaacctaatgtc-3'	200
	Reverse: 5'-tgtaaaacgacggccagtttggaggaatgagtagggcatt-3	
11	Forward: 5'-caggaaacagctatgaccacagggaacataaactctgatcc-3'	338
	Reverse: 5'-tgtaaaacgacggccagtcaacacaccaggcaccttcaga-3'	
12	Forward: 5'-caggaaacagctatgaccgtttgggaatgcgtgtttt-3'	290
	Reverse: 5'-tgtaaaacgacggccagtagaattagaaaatgaaggtagaca-3'	

[a]M13 universal and reverse sequences are underlined.

3. ABI Dye Terminator Cycle Sequencing Ready Reaction Kit (Perkin-Elmer).
4. M13 universal primer (5'-CAGGAAACAGCTATGACC-3' and M13 reverse primer (5'-TGTAAAACGACGGCCAGT-3').
5. Loading buffer: deionized formamide and 25 m*M* EDTA, pH 8.0, in 50 mg/mL, 5/1 v/v.
6. Thermal cycler machine.
7. Sequence analyzer ABI 373.

2.3. Haplotype Analysis

1. Primers: These are the microsatellite markers covering the AR-JP locus and are listed in **Table 4**. Marker D6S437 is 3.0 c*M* apart from D6S305. Markers D6S305, D6S1579, D6S305, and D6S411 are located within 0 c*M* apart from each other. D6S253 is 5.0 c*M* apart from D6S305. These markers cover an 8.0 c*M* region

Table 4
Primers for Haplotype Analysis

Marker	Primer sequences	Product length (bp)
D6S305	Left: FITC-CACCAGCGTTAGAGACTGC Right: GCAAATGGAGCATGTCACT	200–250
D6S411	Left: FITC-TGGTTGATTGACCCACTTAT Right: TCACAGTGCCTGGTCC	150–200
D6S1579	Left: FITC-TACTCACACATGCACAGGC Right: CTTCCTACCCACATGCAG	100–200
D6S437	Left: FITC-TGTCCTGGTGGAGGCA Right: GGTACAGTGTTTGACCCTAAGA	100–200
D6S253	Left: FITC-GATCTGGGTTCACTTTGTC Right: GATCACCAAGGGAAACTGG	200–300

spanning the *parkin* gene. D6S305 is an intragenic marker, which is located in intron 7 of the *parkin* gene ***(5,6)***.

2. Electrophoresis buffer (10X TBE): 1 *M* Tris base, 0.83 *M* boric acid, 10 m*M* EDTA (filtered through a 0.45-µm filter).
3. Polyacrylamide gel (0.5 mm thick) solution: 6% (w/v) acrylamine/bisacrylamide monomers (99:1), 100 mM Tris-borate (pH 8.3), 1 mM Na_2EDTA, and 7 M ALF grade urea filtered throught a 0.22-µm filter.
4. Ammonium persulfate: 10% (w/v) solution.
5. Tetramethyl ethylenediamine (TEMED).
6. Formamide loading dye: 100% deionized formamide and 5 mg/mL dextran blue 2000.
7. Sizer 50–500, 100, 200, 300 (Pharmacia): Fluorescein-labeled double-stranded DNA fragment (5 fmol/µL in TE buffer).
8. AmpliTaq DNA polymerase (Perkin-Elmer, Applied Biosystems Division).
9. 10 m*M* dNTPs.
10. 10X PCR buffer solution: 100 m*M* Tris-HCl at pH 8.3, 500 m*M* KCl, 15 m*M* $MgCl_2$, 0.01% gelatin.
11. Pharmacia ALF2 autosequencer.
12. Fragment manager software (Pharmacia)

3. Methods

3.1. Exon Deletions

1. Using primers shown in **Table 3**, prepare the following PCR mixture: 100–500 ng genomic DNA, 10 pmol each primer, 10 nmol dNTPs, 50 m*M* KCl, 10 m*M* $MgCl_2$, 0.01% gelatin, and 2.5 U Ampli Taq Gold DNA polymerase (Perkin-Elmer, Applied Biosystems Division) in 25 µL.
2. Follow the PCR menus shown in **Table 5**. These should yield single PCR products (*see* **Note 5**).

Table 5
PCR Menus for Exon PCR

Exon 1
Initial denaturation
94°C for 10 min
40 cycles of:
96°C for 30 s
60°C for 30 s
72°C for 45 s
Final extension
72°C for 10 min
Exons 2, 3, 6–9, and 10
Initial denaturation
94°C for 10 min
40 cycles of:
94°C for 30 s
60°C for 30 s
72°C for 45 s
Final extension
72°C for 10 min
Exon 4
Initial denaturation
94°C for 10 min
40 cycles of:
94°C for 30 s
53°C for 45 s
72°C for 45 s
Final extension
72°C for 10 min
Exons 5 and 12
Initial denaturation
94°C for 10 min
40 cycles of:
94°C for 30 s
55°C for 30 s
72°C for 45 s
Final extension
72°C for 10 min
Exon 11
Initial denaturation
94°C for 10 min
40 cycles of:
94°C for 30 s
62°C for 30 s
72°C for 45 s
Final extension
72°C for 10 min

3. Electrophorese and visualize the PCR product on 2–3% agarose gel containing ethidium bromide (0.5 µg/mL).
4. Add a negative control sample with no DNA template in each experiment in order to exclude possible DNA contamination. Repeat the PCR studies at least twice to confirm the results.
5. When no exonic deletions are detected, proceed to exon sequencing.

3.2. Exon Sequencing

1. Following exon PCR (discussed above in **Subheading 3.1.**), use M13 universal and reverse primers for exon sequencing when no exonic deletions are detected.
2. Remove excess primers and dNTPs by using an Ultrafree-MC centrifugal filter (Millipore, Tokyo, Japan).
3. Perform the sequencing reaction according to the manufacturer's protocol for the ABI Dye Terminator Cycle Sequencing Ready Reaction Kit (Perkin-Elmer).
   Sequencing Reaction mixture:
      Terminator Ready Reaction Mix 8.0 µL
      PCR template 100–200 ng
      M13 universal or reverse primer 3.2 pmol
      Add dH_2O to a final reaction volume of 20 µL
   PCR conditions for the DNA Thermal Cycler are 25 cycles of:
      96°C for 30 s
      50°C for 15 s
      60°C for 4 min
4. Purify the PCR products with Centri-Sep spin columns as described in the protocol supplied by the manufacturer.
5. Add the loading buffer, denature at 90°C for 2 min, chill on ice, electrophorese, and analyze the sequence with an ABI 373 Sequence Analyzer (*see* **Note 6**).

3.3. Haplotype Analysis

1. Label one of the primer pairs (sense or antisense primer) for microsatellite markers (**Table 4**) with fluorescein (FITC-labeled).
2. Prepare PCR mix: 10 µL reaction solution, 100 ng genomic DNA, 2.5 pmol of each primer, 2.0 nmol of dNTPs in 10 m*M* Tris-HCl, pH 8.3, 50 m*M* KCl, 1.5 m*M* $MgCl_2$, 0.001% gelatin, and 0.5 U AmpliTaq DNA polymerase.
3. Run the PCR menu as follows:
   An initial denaturation for 5 min at 95°C, followed by 35 cycles of:
      94°C for 0.5 min
      50°C for 0.5 min
      72°C for 0.5 min
   A final extension at 72°C for 5 min.
4. Dilute the PCR product 10–20-fold with loading dye (*see* **Note 7**).
5. Add 5 fmol (1 µL) of 100-, 200-, and 300-bp fluorescein-labeled fragments (Sizer 100, 200, and 300 from Pharmacia), which encompass the size range of PCR

products to 3–4 μL of diluted samples (*see* **Note 8**). Sizer 50–500 (Pharmacia) is applied in one lane per 4–8 lanes and is used as an external standard (*see* **Note 8**).

6. Denature the samples at 94°C for 3 min.
7. Chill on ice.
8. Apply this mixture (5–6 μL) onto a 0.5-mm-thick 6% polyacrylamide gel with 0.6X TBE electrophoresis buffer.
9. Run the gel in 0.6X TBE electrophoresis buffer using a Pharmacia ALF2 fluorescence automated sequence analyzer.
10. Set the running condition at 1500 V, 38 mA, 34 W, and 45 Å. Set the Lazer power and interval at 3 mW power and 2 s, respectively.
11. After running the gel, analyze the PCR products by Fragment manager software (Pharmacia) (*see* **Figs. 3** and **4**).

4. Notes

1. A recessive disease is caused by the presence of two mutations, each of which has occurred in the same gene residing on homologous chromosomes. A compound heterozygote is a patient who has two different mutations on each of homologous chromosomes. As each of the mutations is derived from a different ancestor of the disease mutation, a compound heterozygote has two different haplotypes (*see* **Note 8**), which originate from different ancestors of the mutation.
2. A haplotype is a set of alleles on one chromosome. Alleles are alternative forms of a gene or marker occupying the same locus on homologous chromosomes. As human cells have two copies of each chromosome (diploid cells), an individual always has a pair of alleles, one from each parent. Accordingly, an individual has two haplotypes. If alleles are very closely linked, haplotypes within a kindred are transmitted as units. However, when alleles are not closely located, recombination by crossing over occurs and haplotypes are changed. Homozygotes have the same alleles or haplotypes on both homologous chromosomes, whereas heterozygotes have different alleles or haplotypes.
3. In a consanguineous pedigree, each parent is usually a carrier of the same mutation, i.e., has a single identical mutation derived from a single person who first acquired the mutation in an earlier generation, i.e., the ancestor of the mutation. Accordingly, if a patient born from a consanguineous marriage has homozygous haplotypes for the markers that flank or reside in a certain gene, this is a strong indication that the patient has two identical mutations in the same gene (theory of homozygosity mapping) ***(18)***. The probability for homozygosity to show true linkage is heavily dependent on the rarity of the alleles or haplotypes showing homozygosity. This is based on the fact that if the frequency of the marker in the control population is rare, the chance for its heterozygosity in the general population as well as in the parents increases. The latter, in turn, increases the power of detection for the single identical allele to be transmitted from each parent to the affected person (homozygosity by descent). On the other hand, if the marker frequency is high in the general population, homozygosity by chance increases and, therefore, homozygosity in the patient by itself is not informative (homozygos-

ity by state). Thus, to substantiate segregation of the haplotype with the disease, especially when only information about the patients' haplotypes is available, knowledge of the allele frequencies of the markers that constitute homozygous haplotypes are important. Analysis of 30–50 DNA samples obtained from normal persons is sufficient to determine allele frequencies of the markers.

4. PCR with primers without M13 universal sequences are also possible. In this case, the extracted DNA can be directly sequenced using internal primer sequences or can be subcloned into the TA-vector plasmid (TA-vector cloning kit, Invitrogen) without filling in the ends of the DNA fragment. The insert in the TA-vector can be sequenced with universal primers (M13 and M13 reverse). Several clones should be assessed to exclude possible PCR- and cloning-based mutations.
5. If extra bands in PCR products are observed in the gel, cutting the band corresponding to the expected size, extraction, and purification of DNA with the Quiaquick Gel extraction kit (Qiagen) is recommended for further sequencing.
6. Single-strand sequencing using T7 polymerase is an alternative method for the sequencing. The major merit of single-strand sequencing with T7 polymerase is uniformity of signal intensity, allowing easy detection of heterozygous mutations. The sequencing kit (Autoread sequencing kit) can be purchased from Pharmacia (Uppsala, Sweden). The single-strand template is recovered from the PCR product by magnetic force. As one of the PCR primers is biotin-labeled, the addition of streptavidin-coated magnetic beads (Dynal) to the PCR product results in their binding to the biotin-labeled DNA strand. Accordingly, the biotin labeled strand is isolated by magnetic force. A sequencing sample is applied in four lanes (A, C, G, and T) of the sequencing gel and analyzed with a Pharmacia ALF2 fluorescence autosequence analyzer. Universal sequences are added to the 5' end of PCR primers and fluorescein isothiocyanate (FITC)-labeled universal primers are used for sequencing. FITC-labeled universal primers are included in the Autoread sequencing kit (5'-CGACGTTTAAAACGACGGCCAGT-3' for M13 primer and 5'-CAGGAGGCAGCTATGAC-3' for M13 reverse primer). Sequencing primers must be derived from the region located at least one nucleotide internal to the site of PCR primers.
7. Scale-out of the peak of the signal occurs when dilution of the sample is insufficient.
8. Two different types of size standards—internal and external—are used. As internal standards, two size markers encompassing the size of the PCR product are loaded in the same lane with the PCR product. For example, Sizers 200 and 300 are loaded with the product whose expected size is between 200 and 300 bp. The molecular size of the peak of the PCR product is determined by reading the retention times of respective peaks of internal standards flanking the PCR product. As external standards, only the sizer markers are loaded in the lane that is called as the reference lane. For each group of sample lanes (usually four to five lanes) with reference lanes on both sides, the standard curves of the reference lanes are calculated. The molecular size of the PCR sample is calculated by first using the external standard and then adjusting the resulting standard curves to the internal reference points.

References

1. Yamamura, Y., Sobue, I., Ando, K., et al. (1973) Paralysis agitans of early onset with marked diurnal fluctuation of symptoms. *Neurology* **23,** 239–244.
2. Ishikawa, A. and Tsuji, S. (1996) Clinical analysis of 17 patients in 12 Japanese families with autosomal-recessive type juvenile parkinsonism. *Neurology* **47,** 160–169.
3. Matsumine, H., Saito, M., Matsubayashi, S., et al. (1997) Localization of a gene for autosomal recessive form of juvenile parkinsonism (AR-JP) to chromosome 6q25.2-27. *Am. J. Hum. Genet.* **60,** 588–596.
4. Matsumine, H., Yamamura, Y., Kobayashi, T., et al. (1998) Early-onset parkinsonism with diurnal fluctuation maps to a locus for juvenile parkinsonism. *Neurology* **50,** 1340–1345.
5. Matsumine, H., Yamamura, Y., Hattori, N., et al. (1998) A microdeletion of D6S305 in a family of autosomal recessive juvenile parkinsonism (PARK2). *Genomics* **49,** 143–146.
6. Kitada, T., Asakawa, S., Hattori, N., et al. (1998) Mutations in the parkin gene cause autosomal recessive juvenile parkinsonism. *Nature* **392,** 605–608.
7. Jones, AC., Yamamura, Y., Almasy, L, et al. (1998) Autosomal recessive juvenile parkinsonism maps to 6q25.2-q27 in four ethnic groups: detailed genetic mapping of the linked region. *Am. J. Hum. Genet.* **63,** 80–87.
8. Tassin, J., Durr, A., Broucker, T., et al. (1998) Chromosome 6-linked autosomal recessive early-onset in European and Algerian families, extension of the clinical spectrum, and evidence of a small homozygous deletion in one family. *Am. J. Hum. Genet.* **63,** 88–94.
9. Hattori, N., Kitada, T., Matsumine, H., et al. (1998) Molecular genetic analysis of a novel Parkin gene in Japanese families with autosomal recessive juvenile parkinsonism: evidence for variable homozygous deletions in the Parkin gene in affected individuals. *Ann. Neurol.* **44,** 935–941.
10 Hattori, N., Matsumine, H., Asakawa, S., et al. (1998) Point mutations (Thr240Arg and Gln311Stop) in the Parkin gene. *Biochem. Biophys. Res. Commun.* **249,** 754–758.
11. Lucking, C. B., Abbas, N., Durr, A., et al. (1998) Homozygous deletions in parkin gene in European and North African families with autosomal recessive juvenile parkinsonism. *Lancet* **352,** 1355–1356.
12. Leroy, E., Anastasopoulos, D., Konitsiotis, S., et al. (1998) Deletions in the Parkin gene and genetic heterogeneity in a Greek family with early onset Parkinson's disease. *Hum. Genet.* **103,** 424–427.
13. Abbas, N., Luckingberg, C. B., Ricard, S., et al. (1999) A wide variety of mutations in the parkin gene are responsible for autosomal recessive parkinsonism in Europe. *Hum. Mol. Genet.* **8,** 567–574.
14. Sunada, Y., Saito, F, Matsumura, K., et al. (1998) Differential expression of the parkin gene in the human brain and peripheral leukocytes. *Neurosci. Lett.* **254,** 180–182.
15. Wang, M., Hattori, N., Matsumine, H., et al. (1999) Polymorphism in the parkin gene in sporadic Parkinson's disease. *Ann. Neurol.* **45,** 655–658.

16. van Ommen, G. J. B., Bakker, E., and den Dannen, J. T. (1999) The human genome project and the future of diagnostic treatment and prevention. *Lancet* **354(Suppl 1),** 5–10
17. Matsumine, H. (1998) A loss-of-function mechanism of nigral neuron death without Lewy body fromation: autosomal recessive juvenile parkinsonism (AR-JP). *J. Neurol.* **245(Suppl 3),** 10–14.
18. Lander, E. S. and Botstein, D. Homozygosity mapping: a way to map human recessive traits with the DNA of inbred children. *Science* **236,** 1567–1570.

II

Molecular Pathogenetic Studies

3

Parkinson's Disease, Dementia with Lewy Bodies, and Multiple System Atrophy as α-Synucleinopathies

Michel Goedert, Ross Jakes, R. Anthony Crowther, and Maria Grazia Spillantini

1. Introduction

Parkinson's disease (PD) is the most common neurodegenerative movement disorder *(1)*. Neuropathologically, it is defined by nerve cell loss in the substantia nigra and the presence of Lewy bodies and Lewy neurites *(2,3)*. In many cases, Lewy bodies are also found in the dorsal motor nucleus of the vagus, the nucleus basalis of Meynert, the locus coeruleus, the raphe nuclei, the midbrain Edinger-Westphal nucleus, the cerebral cortex, the olfactory bulb, and some autonomic ganglia *(4)*.

Besides the substantia nigra, nerve cell loss is also found in the dorsal motor nucleus of the vagus, the locus coeruleus, and the nucleus basalis of Meynert. Ultrastructurally, Lewy bodies and Lewy neurites consist of abnormal filamentous material *(5)*. Lewy bodies and Lewy neurites also constitute the defining neuropathologic characteristics of dementia with Lewy bodies (DLB), a common late-life dementia that exists in a pure form or overlaps with the neuropathologic characteristics of Alzheimer's disease (AD) *(6–9)*.

Unlike PD, DLB is characterized by large numbers of Lewy bodies in cortical brain areas, such as the entorhinal and cingulate cortices. However, Lewy bodies and Lewy neurites are also present in the substantia nigra in DLB, whereas hippocampal Lewy neurites are found in a proportion of individuals who have PD with a severe cognitive impairment. Disorders with Lewy bodies and Lewy neurites thus present as a clinical and neuropathologic spectrum. Classical PD with minor cognitive impairment and minimal cortical pathology

From: *Methods in Molecular Medicine, vol. 62: Parkinson's Disease: Methods and Protocols*
Edited by: M. M. Mouradian © Humana Press Inc., Totowa, NJ

is at one end of the spectrum, and severe dementia with or without antecedent parkinsonism, but with a severe Lewy body and Lewy neurite pathology is at the other end. The Lewy body was first described in 1912, but its biochemical composition remained unknown until the middle of 1997.

The discovery of a point mutation in the α-*synuclein* gene as a rare cause of familial PD has led us to the finding that α-*synuclein* is the major component of Lewy bodies and Lewy neurites in idiopathic PD and DLB ***(10–12)***. The Lewy body pathology that is sometimes associated with other neurodegenerative diseases, such as sporadic and familial AD, Down's syndrome and neurodegeneration with brain iron accumulation type 1 (Hallervorden-Spatz syndrome) has also been shown to be α-synuclein positive ***(12–18)***. Moreover, the filamentous glial and neuronal inclusions of multiple system atrophy (MSA) have been found to be made of α-synuclein ***(19–22)***. Taken together, this work has shown that PD, DLB, and MSA are α-synucleinopathies. Here we first review the field of synucleins, with the emphasis on the role played by α-synuclein in neurodegenerative diseases. We then describe some of the experimental protocols that were instrumental in unravelling that role.

1.1. The Synuclein Family

The first synuclein nucleotide and amino acid sequences were reported in 1988 by Maroteaux et al. from the electric organ of the Pacific electric ray (*Torpedo californica*) ***(23)***. The protein was named synuclein, because of its apparent localization in presynaptic nerve terminals and portions of the nuclear envelope. All subsequent studies have shown the presence of synucleins in nerve terminals but have failed to confirm a nuclear localization. Nonetheless, for historical reasons, the original name has survived.

In 1991, Maroteaux et al. reported cDNA sequences from rat brain that were homologous to the synuclein sequence from *T. californica* ***(24)***. In 1992, Tobe et al. reported the amino acid sequence of an abundant protein from rat brain that they called phosphoneuroprotein-14 ***(25)***. In 1993, Uéda et al. reported the amino acid sequence of a protein from human brain that they named "non-amyloid-β component precursor" (NACP), because of the apparent localization of a portion of this protein in some amyloid plaques from AD brain ***(26)***. However, more recent studies using new antibodies have been unable to reproduce this original finding, which may have resulted from antibody crossreactivity with the β-amyloid protein Aβ ***(27,28)***. In 1994, Jakes et al. reported the amino acid sequences of two homologous proteins from human brain that were identified because they reacted with an antibody raised against paired helical filament preparations from AD brain ***(29)***. The first protein was identical to NACP, whereas the second protein was the human homolog of rat phosphoneuroprotein-14. We noticed that both proteins were similar to each other and to synuclein from *T. californica* and consequently named them α-synuclein and β-synuclein, respectively. Human α-synuclein is 140 amino acids in length, and β-synuclein is 134 amino acids long. In 1995, George et al. reported the amino acid sequence of a protein from zebra finch brain that they called synelfin ***(30)***. Synelfin is the zebra finch homolog of α-synuclein.

Human α- and β-synucleins are 62% identical in amino acid sequence and share a similar domain organization (**Fig. 1**). The amino-terminal half of each protein is taken up by imperfect amino acid repeats, with the consensus sequence KTKEGV. Individual repeats are separated by an interrepeat region of five to eight amino acids. Depending on the alignment, α-synuclein has five to seven repeats, whereas β-synuclein has five repeats. The repeats are followed by a hydrophobic middle region and a negatively charged carboxy-terminal region, although both proteins have an identical carboxy-terminus. The human α-synuclein gene maps to chromosome 4q21, whereas the β-synuclein gene maps to chromosome 5q35 ***(31–35)***. Their genes are composed of five coding exons of similar sizes, with the overall organization of these genes being well conserved. Alternative mRNA splicing has been observed for exons 4 and 6 of the human α-synuclein gene ***(36)***. Similarly, the rat cDNAs SYN1, SYN2, and SYN3 appear to be splice variants of the same synuclein gene ***(24)***. However, at the protein level, there is no evidence to suggest the existence of multiple α-synuclein isoforms. So far, no splice variants have been described for β-synuclein. The α- and β-synuclein sequences from several vertebrate species are very similar. No synuclein homolog have been identified in *Saccharomyces cerevisiae* and *Caenorhabditis elegans*, suggesting that the presence of synucleins may be limited to vertebrates.

By Northern blotting, α– and β-*synuclein* mRNAs are expressed at highest levels in the nervous system, with lower transcript levels in other tissues ***(26,29)***. By immunohistochemistry, both proteins are concentrated in nerve terminals, with little staining of nerve cell bodies and dendrites. Ultrastructurally, they are found in nerve terminals, in close proximity to synaptic vesicles ***(24,29)***. The physiologic functions of α-synuclein and β-synuclein are unknown. Both are abundant brain proteins and it has been estimated that they make up 0.1–0.2% of total brain protein.

Biophysical studies have shown that α-synuclein is monomeric, has little secondary structure, and is natively unfolded, in keeping with its heat stability ***(37)***. As a result, α- and β-synuclein have an apparent molecular mass of 19 kDa on sodium dodecyl sulfate polyacrylmide gel electrophoresis (SDS-PAGE), with α-synuclein running slightly faster than β-synuclein (**Fig. 2**). It appears likely that α-synuclein is normally bound to cellular constituents through its repeats and that it becomes structured as a result. Experimental studies have shown that α-synuclein can bind to lipid membranes through its

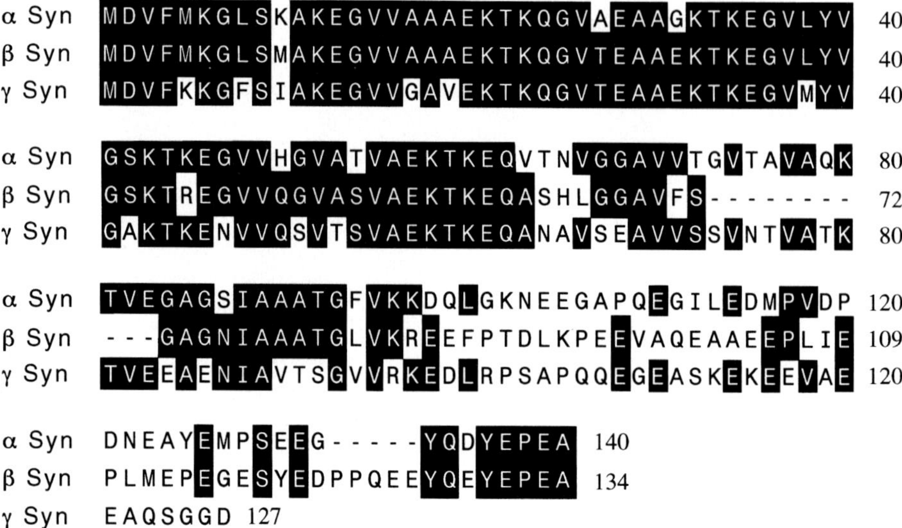

Fig. 1. Sequence comparison of human α-synuclein (α Syn), β-synuclein (β Syn), and γ-synuclein (γ Syn). Amino acid identities between at least two of the three sequences are indicated by black bars. As a result of a common polymorphism, residue 110 of γ-synuclein is either E or G.

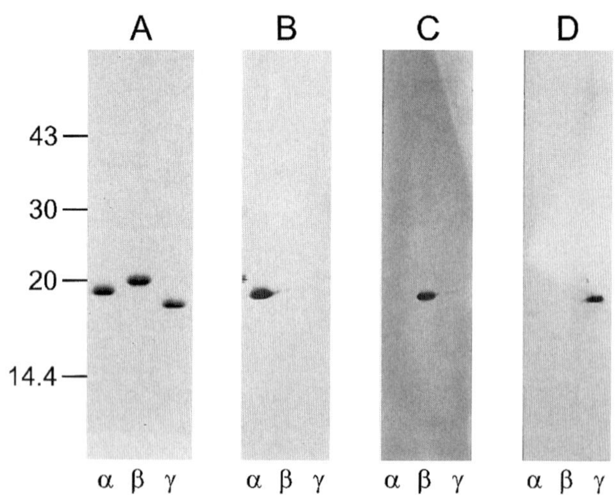

Fig. 2. SDS-PAGE and immunoblotting of recombinant human synuclein proteins. **(A)** Coomassie-stained gel of purified recombinant human α-, β-, and γ-synuclein. **(B)** Immunoblotting using the α-synuclein-specific antibody LB509. **(C)** Immunoblotting using the β-synuclein-specific antibody SYN207. **(D)** Immunoblotting using the γ-synuclein-specific antibody PER5.

amino-terminal repeats, suggesting that it may be a lipid-binding protein *(38,39)*. Both synucleins have been shown to inhibit phospholipase D2 selectively *(40)*. This isoform of phospholipase D localizes to the plasma membrane, where it may play a role in signal-induced cytoskeletal regulation and endocytosis *(41)*. It is therefore possible that α- and β-synuclein regulate vesicular transport processes. Little is known about posttranslational modifications of synucleins in brain. In transfected cells, α-synuclein becomes constitutively phosphorylated at serine residues 87 and 129 *(42)*.

In 1997, Ji et al. reported the amino acid sequence of a 127-amino acid protein that they named breast cancer-specific gene-1 (BCSG-1) protein, because of its presence in large amounts in human breast cancer tissue *(43)*. BCSG1 shares 55% sequence identity with human α-synuclein and has therefore been renamed γ-synuclein *(44)* (**Fig. 1**). It was independently discovered by Buchman et al., who named it persyn *(45)*. The synuclein that was originally identified in *T. californica* *(23)* was probably a γ-synuclein homolog.

γ-Synuclein has the same general domain organization as α-synuclein and β-synuclein and is also encoded by five exons *(46,47)*. The human γ-synuclein gene maps to chromosome 10q23. By Northern blotting, γ-synuclein mRNA is expressed at highest levels in the nervous system and the heart, with lower transcript levels in other tissues. By immunohistochemistry, it appears to be present throughout nerve cells, unlike α- and β-synuclein, which are concentrated in presynaptic nerve terminals. γ-Synuclein is heat stable and runs with an apparent molecular mass of 18 kDa on SDS-PAGE, ahead of both α- and β-synuclein (**Fig. 2**). In 1999, Surguchov et al. reported the sequence of a 127-amino acid protein that they named synoretin because of its expression in the retina *(48)*. At the amino acid level, synoretin is 87% identical to γ-synuclein. By Northern blotting, it shows the same tissue distribution as β-*synuclein* mRNA. A curious feature of the synoretin sequence is that its 5' untranslated region is identical to that of γ-*synuclein*. Future experiments will show whether synoretin is a *bona fide* synuclein.

1.2. α-Synuclein in Parkinson's Disease and Dementia with Lewy Bodies

In 1912, Friederich Lewy described serpentine or elongated intracytoplasmic bodies in the dorsal motor nucleus of the vagus nerve and in the substantia innominata from patients with PD *(2)*. Trétiakoff first described the presence of "corps de Lewy" in the substantia nigra in 1919 and proposed that they constitute a form of nigral pathology that is specific to PD *(3)*.

The light microscopic appearance of the Lewy body is characteristic. Classical brainstem Lewy bodies appear as intracytoplasmic circular inclusions, 5–25 μm in diameter, with a dense eosinophilic core and a clearer surrounding halo

(4). Lewy bodies can extend into nerve cell processes or lie free in the neuropil (extracellular Lewy bodies). The ultrastructure of the brainstem Lewy body is also characteristic in that it is composed of a dense core of filamentous and granular material surrounded by radially orientated filaments of 10–20 nm in diameter *(5)*.

The term "cortical Lewy body" refers to the less well-defined spherical inclusion seen in cortical areas *(6,7)*. It lacks a distinctive core and halo but is made of filaments with similar morphologies to those from brainstem Lewy bodies. The Lewy neurites constitute an important part of the pathology of PD and DLB. They correspond to abnormal neurites that have the same immunohistochemical staining profile as Lewy bodies and contain abnormal filaments similar to those found in Lewy bodies.

The Lewy body constitutes the second most common nerve cell pathology, after the neurofibrillary lesions of AD. Until recently, our understanding of the biochemical composition of the Lewy body filaments was at the same stage as was our understanding of the composition of the paired helical filaments of AD some 15 years ago. Immunohistochemical studies had shown that Lewy bodies stain to various extents with ubiquitin and neurofilament antibodies. Moreover, antibodies against some 30 different proteins had been reported to stain the halo of brainstem Lewy bodies. However, purification of Lewy body filaments to homogeneity had not been achieved. In PD and DLB the density of Lewy bodies and Lewy neurites is much lower than that of neurofibrillary lesions in AD. This renders purification and chemical analysis of the insoluble filaments a daunting task.

Most cases of PD are idiopathic, without an obvious family history. However, a small percentage of cases are familial and inherited in an autosomal-dominant manner. In 1996, Polymeropoulos et al. established genetic linkage of levodopa-responsive parkinsonism with autopsy-confirmed Lewy bodies in a large Italian-American kindred (the Contursi family) to chromosome 4q21-23 *(49,50)*. This was followed in 1997 by the discovery of a point mutation in the α-synuclein gene in this family and in three Greek families that share a common founder with the Contursi family *(10,51)*. The mutation lies in exon 4 and consists of a G to A transition at position 157 of the coding region of α-synuclein, which changes alanine residue 53 to threonine (A53T); it lies in the linker region between repeats 4 and 5 of α-synuclein (**Fig. 3**). β-Synuclein also carries an alanine at this position, whereas γ-synuclein has a threonine at the equivalent position. To date, there is no evidence suggesting an involvement of β-synuclein or γ-synuclein in the etiology of familial PD *(52–54)*.

Somewhat surprisingly, rodent and zebra finch α-synucleins carry a threonine residue at position 53, like the mutated human protein *(24,30)*. This, together with the common founder effect of the A53T mutation *(51)*, led some

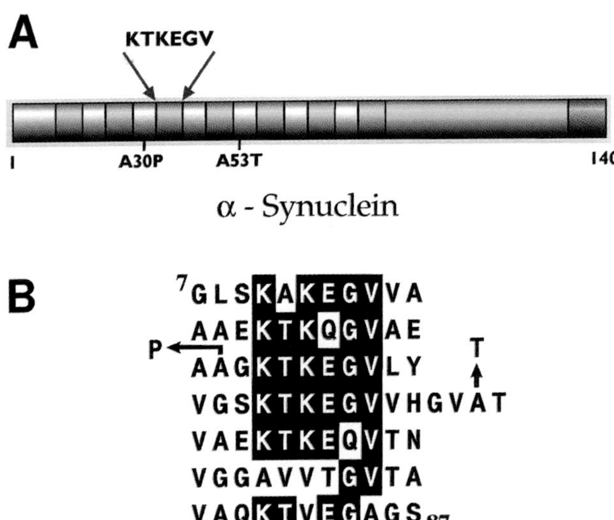

Fig. 3. Mutations in the α-synuclein gene in familial Parkinson's disease. **(A)** Schematic diagram of human α-synuclein. The seven repeats with the consensus sequence KTKEGV are shown as green bars. The hydrophobic region is shown in blue and the negatively charged C-terminus in yellow. The two known missense mutations are indicated. **(B)** Repeats in human α-synuclein. Residues 7–87 of the 140-residue protein are shown. Amino acid identities between at least five of the seven repeats are indicated by black bars. The A to P mutation at residue 30 between repeats two and three and the A to T mutation at residue 53 between repeats four and five are shown.

to propose that the A53T change may be nothing more than a rare, benign polymorphism. However, the discovery of a second mutation in *α-synuclein* in a family with PD of German descent has settled this controversy in favor of the relevance of α-synuclein for the etiology and pathogenesis of at least some familial cases of PD *(55)*. The second mutation lies in exon 3 and consists of a G to C transversion at position 88 of the coding region of *α-synuclein*, which changes alanine residue 30 to proline (A30P); it lies in the linker region between repeats 2 and 3 of α-synuclein (**Fig. 3**). Unlike residue 53, which, depending on the species, is alanine or threonine, residue 30 of α-synuclein is an alanine in all species examined. β-Synuclein and γ-synuclein also have alanine at this position.

Although the A53T mutation in α-synuclein accounts for only a small percentage of familial cases of PD, its identification was quickly followed by the discovery that α-synuclein is the major component of Lewy bodies and Lewy neurites in all cases of PD and DLB (**Figs. 4** and **5**) *(11)*. Full-length, or close to full-length, α-synuclein has been found in Lewy bodies and Lewy neurites,

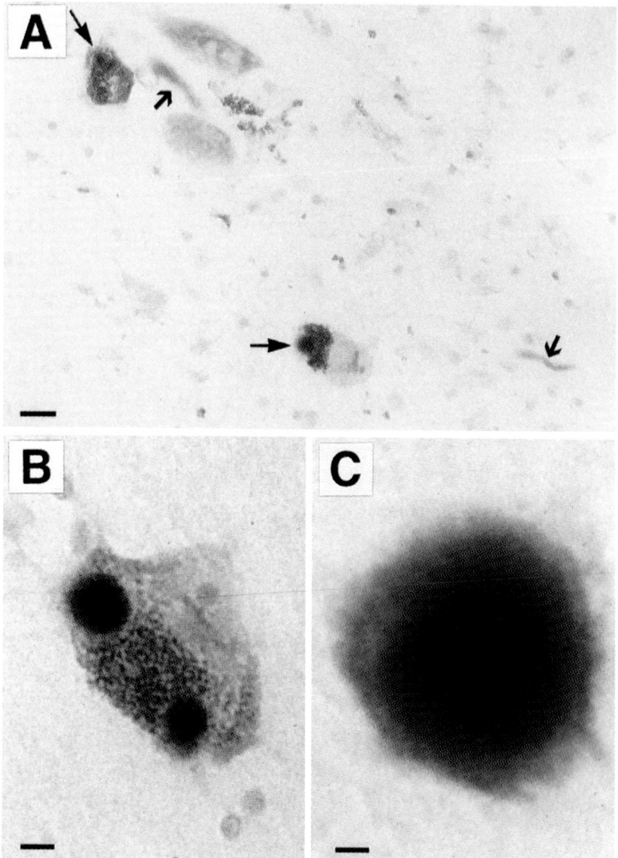

Fig. 4. Substantia nigra from patients with Parkinson's disease immunostained for α-synuclein. **(A)** Two pigmented nerve cells, each containing an α-synuclein-positive Lewy body (large arrows) stained with an antibody recognising the carboxy-terminal region of α-synuclein (antibody PER2). Lewy neurites (small arrows) are also immunopositive. Scale bar, 20 μm. **(B)** Pigmented nerve cell with two α-synuclein-positive Lewy bodies. Scale bar, 8 μm. **(C)** α-Synuclein-positive extracellular Lewy body. Scale bar, 4 μm.

with both the core and the corona of the Lewy body being stained. Staining for α-synuclein has been found to be more extensive than staining for ubiquitin, which was until then the most sensitive marker for Lewy bodies and Lewy neurites ***(12)***. In transfected cells, α-synuclein is degraded by the proteasome-ubiquitin pathway, with the A53T mutation conferring a longer half-life to the transfected protein ***(56)***. The Lewy body pathology does not stain for β-synuclein or γ-synuclein ***(12)***. Thus, of the three brain synucleins, only α-synuclein is of

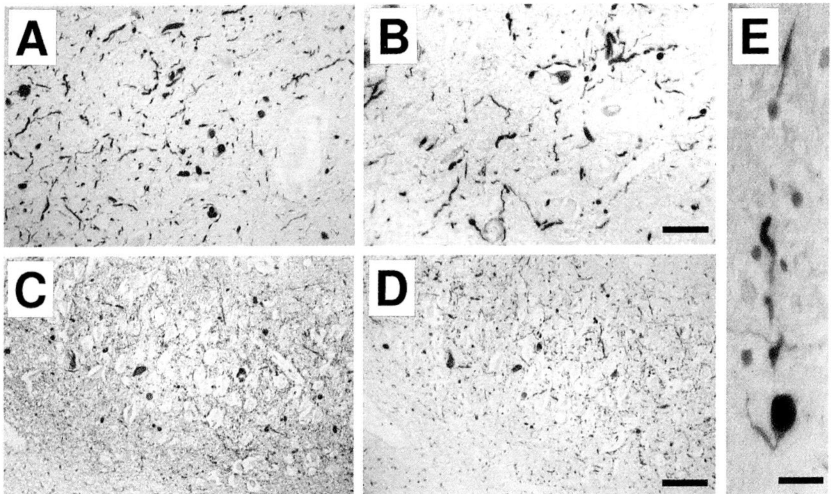

Fig. 5. Brain tissue from patients with dementia with Lewy bodies immunostained for α-synuclein. **(A,B)** α-Synuclein-positive Lewy bodies and Lewy neurites in substantia nigra stained with antibodies recognizing the amino-terminal (antibody PER1) (A) or the carboxy-terminal (antibody PER2) (B) region of α-synuclein. Scale bar = 100 μm in B; applies to A and B. **(C,D)** α-Synuclein-positive Lewy neurites in serial sections of hippocampus stained with antibodies recognizing the amino-terminal (C) or the carboxy-terminal (D) region of α-synuclein. Scale bar = 80 μm in D; applies to C and D. **(E)** α-Synuclein-positive intraneuritic Lewy body in a Lewy neurite in substantia nigra stained with an antibody recognizing the carboxy-terminal region of α-synuclein. Scale bar = 40 μm.

relevance in the context of PD and DLB. The original finding that α-synuclein is present in Lewy bodies and Lewy neurites ***(11)*** was rapidly confirmed and extended ***(12–18,57–65)***.

This work suggested, but did not prove, that α-synuclein is the major component of the abnormal filaments that make up Lewy bodies and Lewy neurites. In DLB, the pathologic changes are particularly numerous in the cingulate cortex, facilitating the extraction of filaments. Isolated filaments were strongly labeled along their entire lengths, demonstrating that they contain α-synuclein as a major component (**Fig. 6**) ***(12)***. Filament morphologies and staining characteristics with several antibodies have led to the suggestion that α-synuclein molecules might run parallel to the filament axis and that the filaments are polar structures. Moreover, under the electron microscope, some filaments and granular material in partially purified Lewy bodies appeared to be labeled by α-synuclein antibodies ***(59)***. Immunoelectron microscopy has shown decoration of Lewy body filaments in tissue sections from brain of individuals with PD and DLB ***(66,67)***.

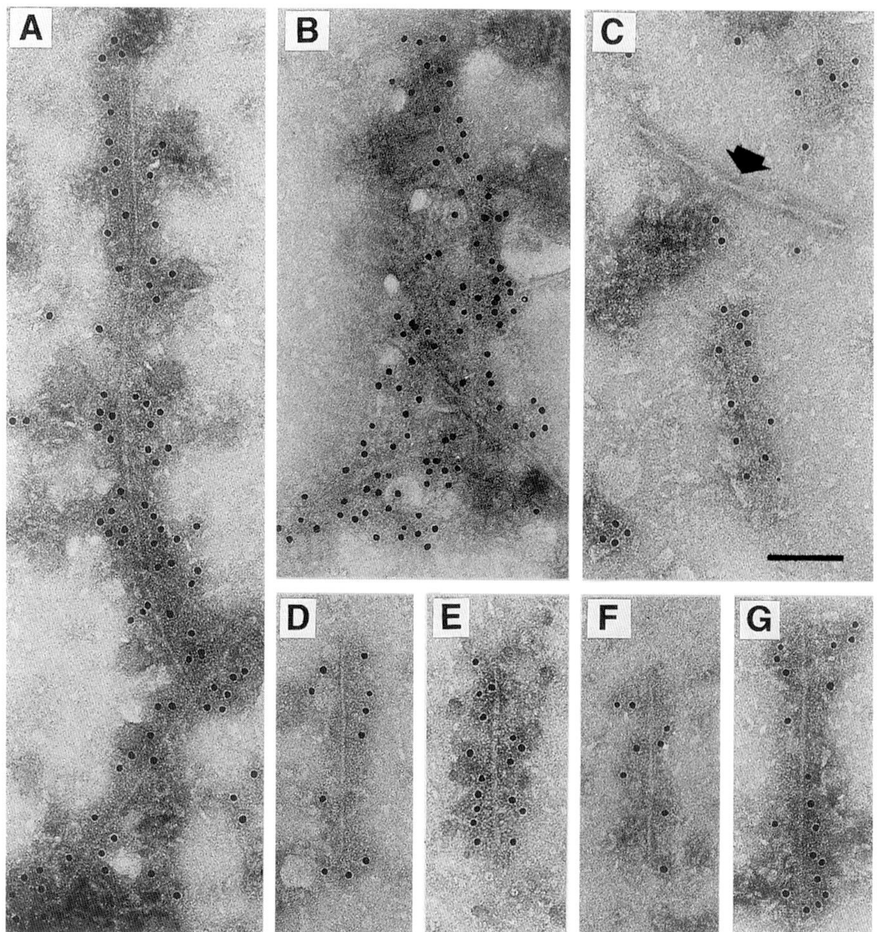

Fig. 6. Filaments from cingulate cortex of patients who had dementia with Lewy bodies immunolabeled for α-synuclein. **(A,B)** Small clumps of α-synuclein filaments. **(C)** A labeled α-synuclein filament and an unlabeled tau protein-containing paired helical filament (arrow). **(D–G)** The labeled filaments have various morphologies, including a 5-nm filament (D), a 10-nm filament with dark stain penetrated center line (E), a twisted filament showing alternating width (F), and a 10-nm filament with slender 5-nm extensions at the ends (G; also C). Antibody PER4, which recognizes the carboxy-terminal region of α-synuclein, was used. The 10-nm gold particles attached to the secondary antibody appear as black dots. Scale bar = 100 nm in C; applies to A–G.

1.3. α-Synuclein in Multiple System Atrophy

MSA is largely a sporadic neurodegenerative disorder that comprises cases of olivopontocerebellar atrophy, striatonigral degeneration, and Shy-Drager syndrome *(68)*. Clinically, it is characterized by a combination of cerebellar, extrapyramidal and autonomic symptoms.

Neuropathologically, glial cytoplasmic inclusions (GCIs), which consist of filamentous aggregates, are the defining feature of MSA *(69)*. They are found mostly in the cytoplasm and, to a lesser extent, in the nucleus of oligodendrocytes. Inclusions are also observed in the cytoplasm and nucleus of some nerve cells, as well as in neuropil threads. They consist of straight and twisted filaments, with reported diameters of 10–30 nm *(70)*. At the light microscopic level, GCIs are immunoreactive for ubiquitin and, to a lesser extent, for cytoskeletal proteins such as tau and tubulin. However, until recently, the biochemical composition of GCI filaments was unknown.

This has changed with the discovery that GCIs are strongly immunoreactive for α-synuclein and that filaments isolated from the brains of patients with MSA are labeled by α-synuclein antibodies (**Figs. 7** and **8**) *(19–22)*. Moreover, in tissue sections, GCI filaments are decorated by α-synuclein antibodies, as are filaments from partially purified GCIs *(65,71,72)*. The morphologies of isolated filaments and their staining characteristics were found to be very similar to those of filaments extracted from the cingulate cortex of patients with DLB *(21)*. As for the latter, staining for α-synuclein was far more extensive than staining for ubiquitin, until then the most sensitive immunohistochemical marker of GCIs *(21)*.

The number of α-synuclein filaments extracted from the MSA brain is higher than that extracted from the DLB brain, in keeping with the larger number of inclusions in MSA *(73)*. To date, there is no genetic evidence implicating α-synuclein in MSA *(74)*. Taken together, this work has demonstrated that α-synuclein is the major component of the GCI filaments and has revealed an unexpected molecular link between MSA and the Lewy body disorders PD and DLB.

1.4. Synthetic α-Synuclein Filaments

The discovery of α-synuclein filaments in Lewy body diseases and MSA has led to attempts aimed at producing synthetic α-synuclein filaments under physiologic conditions. A first study reported that removal of the C-terminal 20–30 residues of α-synuclein leads to spontaneous assembly into filaments within 24–48 h at 37°C, with morphologies and staining characteristics indistinguishable from those of Lewy body filaments (**Fig. 9**) *(75)*. This indicates that the packing of α-synuclein molecules in the filaments in vitro is very similar to that of filaments extracted from brain. A proportion of α-synuclein extracted from partially purified Lewy bodies and GCI filaments has been found to be truncated *(59,72)*. It remains to be seen whether truncation occurs before or after assembly of α-synuclein into filaments. Two subsequent studies

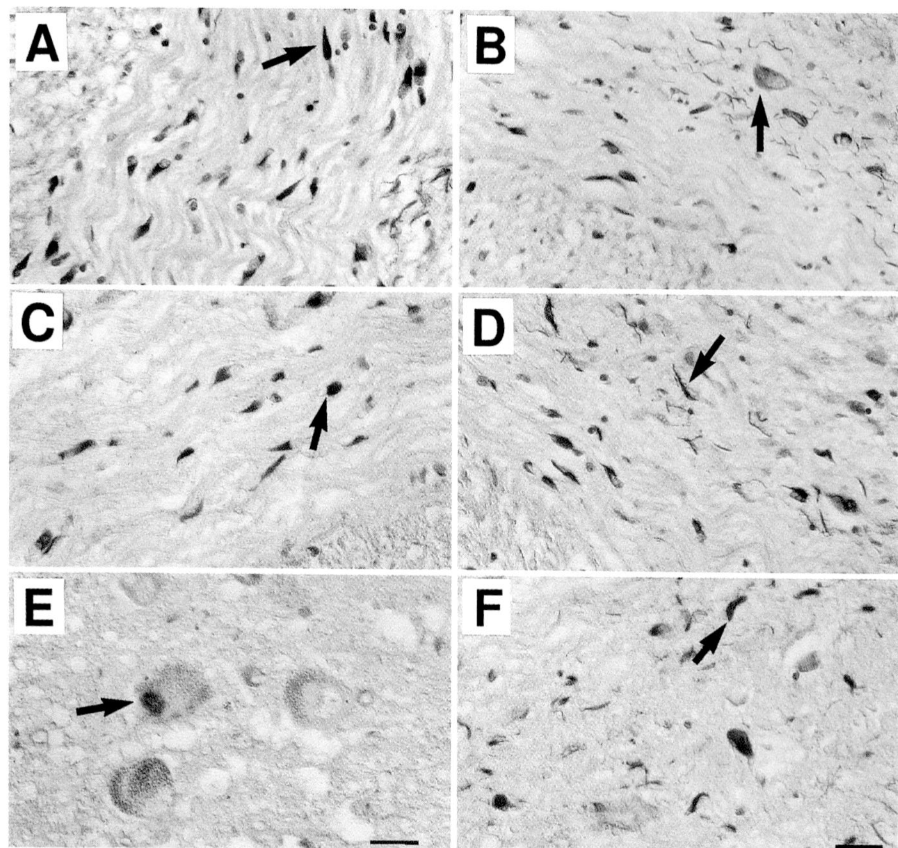

Fig. 7. White matter of pons and cerebellum and gray matter of pons and frontal cortex from patients with multiple system atrophy immunostained for α-synuclein. **(A–D)** α-Synuclein-immunoreactive oligodendrocytes and nerve cells in white matter of pons (A, B, D) and cerebellum (C) identified with antibodies recognizing the amino-terminal (antibody PER1) (A, C) or the carboxy-terminal (antibody PER2) (B, D) region of α-synuclein. **(E, F)** α-Synuclein-immunoreactive oligodendrocytes and nerve cells in gray matter of pons (E) and frontal cortex (F) identified with antibodies recognizing the amino-terminal (E) or the carboxy-terminal (F) region of α-synuclein. Arrows identify representative examples of each of the characteristic lesions stained for α-synuclein: cytoplasmic oligodendroglial inclusions (in A and F), cytoplasmic nerve cell inclusion (in B), nuclear oligodendroglial inclusion (in C), neuropil threads (in D), and nuclear nerve cell inclusion (in E). Scale bars = 33 μm in E; 50 μm in F (applies to A–D, F).

reported filament assembly from full-length α-synuclein after incubations ranging from 1 wk to 3 mo at 37°C ***(76,77)***. The A53T mutation was shown to

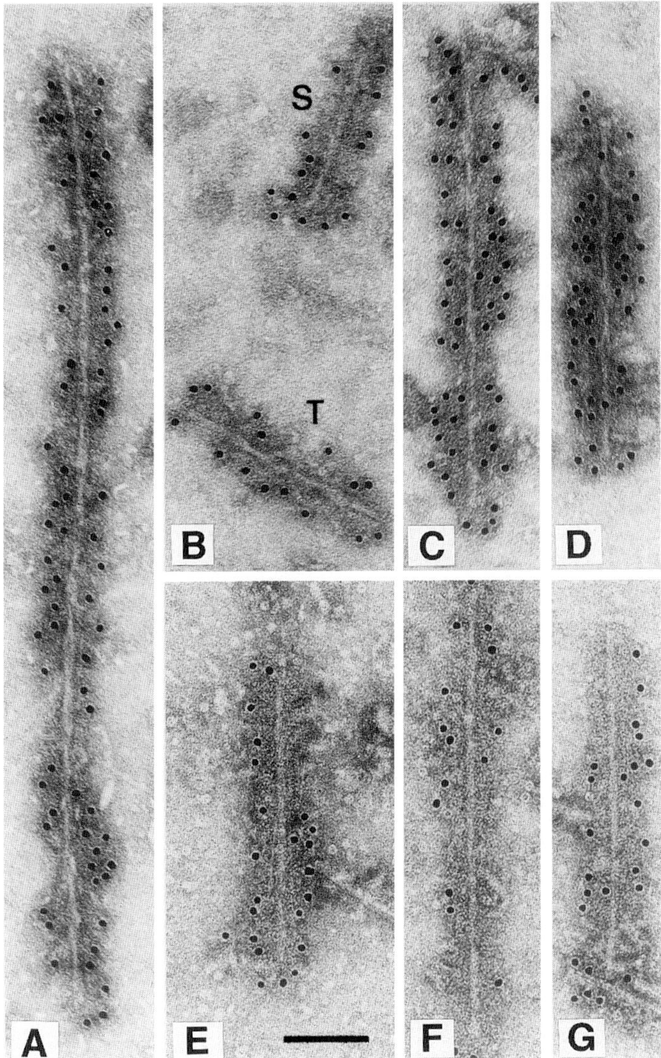

Fig. 8. Filaments from frontal cortex and cerebellum of patients with multiple system atrophy immunolabeled for α-synuclein. **(A, C, D)** Examples of twisted filaments. **(E–G)** Straight filaments. **(B)** Both a twisted (T) and a straight (S) filament. Antibody PER4, which recognizes the carboxy-terminal region of α-synuclein, was used. The 10-nm gold particles attached to the secondary antibody appear as black dots. Scale bar = 100 nm.

increase the rate of filament assembly *(77)*. However, based on the evidence presented, one could not exclude the possibility that the recombinant α-synuclein became truncated during the long incubation times.

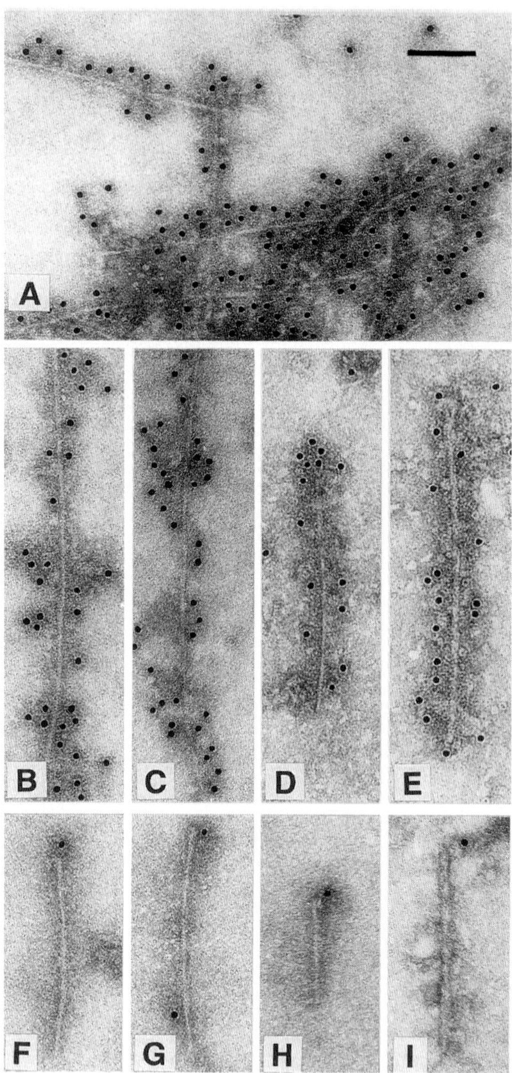

Fig. 9. Immunolabeling of synthetic α-synuclein(1–120) filaments and filaments extracted from dementia with Lewy bodies and multiple system atrophy brains. Filaments are labelled with an antibody that recognizes the carboxy-terminal (antibody PER4) **(A–E)** or the amino-terminal region of α-synuclein (antibody PER 1) (F–I). (A-C) α-Synuclein(1–120) filaments showing a labelled clump and individual filaments. (D, E) Filaments extracted from brains with Lewy body dementia (D) or multiple system atrophy (E). **(F–I)** End-labeled filaments, showing α-synuclein(1–120) filaments (F–H) and a filament from a brain with multiple system atrophy (I). The 10-nm gold particles attached to the secondary antibody appear as black dots. Scale bar = 100 nm.

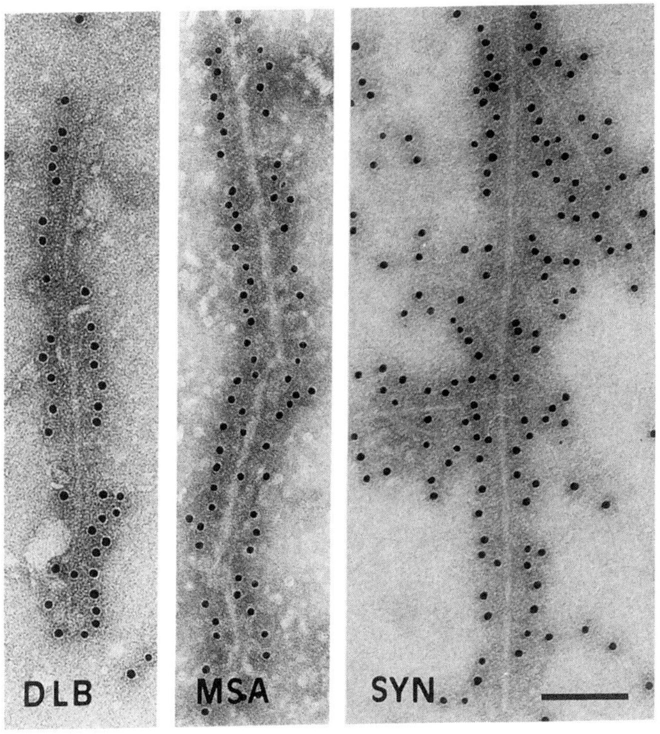

Fig. 10. Immunolabeling of synthetic α-synuclein(1–140) filaments (SYN) and filaments extracted from dementia with Lewy bodies (DLB) and multiple system atrophy (MSA) brains. Filaments are labeled with an antibody that recognizes the carboxy-terminal 10 amino acids of human α-synuclein (antibody H3C). The 10-nm gold particles attached to the secondary antibody appear as black dots. Scale bar = 100 nm.

More recently, improved methods requiring much shorter incubation times have shown unambigously that full-length α-synuclein assembles into filaments ***(78–81)***. The synthetic filaments were decorated by an antibody that recognizes the carboxy-terminal 10 amino acids of α-synuclein, as were filaments extracted from DLB and MSA brains (**Fig. 10**) ***(81)***. These experiments have also shown that the A53T mutation and carboxy-terminal truncation, as in α-synuclein(1–87) and α-synuclein(1–120), produce markedly increased rates of filament assembly. α-Synuclein thus assembles through its repeat-containing amino-terminal half. Earlier work had shown that a synthetic peptide comprising amino acids 61–95 of human α-synuclein readily assembles into filaments ***(82)***. Interestingly, residues 66–73 of α-synuclein (VGGAVVTG) resemble residues 36–42 of amyloid Aβ (VGGVVIAT) and residues 117–124 of the prion protein (AAGAVVGG).

Depending on the studies, the effect of the A30P mutation on the rate of filament assembly was either small *(79)* or absent *(81)*. Increased fibrillogenesis of mutant α-synuclein may therefore not be a feature shared by the two familial PD mutations. Unlike recombinant α-synuclein with the A53T mutation, α-synuclein with the A30P mutation has been shown to be devoid of significant vesicle-binding activity, suggesting that this may be its primary effect *(39)*. Rodent and zebra finch α-synuclein readily assembled into filaments, consistent with the presence of a threonine residue at position 53 *(81)*. Circular dichroism spectroscopy indicated that α-synuclein undergoes a conformational change from random coil to β-sheet structure during assembly *(81)*. By X-ray diffraction and electron diffraction, the various synthetic α-synuclein filaments showed a cross-β conformation characteristic of amyloid *(81)*. Upon shaking, filaments formed within 48 h at 37°C. β-Synuclein and γ-synuclein only assembled after several weeks of incubation, in keeping with the finding that antibodies directed against β-synuclein and γ-synuclein do not stain the pathologic inclusions of PD, DLB, and MSA.

2. Materials

2.1. Detection of α-Synuclein Inclusions by Immunohistochemistry

2.1.1. Antibodies

Here we show results obtained with the anti-synuclein antibodies PER1 *(11,12)*, PER2 *(11,12,29)*, PER4 *(12,21)*, PER5 *(12)*, LB509 *(59,64)*, SYN207 *(16,65)*, and H3C *(30)*. PER1 and PER2 are polyclonal antibodies that were raised against synthetic peptides corresponding to amino acids 11–34 and 117–131 of human α-synuclein, respectively. PER4 is a polyclonal antibody that was raised against recombinant human α-synuclein and recognizes the carboxy-terminal half of α-synuclein. PER5 is a polyclonal antibody that was raised against recombinant γ-synuclein. LB509 is a monoclonal antibody that was raised against partially purified Lewy bodies. It recognizes residues 117–124 of human α-synuclein. SYN207 is a monoclonal antibody that was raised against recombinant human β-synuclein. H3C is a monoclonal antibody that was raised against a synthetic peptide corresponding to residues 129–143 of zebra finch α-synuclein (synelfin) (*see* **Note 1**).

2.1.2. Tissue Processing

1. Phosphate-buffered saline (PBS): 0.13 *M* NaCl, 7 m*M* Na_2HPO_4, and 7 m*M* NaH_2PO_4 in water.
2. Paraformaldehyde solution: Four grams of paraformaldehyde are weighed out in a hood and added to 100 mL PBS. The solution is stirred and heated to 50°C. After 15–20 min, a few drops of 2 *M* NaOH are added, to clear the solution,

which is then filtered through Whatman filter paper. Paraformaldehyde is always prepared fresh.

3. Sucrose solutions: Five or 30 g sucrose are added to 100 mL PBS and stirred until dissolved (to give 5 and 30% solutions, respectively).

2.1.3. Immunohistochemistry

1. Methanol/hydrogen peroxide solution: Add 10 mL methanol and 10 mL hydrogen peroxide to 80 mL water.
2. 3,3-Diaminobenzidine (DAB) and 4-chloro-1-naphthol solutions: We routinely use the Vectastain Elite kit (Vector) and develop the staining with DAB and horseradish peroxidase (Vector) or with 4-chloro-1-naphthol (Sigma). The DAB solution is prepared by adding two drops of buffer solution, three drops of DAB solution, and two drops of hydrogen peroxide to 5 mL water. The 4-chloro-1-naphthol solution is prepared by adding 50 mg 4-chloro-1-naphthol to 100 mL absolute ethanol, followed by addition of 100 mL 250 m*M* Tris-HCl, pH 7.4, and 15 μL 30% hydrogen peroxide.
3. Cresyl violet: A stock solution of 1% cresyl violet (British Drug House) in water is diluted tenfold.

2.2. Extraction of Isolated α-Synuclein Filaments

1. Frozen brain tissue from individuals with PD, DLB, and MSA is used. The tissue is removed at autopsy (4–16 h after death) and kept at –70°C until use (*see* **Note 2**). Filaments are extracted using a procedure developed for the extraction of dispersed tau filaments from AD brain ***(83,84)*** (*see* **Subheading 3.2.**).
2. Homogenization buffer: 10 m*M* Tris-HCl, pH 7.4, 0.8 *M* NaCl, 1 m*M* ethylene glycol bis(β-aminoethyl ether)N,N,N',N'-tetra-acetic acid (EGTA), 10% sucrose in water.
3. Sarcosyl solution: Prepare a 10% solution of *N*-lauroylsarcosinate (w/v, Sigma) in water.

2.3. Electron Microscopy

Lithium phosphotungstate: Prepare a 1% solution of dodeca-tungstophosphoric acid (British Drug House) in water. Use 1 *M* lithium hydroxide to bring pH to 6.5.

2.4. Expression and Purification of Recombinant Synucleins

1. cDNA fragments encoding α-, β-, or γ-synuclein are amplified by polymerase chain reaction (PCR), verified by DNA sequencing, and subcloned into a bacterial expression vector. Our work makes use of the expression vector pRK172, into which human α- and β-synuclein are subcloned as *Nde*I/*Hin*dIII fragments and human γ-synuclein as an *Nde*I/*Eco*RI fragment ***(12,29)***.
2. Buffer 1: 50 m*M* Tris-HCl, pH 7.4, 0.5 m*M* ethylenediamine tetraacetic acid (EDTA), 0.1 m*M* dithiothreitol (DTT), 0.1 m*M* phenylmethylsulphonyl fluoride (PMSF).
3. Buffer 2: 50 m*M* Tris-HCl, pH 8.25, 50 m*M* NaCl, 0.1 m*M* DTT, 0.1 m*M* PMSF.

2.5. Filament Assembly of Recombinant α-Synuclein

Assembly buffer: 30 m*M* 3-[*N*-morpholino]propanesulphonic acid (MOPS), pH 7.2, containing 0.02% sodium azide.

3. Methods

3.1. Detection of α-Synuclein Inclusions by Imunohistochemistry

3.1.1. Antibodies

Prior to use, antibodies are diluted in PBS. The dilutions usually range from 1:500 to 1:5,000 and depend on the antibody titer. The optimal dilution of a given antibody is determined empirically.

3.1.2. Tissue Processing

1. For immunohistochemistry of synucleins, we use fixed free-floating or deparaffinized tissue sections ***(11,12,21)***. Fresh-frozen tissue (1 g) is immersion-fixed for 12 h in 20 mL 4% paraformaldehyde.
2. The fixed tissue is then transferred into 30% sucrose and left at 4°C until it has sunk to the bottom of the vial.
3. Sections (40 μm) are cut on a freezing microtome and kept at 4°C in 5% sucrose + 0.002% sodium azide until use.
4. Immunostaining is performed in either 1.5-mL Eppendorf tubes or 24-well microtiter dishes.
5. For paraffin embedding, the fixed tissue is dehydrated by passing through distilled water for 5 min and successively for 10 min through 50, 70, and 95% ethanol, followed by 2 × 10 min in absolute ethanol.
6. The dehydrated tissue is then immersed for 10 h in chloroform and embedded in hot, melted paraffin wax and left in a vacuum oven at 60°C for 1 h.
7. The paraffin solution is changed twice, and the tissue is transferred into a mold in water, where the paraffin solidifies. The wax block is kept at room temperature or at 4°C.
8. Sections (7–10 μm) are cut on a microtome, and the cut ribbons are placed in a 50°C water bath from which they are collected onto glass slides pretreated with poly-L-lysine (0.01%) or with poly-L-lysine and gelatin.
9. Prior to immunostaining, paraffin is removed by heating the sections to 60°C for 15 min, followed by immersion in xylene for 30 min.
10. The tissue sections are then rehydrated through an ascending alcohol series and dipped in water and PBS.

3.1.3. Immunohistochemistry

1. Immerse tissue sections in 10% methanol/10% hydrogen peroxide for 10 min at room temperature, to block endogenous peroxidase activity.
2. Incubate sections for 30 min at room temperature in 30% goat or horse serum, depending on whether the secondary antibody is anti-rabbit raised in goat or anti-mouse raised in horse.
3. Incubate sections in diluted primary antibody at 4°C for 16 h.

4. Wash sections 3 × 10 min in PBS at room temperature.
5. Incubate sections for 2 h at room temperature in biotinylated secondary antibody (diluted 1:200).
6. Wash sections 3 × 10 min in PBS at room temperature.
7. Incubate sections in avidin-conjugated horseradish peroxidase for 1 h at room temperature.
8. Wash sections 3 × 10 min in PBS at room temperature.
9. Development of the reaction product with DAB is done according to the manufacturer's (Vector) instructions. Development of the brown color is followed under the microscope and the reaction stopped by rinsing the sections in water.
10. Double-staining immunohistochemistry follows the above protocol, except that the steps prior to incubation with the primary antibody are omitted. Staining with the second primary antibody is revealed using 4-chloro-1-naphthol. Development of the blue color is followed under the microscope and stopped by rinsing the sections in water.
11. Following the staining, the free-floating sections are mounted onto microscope slides coated with poly-L-lysine and left to air-dry.
12. Single-stained sections that were developed using DAB are counterstained with cresyl violet (British Drug House), dehydrated through an ascending alcohol series, left in xylene for 30 min, and mounted in DPX Mountant (British Drug House). Double-stained sections or single-stained sections developed using 4-chloro-1-naphthol are not counterstained but mounted directly using gelatin or aqueous mountant, since the blue color is soluble in ethanol.

3.2. Extraction of Isolated α-Synuclein Filaments

1. Homogenize brain tissue with a Polytron (30 s at setting 7) in 10 volumes (w/v) of homogenization buffer.
2. Spin for 20 min at 20,000*g* and retain the supernatant.
3. Rehomogenize the pellet in 5 vol of homogenization buffer and recentrifuge.
4. Bring combined supernatants to 1% *N*-lauroylsarcosinate and incubate for 1 h at room temperature while shaking.
5. Spin for 1 h at 100,000*g* and discard supernatant.
6. Resuspend the sarcosyl-insoluble pellet in 50 m*M* Tris-HCl, pH 7.4, 0.1 m*M* PMSF (0.2 mL/g starting material) and store at 4°C. This material is used for electron microscopy and immunoblotting.

3.3. Electron Microscopy

1. Place a small droplet of resuspended sarcosyl-insoluble pellet on carbon-coated copper grid (400 mesh) and allow to evaporate partially.
2. Unlabeled filaments are stained with a few drops of 1% lithium phosphotungstate and allowed to air dry.
3. For antibody labeling, place the grid with adsorbed specimen on a drop of 0.1% gelatin in PBS and block for 5–10 min.
4. Lift grid, blot excess solution, and place grid on a solution of primary antibody for 1 h at room temperature (*see* **Note 3**).

5. Wash grid with a few drops of 0.1% gelatin in PBS, blot, and place on a solution of secondary antibody conjugated to gold (1:100, Sigma) for 1 h at room temperature.
6. Wash grid with a few drops of gelatin solution, blot, and stain with a few drops of 1% lithium phosphotungstate. Allow to air dry.
7. Micrographs are recorded at a nominal magnification of ×40,000 on a Philips model EM208S microscope.

3.4. Expression and Purification of Recombinant Synucleins

1. Transform expression plasmids into *Escherichia coli* strain BL21(DE3) and grow to an optical density (at 600 nm) of 0.6–1.0 at 37°C.
2. Add isopropyl β-D-thiogalactopyranoside (IPTG) to 0.4 m*M* and grow for a further 3 h.
3. Spin bacteria for 15 min at 3,000*g* and quick-freeze in liquid nitrogen. Keep at –20°C until use.
4. Resuspend bacterial paste from 1 L culture in 30 mL buffer 1 and sonicate using a Kontes Micro Ultrasonic Cell Disrupter (3 × 30 s bursts). Spin for 15 min at 10,000*g*.
5. Pass supernatant over a DEAE column (25 × 80 mm) and step-elute with 10-mL aliquots of buffer 1 containing increasing amounts of NaCl. The three human synucleins elute at the following NaCl concentrations: 180 m*M* for γ-synuclein, 225 m*M* for α-synuclein, and 250 mM for β-synuclein.
6. Precipitate samples with 50% ammonium sulphate and redissolve in a small volume of buffer 2. Pass over a Sephacryl S-200 column (1.4 × 100 cm) equilibrated in buffer 2.
7. Apply peak fractions to a Pharmacia MonoQ column and elute proteins using a 0–500 m*M* NaCl gradient in buffer 2 at a flow rate of 1 mL/min. The synucleins elute at about 200 m*M* NaCl.
8. Dialyze the purified proteins overnight against 5 m*M* ammonium bicarbonate using Spectrapor dialysis tubing (cutoff 2000 molecular mass), shell-freeze, freeze-dry, and resuspend in water at approximately 10 mg/mL. The exact protein concentrations are determined by quantitative amino acid analysis. All purification steps are monitored by SDS/PAGE.

3.5. Filament Assembly of Recombinant α-Synuclein

1. Purified recombinant α-synuclein of known concentration is kept at 4°C until use.
2. Assembly is performed at 37°C in plastic or glass tubes placed in a shaking bacterial incubator (G24 Environmental Incubator Shaker, New Brunswick Scientific, speed setting of 450) ***(81)***.
3. Full-length human α-synuclein is used at 7 mg/mL (400 μ*M*) in assembly buffer. Bulk assembly into filaments is reliably observed after 48 h (*see* **Note 4**).
4. α-Synuclein filaments are detected by electron microscopy and their identity confirmed by immunoelectron microscopy (*see* above for Methods).

4. Notes

1. Various rabbit polyclonal antibodies that were raised against either synthetic peptides of α-synuclein (such as residues 11–34 or 117–131) or against purified recombinant α-synuclein have been used to detect α-synuclein inclusions in tissue sections ***(11,12,21,29)***. A number of monoclonal anti-α-synuclein antibodies have been produced, using synthetic peptides, recombinant proteins, or partially purified Lewy bodies as antigens ***(30,59,65)***. Some antibodies are specific for α-synuclein and fail to recognize β- or γ-synuclein ***(21,29,59,65)***. Several antibodies recognize human α-synuclein but not rodent or zebra finch α-synuclein ***(64,65)***. Antibodies specific for β- and γ-synuclein have also been produced ***(12,29,65)***. The epitopes of synuclein antibodies can be determined by immunoblotting of full-length and truncated recombinant proteins ***(12,29,64,65)***. Monoclonal antibodies are stored at 4°C as culture medium or ascites. Antisera are stored undiluted at –20°C. Several synuclein antibodies are commercially available.
2. The larger the number of pathologic inclusions, the higher the yield of isolated α-synuclein filaments. We have obtained the best results using cingulate cortex from patients with DLB or frontal cortex and cerebellum from patients with MSA ***(12,21)***. The filament yield is especially good in MSA brain, in keeping with the high density of pathology ***(73)***.
3. Antibodies for electron microscopy are used at approximately tenfold higher concentration than for light microscopic immunohistochemical staining.
4. Assembly is strongly concentration dependent and occurs after a lag phase, indicating a nucleation-dependent process. Filament morphologies closely resemble those of isolated filaments from DLB and MSA brain ***(81)***. Recombinant α-synuclein with the familial PD mutations assembles under the same conditions. This method also works for human α-synuclein fragments, such as 1–87 and 1–120, and for rat and zebra finch α-synuclein. Under these conditions, recombinant human β- and γ-synuclein only form filaments after several weeks of incubation ***(81)***.

References

1. Parkinson, J. (1817) *An Essay on the Shaking Palsy*. Sherwood, Neely, and Jones. London.
2. Lewy, F. H. (1912) Paralysis agitans. I. Pathologische Anatomie, in *Handbuch der Neurologie,* vol. 3 (Lewandowsky, M. and Abelsdorff, G., eds.), Springer, Berlin, pp. 920–933.
3. Trétiakoff, M. C. (1919) Thesis, University of Paris.
4. Forno, L. S. (1996) Neuropathology of Parkinson's disease. *J. Neuropathol. Exp. Neurol.* **55,** 259–272.
5. Duffy, P. E. and Tennyson, V. M. (1965) Phase and electron microscopic observations on Lewy bodies and melanin granules in the substantia nigra and locus coeruleus in Parkinson's disease. *J. Neuropathol. Exp. Neurol.* **24,** 398–414.
6. Okazaki, H., Lipkin, L. E., and Aronson, S. M. (1961) Diffuse intracytoplasmic ganglionic inclusions (Lewy type) associated with progressive dementia and quadriparesis in flexion. *J. Neuropathol. Exp. Neurol.* **21,** 442–449.

7. Kosaka, K. (1978) Lewy bodies in cerebral cortex. Report of three cases. *Acta Neuropathol.* **42,** 127–134.
8. Hansen, L. A., Salmon, D., Galasko, D., Masliah, E., Katzman, R., DeTeresa, L., et al. (1990) The Lewy body variant of Alzheimer's disease: a clinical and pathological entity. *Neurology* **40,** 1–8.
9. Perry, R. H., Irving, D., Blessed, G., Fairbairn, A., and Perry, E. K. (1990) Senile dementia of the Lewy body type. A clinically and neuropathologically distinct form of Lewy body dementia in the elderly. *J. Neurol. Sci.* **85,** 119–139.
10. Polymeropoulos, M. H., Lavedan, C., Leroy, E., Ide, S. E., Dehejia, A., Dutra, A., et al. (1997) Mutation in the α-synuclein gene identified in families with Parkinson's disease. *Science* **276,** 2045–2047.
11. Spillantini, M. G., Schmidt, M. L., Lee, V. M.-Y., Trojanowski, J. Q., Jakes, R., and Goedert, M. (1997) α-Synuclein in Lewy bodies. *Nature* **388,** 839–840.
12. Spillantini, M. G., Crowther, R. A., Jakes, R., Hasegawa, M. and Goedert M. (1998) α-Synuclein in filamentous inclusions of Lewy bodies from Parkinson's disease and dementia with Lewy bodies. *Proc. Natl. Acad. Sci. USA* **95,** 6469–6473.
13. Lippa, C. F., Fujiwara, H., Mann, D. M. A., Giasson, B., Baba, M., Schmidt, M. L., et al. (1998) Lewy bodies contain altered α-synuclein in brains of many familial Alzheimer's disease patients with mutations in presenilin and amyloid precursor protein genes. *Am. J. Pathol.* **153,** 1365–1370.
14. Lippa, C. F., Schmidt, M. L., Lee, V. M.-Y., and Trojanowski, J. Q. (1999) Antibodies to α-synuclein detect Lewy bodies in many Down's syndrome brains with Alzheimer's disease. *Ann. Neurol.* **45,** 353–357.
15. Spillantini, M. G., Tolnay, M., Love, S., and Goedert, M. (1999) Microtubule-associated protein tau, heparan sulphate and α-synuclein in several neurodegenerative diseases with dementia. *Acta Neuropathol.* **97,** 585–594.
16. Tu, P.-H., Galvin, J. E., Baba, M., Giasson, B., Tomita, T., Leight, S., et al. (1998) Glial cytoplasmic inclusions in white matter oligodendrocytes of multiple system atrophy brains contain insoluble α-synuclein. *Ann. Neurol.* **44,** 415–422.
17. Arawaka, S., Saito, Y., Murayama, S. and Mori, H. (1998) Lewy body in neurodegeneration with brain iron accumulation type 1 is immunoreactive for α-synuclein. *Neurology* **51,** 887–889.
18. Wakabayashi, K., Yoshimoto, M., Fukushima, T., Koide, R., Horikawa, Y., Morita, T., and Takahashi, G. H. (1999) Widespread occurrence of α-synuclein/NACP-immunoreactive neuronal inclusions in juvenile and adult-onset Hallervorden-Spatz disease with Lewy bodies. *Neuropathol. Appl. Neurobiol.* **25,** 363–368.
19. Wakabayashi, K., Yoshimoto, M., Tsuji, S., and Takahashi, H. (1998) α-Synuclein immunoreactivity in glial cytoplasmic inclusions in multiple system atrophy. *Neurosci. Lett.* **249,** 180–182.
20. Mezey, E., Dehejia, A., Harta, G., Papp, M. I., Polymeropoulos, M. H., and Brownstein, M. J. (1998) Alpha synuclein in neurodegenerative disorders: Murderer or accomplice? *Nature Med.* **4,** 755–757.
21. Spillantini, M. G., Crowther, R. A., Jakes, R., Cairns, N. J., Lantos, P. L., and Goedert, M. (1998) Filamentous α-synuclein inclusions link multiple system

atrophy with Parkinson's disease and dementia with Lewy bodies. *Neurosci. Lett.* **251,** 205–208.

22. Gai, W. P., Power, J. H. T., Blumbergs, P. C., and Blessing, W. W. (1998) Multiple system atrophy: a new α-synuclein disease? *Lancet* **352,** 547–548.
23. Maroteaux, L., Campanelli, J. T., and Scheller, R. H. (1988) Synuclein: A neuron-specific protein localized to the nucleus and presynaptic nerve terminal. *J. Neurosci.* **8,** 2804–2815.
24. Maroteaux, L. and Scheller, R. H. (1991) The rat brain synucleins; family of proteins transiently associated with neuronal membrane. *Mol. Brain Res.* **11,** 335–343.
25. Tobe, T., Nakajo, S., Tanaka, A., Mitoya, A., Omata, K., Nakaya, K., et al. (1992) Cloning and characterization of the cDNA encoding a novel specific 14-kDa protein. *J. Neurochem.* **59,** 1624–1629.
26. Uéda, K., Fukushima, H., Masliah, E., Xia, Y., Iwai, A., Yoshimoto, M., et al. (1993) Molecular cloning of cDNA encoding an unrecognized component of amyloid in Alzheimer disease. *Proc. Natl. Acad. Sci. USA* **90,** 11,282–11,286.
27. Bayer, T. A., Jäkälä, P., Hartmann, T., Havas, L., McLean, C., Culvenor, J. G., et al. (1999) α-Synuclein accumulates in Lewy bodies in Parkinson's disease and dementia with Lewy bodies but not in Alzheimer's disease β-amyloid cores. *Neurosci. Lett.* **266,** 213–216.
28. Culvenor, J. G., McLean, C. A., Cutt, S., Campbell, B. C. V., Maher, F., Jäkälä, P., et al. (1999) Non-Aβ component of Alzheimer's disease amyloid (NAC) revisited. NAC and α-synuclein are not associated with Aβ amyloid. *Am. J. Pathol.* **155,** 1173–1881.
29. Jakes, R., Spillantini, M. G., and Goedert, M. (1994) Identification of two distinct synucleins from human brain. *FEBS Lett.* **345,** 27–32.
30. George, J. M., Jin, H., Woods, W. S., and Clayton, D. F. (1995) Characterization of a novel protein regulated during the critical period for song learning in the zebra finch. *Neuron* **15,** 361–372.
31. Campion, D., Martin, C., Heilig, R., Charbonnier, F., Moreau, V., Flaman, J. M., et al. (1995) The NACP/synuclein gene: Chromosomal assignment and screening for alterations in Alzheimer disease. *Genomics* **26,** 254–257.
32. Chen, X., de Silva, H. A. R., Pettenati, M. J., Rao, P. N., St. George-Hyslop, P., Roses, A. D., et al. (1995) The human NACP/α-synuclein gene: chromosome assignment to 4q21. 3-q22 and *TaqI* RFLP analysis. *Genomics* **26,** 425–427.
33. Spillantini, M. G., Divane, A., and Goedert, M. (1995) Assignment of human α-synuclein (SNCA) and β-synuclein (SNCB) genes to chromosomes 4q21 and 5q35. *Genomics* **27,** 379–381.
34. Shibasaki, Y., Baillie, D. A. M., St. Clair, D., and Brookes, A. J. (1995) High-resolution mapping of SNCA encoding α-synuclein, the non-Aβ component of Alzheimer's disease precursor, to human chromosome 4q21.3-q22 by fluorescence in situ hybridization. *Cytogenet. Cell. Genet.* **71,** 54,55.

35. Lavedan, C., Leroy, E., Torres, R., Dehejia, A., Dutra, A., Buchholtz, S., et al. (1998) Genomic organization and expression of the human β-synuclein gene (SNCB). *Genomics* **54,** 173–175.
36. Uéda, K., Saitoh, T., and Mori, H. (1994) Tissue-dependent alternative splicing of mRNA for NACP, the precursor of non-Aβ component of Alzheimer's disease amyloid. *Biochem. Biophys. Res. Commun.* **205,** 1366–1372.
37. Weinreb, P. H., Zhen, W., Poon, A. W., Conway, K. A., and Lansbury, P. T. (1996) NACP, a protein implicated in Alzheimer's disease and learning, is natively unfolded. *Biochemistry* **35,** 13,709–13,715.
38. Davidson, W. S., Jonas, A., Clayton, D. F., and George, J. M. (1998) Stabilization of α-synuclein secondary structure upon binding to synthetic membranes. *J. Biol. Chem.* **273,** 9443–9449.
39. Jensen, P. H., Nielsen, M. H., Jakes, R., Dotti, C. G., and Goedert, M. (1998) Binding of α-synuclein to rat brain vesicles is abolished by familial Parkinson's disease mutation. *J. Biol. Chem.* **273,** 26,292–26,294.
40. Jenco, J. M., Rawlingson, A., Daniels, B., and Morris, A. J. (1998) Regulation of phospholipase D2: Selective inhibition of mammalian phospholipase D isoenzymes by α- and β-synucleins. *Biochemistry* **37,** 4901–4909.
41. Colley, W. C., Sung, T.-C., Roll, R., Jenco, J., Hammond, S. M., Altshuller, Y., et al. (1997) Phospholipase D2, a distinct phospholipase D isoform with novel regulatory properties that provokes cytoskeletal reorganization. *Curr. Biol.* **7,** 191–201.
42. Okochi, M., Walter, J., Koyama, A., Nakajo, S., Baba, M., Iwatsubo, T., et al. (2000) Constitutive phosphorylation of the Parkinson's disease-associated α-synuclein. *J. Biol. Chem.* **275,** 390–397.
43. Ji, H., Liu, Y. E., Jia, T., Wang, M., Liu, J., Xiao, G., et al. (1997) Identification of a breast cancer-specific gene, *BCSG1*, by direct differential cDNA sequencing. *Cancer Res.* **57,** 759–764.
44. Goedert, M., Jakes, R., and Spillantini, M. G. (1998) Alpha-synuclein and the Lewy body. *NeuroSci. News* **1,** 47–52.
45. Buchman, V. L., Hunter, H. J. A., Pinon, L. G. P., Thompson, J., Privalova, E. M., Ninkina, N. N., et al. (1998) Persyn, a member of the synuclein family, has a distinct pattern of expression in the developing nervous system. *J. Neurosci.* **18,** 9335–9341.
46. Lavedan, C., Leroy, E., Dehejia, A., Buchholtz, S., Dutra, A., Nussbaum, R. L., et al. (1998) Identification, localization and characterization of the human γ-synuclein gene. *Hum. Genet.* **103,** 106–112.
47. Ninkina, N. N., Alimova-Kost, M. V., Paterson, J. W. E., Delaney, L., Cohen, B. B., Imreh, S., et al. (1998) Organization, expression and polymorphism of the human *persyn* gene. *Hum. Mol. Genet.* **7,** 1417–1424.
48. Surguchov, A., Surgucheva, I., Solessio, E., and Baehr, W. (1999) Synoretin—a new protein belonging to the synuclein family. *Mol. Cell. Neurosci.* **13,** 95–103.
49. Golbe, L. I., Di Iorio, G., Bonavita, V., Miller, D. C., and Duvoisin, R. C. (1990) A large kindred with autosomal dominant Parkinson's disease. *Ann. Neurol.* **27,** 276–282.

50. Polymeropoulos, M. H., Higgins, J. J., Golbe, L. I., Johnson, W. G., Ide, S. E., Di Iorio, G., et al. (1996) Mapping of a gene for Parkinson's disease to chromosome 4q21-q23. *Science* **274,** 1197–1199.
51. Athanassiadou, A., Voutsinas, G., Psiouri, L., Leroy, E., Polymeropoulos, M. H., Ilias, A., Maniatis, G. M., and Papapetropoulos, T. (1999) Genetic analysis of families with Parkinson disease that carry the Ala53Thr mutation in the gene encoding α-synuclein. *Am. J. Hum. Genet.* **65,** 555–558.
52. Lincoln, S., Gwinn-Hardy, K., Goudreau, J., Chartier-Harlin, M. C., Baker, M., Mouroux, V., et al. (1999) No pathogenic mutations in the persyn gene in Parkinson's disease. *Neurosci. Lett.* **259,** 65,66.
53. Lincoln, S., Crook, R., Chartier-Harlin, M. C., Gwinn-Hardy, K., Baker, M., Mouroux, V., et al. (1999) No pathogenic mutations in the β-synuclein gene in Parkinson's disease. *Neurosci. Lett.* **269,** 107–109.
54. Flowers, J. M., Leigh, P. N., Davies, A. M., Ninkina, N. N., Buchman, V. L., Vaughan, J., et al. (1999) Mutations in the gene encoding human persyn are not associated with amyotrophic lateral sclerosis or familial Parkinson's disease. *Neurosci. Lett.* **274,** 21–24.
55. Krüger, R., Kuhn, W., Müller, T., Woitalla, D., Graeber, M., Kösel, S., et al. (1998) Ala30Pro mutation in the gene encoding α-synuclein in Parkinson's disease. *Nature Genet.* **18,** 106–108.
56. Bennett, M. C., Bishop, J. F., Leng, Y., Chock, P. B., Chase, T. N., and Mouradian, M. M. (1999) Degradation of α-synuclein by proteasome. *J. Biol. Chem.* **274,** 33,855–33,858.
57. Wakabayashi, K., Matsumoto, K., Takayama, K., Yoshimoto, M., and Takahashi, H. (1997) NACP, a presynaptic protein, immunoreactivity in Lewy bodies in Parkinson's disease. *Neurosci. Lett.* **239,** 45–48.
58. Takeda, A., Mallory, M., Sundsmo, M., Honer, W., Hansen, L., and Masliah, E. (1998) Abnormal accumulation of NACP/α-synuclein in neurodegenerative disorders. *Am. J. Pathol.* **152,** 367–372.
59. Baba, M., Nakajo, S., Tu, P.-H., Tomita, T., Nakaya, K., Lee, V. M.-Y., et al. (1998) Aggregation of α-synuclein in Lewy bodies of sporadic Parkinson's disease and dementia with Lewy bodies. *Am. J. Pathol.* **152,** 879–884.
60. Irizarry, M. C., Growdon, W., Gomez-Isla, T., Newell, K., George, J. M., Clayton, D. F., et al. (1998) Nigral and cortical Lewy bodies and dystrophic nigral neurites in Parkinson's disease and cortical Lewy body disease contain α-synuclein immunoreactivity. *J. Neuropathol. Exp. Neurol.* **57,** 334–337.
61. Mezey, E., Dehejia, A. M., Harta, G., Suchy, S. F., Nussbaum, R. L., Brownstein, M. J., et al. (1998) Alpha synuclein is present in Lewy bodies in sporadic Parkinson's disease. *Mol. Psychiat.* **3,** 493–499.
62. Arai, T., Uéda, K., Ikeda, K., Akiyama, H., Haga, C., Kondo, H., et al. (1999) Argyrophilic glial inclusions in the midbrain of patients with Parkinson's disease and diffuse Lewy body disease are immunopositive for NACP/α-synuclein. *Neurosci. Lett.* **259,** 83–86.

63. Braak, H., Sandmann-Keil, D., Gai, W. P., and Braak, E. (1999) Extensive axonal Lewy neurites in Parkinson's disease: a novel pathological feature revealed by α-synuclein immunocytochemistry. *Neurosci. Lett.* **265,** 67–69.
64. Jakes, R., Crowther, R. A., Lee, V. M.-Y., Trojanowski, J. Q., Iwatsubo, T., and Goedert, M. (1999) Epitope mapping of LB509, a monoclonal antibody directed against human α-synuclein. *Neurosci. Lett.* **269,** 13–16.
65. Giasson, B. I., Jakes, R., Goedert, M., Duda, J. E., Leight, S., Trojanowski, J. Q., et al. (2000) A panel of epitope-specific antibodies detects protein domains distributed throughout human α-synuclein in Lewy bodies of Parkinson's disease. *J. Neurosci. Res.* **59,** 528–533.
66. Wakabayashi, K., Hayashi, S., Kakita, A., Yamada, M., Toyoshima, Y., Yoshimoto, M., et al. (1998) Accumulation of α-synuclein/NACP is a cytopathological feature common to Lewy body disease and multiple system atrophy. *Acta Neuropathol.* **96,** 445–452.
67. Arima, K., Uéda, K., Sunohara, N., Hirai, S., Izumiyama, Y., Tonozuka-Uehara, H., et al. (1998) Immunoelectron-microscopic demonstration of NACP/α-synuclein-epitopes on the filamentous component of Lewy bodies in Parkinson's disease and in dementia with Lewy bodies. *Brain Res.* **808,** 93–100.
68. Graham, J. C. and Oppenheimer, D. R. (1969) Orthostatic hypotension and nicotine sensitivity in a case of multiple system atrophy. *J. Neurol. Neurosurg. Psychiat.* **32,** 28–34.
69. Papp, M. I., Kahn, J. E., and Lantos, P. L. (1989) Glial cytoplasmic inclusions in the CNS of patients with multiple system atrophy. *J. Neurol. Sci.* **94,** 79–100.
70. Kato, S. and Nakamura, H. (1990) Cytoplasmic argyrophilic inclusions in neurons of pontine nuclei in patients with olivopontocerebellar atrophy: Immunohistochemical and ultrastructural studies. *Acta Neuropathol.* **79,** 584–594.
71. Arima, K., Uéda, K., Sunohara, N., Arakawa, K., Hirai, S., Nakamura, M., et al. (1998) NACP/α-synuclein immunoreactivity in fibrillary components of neuronal and oligodendroglial cytoplasmic inclusions in the pontine nuclei in multiple system atrophy. *Acta Neuropathol.* **96,** 439–444.
72. Gai, W. P., Power, J. H. T., Blumbergs, P. C., Culvenor, J. G., and Jensen, P. H. (1999) α-Synuclein immunoisolation of glial inclusions from multiple system atrophy brain reveals multiprotein components. *J. Neurochem.* **73,** 2093–2100.
73. Dickson, D. W., Liu, W.-K., Hardy, J., Farrer, M., Mehta, N., Uitti, R., et al. (1999) Widespread alterations of α-synuclein in multiple system atrophy. *Am. J. Pathol.* **155,** 1241–1251.
74. Ozawa, T., Takano, H., Onodera, O., Kobayashi, H., Ikeuchi, T., Koide, R., et al. (1999) No mutation in the entire coding region of the α-synuclein gene in pathologically confirmed cases of multiple system atrophy. *Neurosci. Lett.* **270,** 110–112.
75. Crowther, R. A., Jakes, R., Spillantini, M. G., and Goedert, M. (1998) Synthetic filaments assembled from C-terminally truncated α-synuclein. *FEBS Lett.* **436,** 309–312.
76. El-Agnaf, O. M. A., Jakes, R., Curran, M. D., and Wallace, A. (1998) Effects of the mutations Ala30 to Pro and Ala53 to Thr on the physical and morphological

properties of α-synuclein protein implicated in Parkinson's disease. *FEBS Lett.* **440,** 67–70.

77. Conway, K. A., Harper, J. D., and Lansbury, P. T. (1998) Accelerated in vitro fibril formation by a mutant α-synuclein linked to early-onset Parkinson disease. *Nature Med.* **4,** 1318–1320.
78. Giasson, B. I., Uryu, K., Trojanowski, J. Q., and Lee, V. M.-Y. (1999) Mutant and wild type human α-synucleins assemble into elongated filaments with distinct morphologies *in vitro*. *J. Biol. Chem.* **274,** 7619–7622.
79. Narhi, L., Wood, S. J., Steavenson, S., Jiang, Y., Wu, G. M., Anafi, D., et al. (1999) Both familial Parkinson's disease mutations accelerate α-synuclein aggregation. *J. Biol. Chem.* **274,** 9843–9846.
80. Wood, S. J., Wypych, J., Steavenson, S., Louis, J.-C., Citron, M., and Biere, A. L. (1999) α-Synuclein fibrillogenesis is nucleation-dependent. *J. Biol. Chem.* **274,** 19,509–19,512.
81. Serpell, L. S., Berriman, J., Jakes, R., Goedert, M., and Crowther, R. A. (2000) Fibre diffraction of synthetic α-synuclein filaments shows amyloid-like cross-β conformation. *Proc. Natl. Acad. Sci. USA* **97,** 4897–4902
82. Han, H., Weinreb, P. H., and Lansbury, P. T. (1995) The core of Alzheimer's peptide NAC forms amyloid fibrils which seed and are seeded by β-amyloid: Is NAC a common trigger or target in neurodegenerative disease? *Chem. Biol.* **2,** 163–169.
83. Greenberg, S. G. and Davies, P. (1990) A preparation of Alzheimer paired helical filaments that displays distinct tau proteins by polyacrylamide gel electrophoresis. *Proc. Natl. Acad. Sci. USA* **87,** 5827–5831.
84. Goedert, M., Spillantini, M. G., Cairns, N. J., and Crowther, R. A. (1992) Tau proteins of Alzheimer paired helical filaments: abnormal phosphorylation of all six brain isoforms. *Neuron* **8,** 159–168.

4

α-Synuclein/Amyloid Interactions

Poul Henning Jensen

1. Introduction

Human α-synuclein was originally identified as the precursor of a peptide named non-Aβ component of Alzheimer's disease (NAC) that was tightly associated to purified Alzheimer's disease amyloid ***(1)***. Senile amyloid plaques consist predominantly of the 39–42 amino acid residue peptide Aβ arranged in β-pleated sheets. Aβ is generated by hydrolysis from the transmembrane amyloid precursor protein APP. The mechanism by which the intracellular presynaptic α-synuclein or its NAC fragment becomes integrated in extracellular senile plaques is still unclear. However, in vitro studies have shown that NAC and α-synuclein have the potential to participate actively in the biology of senile plaques since NAC can (1) interact with Aβ ***(2)***, (2) form amyloid fibrils ***(3)***, and (3) stimulate the aggregation of Aβ ***(4)***. α-synuclein can also stimulate Aβ aggregation and interact with senile plaques *in situ* ***(5)***. The techniques described in this chapter allow the study of interactions of α-synuclein with senile plaques in brain sections and with Aβ peptides in solution. Information on the following points are found in Jensen et al. ***(5)*** and references therein: (1) Expression and purification of recombinant human α-synuclein; (2) methodology for performing sodium dodecyl sulfate (SDS) gel electrophoresis and fluorography; and (3) standard histologic techniques for fixing, sectioning, and handling of human brain tissue.

2. Materials

2.1. Biotinylation

1. Biotin-*N*-hydroxysuccinimide (Sigma).
2. Dimethylformamide.
3. 0.1 *M* $NaHCO_3$, pH 8.0.

From: *Methods in Molecular Medicine, vol. 62: Parkinson's Disease: Methods and Protocols*
Edited by: M. M. Mouradian © Humana Press Inc., Totowa, NJ

4. 0.1 *M* Tris-HCl, pH 7.4
5. Dialysis tubing (Spectrapor 7, cutoff 3500 kDa, Spectrum).

2.2. Assay for Binding of Biotin-α-Synuclein to Brain Tissue

1. Sections (10 μm) from paraffin embedded hippocampal brain tissue from Alzheimer's disease patients. (We obtained the tissue from The Netherlands Brain bank.)
2. Biotin-α-synuclein.
3. Mixture of streptavidin and biotinylated horseradish peroxidase (StreptABComplex HRP kit; DAKO).
4. Phosphate-buffered saline (PBS): 150 m*M* NaCl, 20 m*M* NaH_2PO_4, pH 7.4.
5. 0.05% 3,3'-diaminobenzidine tetrahydrochloride/0.1% H_2O_2 in PBS.

2.3. Iodination

1. Aβ(1–40) was synthesized at Schaefer N, Denmark but can be bought from many sources, e.g., Bachem, Switzerland.
2. ^{125}I (2.0 Ci/μmol; Amersham).
3. 0.2 *M* phosphate buffer, pH 8.0.
4. Chloramine-T, 0.5 mg/ml in water.
5. 1 *M* HEPES, pH 6.3, 0.25% 3-[(3-cholamidopropyl)dimethylammonio]-1-propanesulfonate (CHAPS).
6. 20 m*M* HEPES, pH 7.0, 0.25% CHAPS.
7. A 2 mL Sephadex G25 column assembled in a 2-mL syringe.
8. Trichloroacetic acid.

2.4. Crosslinking Assay

1. Binding buffer: 150 NaCl, 1 m*M* $CaCl_2$, 10 m*M* HEPES, pH 7.4.
2. 50 mM bis(sulphosuccinimidyl)suberate (BS_3; Pierce) in water.
3. 2X loading buffer: 40 m*M* Tris-HCl, pH 6.8, 40% glycerol, 4% SDS, 40 m*M* dithioerythreitol, bromophenol blue.

3. Methods

All procedures are carried out at 20°C unless otherwise stated.

3.1. Binding of Biotin-α-Synuclein to Brain Tissue

1. Make a 5 m*M* stock solution of biotin-*N*-hydroxysuccinimide in dimethylformamide. This solution can be stored for years at –20°C.
2. Dialyze α-synuclein (1 mg/mL) against 0.1 *M* $NaHCO_3$, pH 8.0.
3. Mix 1 mL α-synuclein and 120 μL biotin-*N*-hydroxysuccinimide and incubate for 1 h. Add 120 μL Tris-HCl, pH 7.4, and dialyze extensively against PBS for 1 h. Supplement the biotin-α-synuclein to 50% glycerol (v/v) and store at –20°C in aliquots. Measure the protein concentration (Bio-Rad Protein Assay). The efficiency of the biotinylation reaction and comparison between different batches is

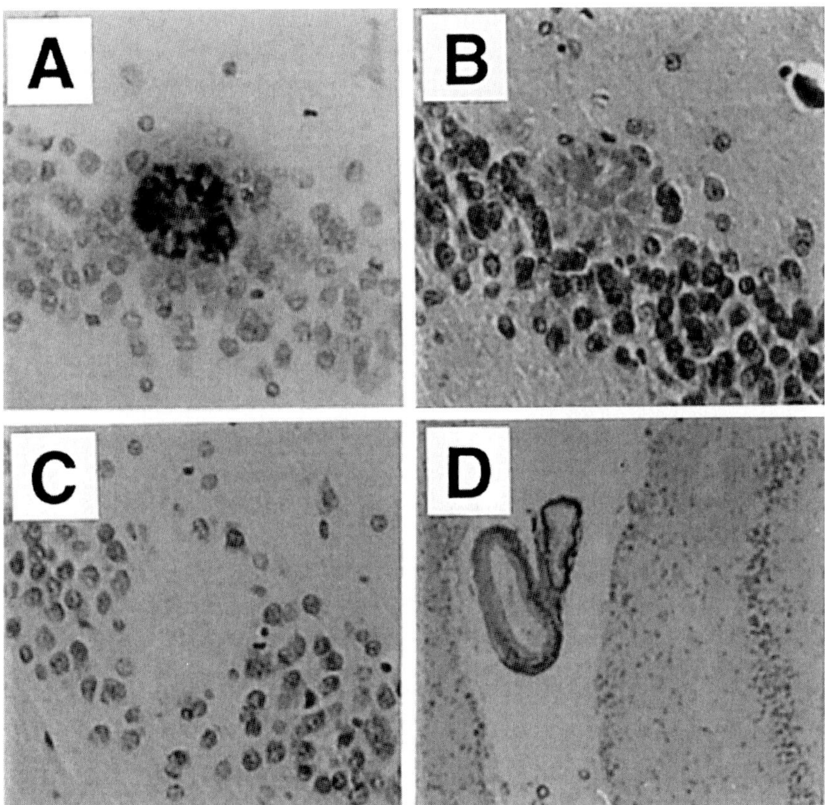

Fig. 1. Binding of biotinylated α-synuclein to AD-amyloid *in situ.* Adjacent tissue sections from a paraformaldehyde-fixed and paraffin-embedded hippocampus of an AD patient were incubated with **(A)** monoclonal antibody against Aβ; **(B)** biotinylated α-synuclein (1 μg/mL); **(C)** biotinylated α-synuclein plus 50 μg/mL unlabeled α-synuclein. Bound antibody and α-synuclein were visualized by a streptavidin/HRP complex using 3,3'diaminobenzidine tetrahydrochloride as chromogen; **(D)** similar to C, but presenting a part of the section with the pia and subpial tissue. Note the positive staining of pia in the presence of excess unlabeled α-synuclein. (Reproduced with permission from **ref. 5**.)

assessed by determining the minimal amount of biotin-α-synuclein that could be detected by dot-blot analysis using HRP-conjugated streptavidin (Boehringer Mannheim) followed by enhanced chemiluminescense (ECL, Amersham).

4. For demonstrating biotin-α-synuclein binding sites in brain tissue, perform all rinsing steps in PBS. Block endogenous peroxides in dewaxed and rehydrated hippocampal tissue by 0.5% H_2O_2 for 10 min. Cover sections with 1 μg/mL biotin-α-synuclein in PBS for 60 min (**Fig. 1B**). Confirm specificity of the tissue

binding of biotin-α-synuclein by competition with 50 μg/mL unlabeled α-synuclein (**Fig. 1C**). Demonstrate tissue-bound biotin-α-synuclein by incubation with streptavidin/biotinylated HRP for 20 min and, after rinsing, 0.05% 3,3'-diaminobenzidine tetrahydrochloride/0.1% H_2O_2 in PBS. Counterstain the tissue by Mayer's hematoxylin, dehydrate, and mount in hydrophobic mounting medium; the sections are then ready for inspection (*see* **Note 1**).

3.2. Analyzing Interactions Between α-Synuclein and ^{125}I-Aβ by Chemical Crosslinking

1. Dilute Aβ(1-40) in water to 1 mg/mL. Store in aliquots at –20°C. Mix 2 μL Aβ, 15 μL 0.2 *M* NaH_2PO_4, pH 8.0, 2 μL ^{125}I equivalent to 200 μCi, and 4 μL chloramine-T (0.5 mg/mL) for 2 min. Stop by adding 50 μL 1 *M* HEPES, pH 6.3, 0.25% CHAPS, and gel filtrate in 20 m*M* HEPES, pH 7.0, 0.25% CHAPS on Sephadex G25 column, to separate free and protein-bound ^{125}I. The incorporation of ^{125}I, as determined by precipitating a sample from the reaction mixture in 20% trichloroacetic acid, is routinely about 60%, thus giving a specific activity about 20 mCi/mg Aβ.
2. Mix 20,000 cpm ^{125}I-Aβ(1–40), 1.5 μg α-synuclein in 40 μL binding buffer and incubate for 16 h at 4°C. Add 1 μL BS_3 stock solution and leave at 20°C for 15 min before quenching the crosslinking reaction with 40 μL 2X loading buffer. Heat to 95°C for 3 min prior to 8–16% gradient SDS-polyacrylamide gel electrophoresis. Dry the gel and lay it on an autoradiography film. The assay can be performed with (1) different α-synuclein fragments to identify binding domains; (2) increasing concentrations of α-synuclein to estimate the affinity of the interaction; and (3) different ^{125}I-Aβ peptides, provided they contain a tyrosine residue, for localizing the reactive segment in Aβ (*see* **Note 2**).

4. Notes

1. The technique described above is also applicable for the study of biotinylated α-synuclein interactions with brain structures other than amyloid plaques, e.g., normal and pathological nerve cell constituents. In all such studies, it is essential to control for the specificity of the interactions by competition with unlabeled α-synuclein to exclude nonspecific absorption, as we noted with the intima of vessel walls and pia mater *(5)*.
2. The interaction between ^{125}I-Aβ and α-synuclein can also be performed in solid phase binding assays *(5,6)*. However, such assays have the inherent risk of artifacts created by the absorption of α-synuclein to the solid support, in contrast to crosslinking assays performed with all the reactants in solution. Potential pit falls in crosslinking assays rely on the chemistry of the crosslinker and the ligand/ receptor surface. The former varies in terms of the length of the spacer and the hydrophilicity. Lee et al. *(7)* have shown that a hydrophobic, rather than a hydrophilic, crosslinker is more suited for visualizing Aβ-stimulated α-synuclein aggregates. It is also possible to reverse the assay and iodinate α-synuclein. However, the α-synuclein tracer will only be separated approximately 4 kDa from the Aβ/^{125}I-α-synuclein complex, in contrast to the approx 20-kDa separation when

Aβ is iodinated. Nevertheless, the ^{125}I-α-synuclein tracer is useful to study its binding to other putative α-synuclein ligands.

References

1. Ueda, K., Fukushima, H., Masliah, E., Xia, Y., Iwai, A., Yoshimoto, M., et al. (1993) Molecular cloning of cDNA encoding an unrecognized component of amyloid in Alzheimer disease. *Proc. Natl. Acad. Sci. USA* **23,** 11,282–11,286.
2. Jensen, P. H., Sorensen, E. S., Petersen, T. E., Gliemann, J., and Rasmussen, L. K. (1995) Residues in the synuclein consensus motif of the alpha-synuclein fragment, NAC, participate in transglutaminase-catalysed cross-linking to Alzheimer-disease amyloid beta A4 peptide. *Biochem. J.* **310,** 91–94.
3. Iwai, A., Yoshimoto, M., Masliah, E., and Saitoh, T. (1995) Non-A beta component of Alzheimer's disease amyloid (NAC) is amyloidogenic. *Biochemistry* **34,** 10,139–10,145.
4. Han, H., Weinreb, P. H., and Lansbury, P. T., Jr. (1995) The core Alzheimer's peptide NAC forms amyloid fibrils which seed and are seeded by beta-amyloid: is NAC a common trigger or target in neurodegenerative disease? *Chem. Biol.* **2,** 163–169.
5. Jensen, P.H., Højrup, P., Hager, H., Nielsen, M.S., Jacobsen, L., Olesen, O.F., Gliemann, J., and Jakes, R. (1997) Binding of Aβ to α- and β-synucleins: identification of segments in α-synuclein/NAC precursor that bind Aβ and NAC. *Biochem. J.* **323,** 539–546.
6. Yoshimoto, M., Iwai, A., Kang, D., Otero, D.A., Xia, Y., and Saitoh, T. (1995) NACP, the precursor protein of the non-amyloid beta/A4 protein (A beta) component of Alzheimer disease amyloid, binds A beta and stimulates A beta aggregation. *Proc. Natl. Acad. Sci. USA* **92,** 9141–9145.
7. Lee, J. H., Shin, H. J., Chang, C. S., and Paik, S. R. (1998) Comparisons of the NACP self-oligomerizations induced by Abeta25-35 in the presence of dicyclohexylcarbodiimide and N-(ethoxycarbonyl)-2-ethoxy-1,2-dihydroquinoline. *Neurochem. Res.* **23,** 1427–1434.

5

Functional Defect Conferred by the Parkinson's Disease-Causing α-Synuclein (Ala30Pro) Mutation

Poul Henning Jensen

1. Introduction

The association of missense mutations in the α-synuclein gene to heritable Parkinson's diesease (PD) indicates that dysfunction of normal α-synuclein metabolism, or novel gain-of-functions by the mutant peptides, can elicit early-onset PD *(1,2)*. The accumulation of α-synuclein in nerve cell Lewy bodies of the common sporadic PD suggests a wider role for α-synuclein in the development of PD *(3)*. However, investigations into the loss and gain of functions caused by the specific mutations have been sparse, although an increased fibrillogenic potential have been reported *(4,5)*. We have shown that a fraction of α-synuclein is moved by fast axonal transport to the synaptic terminus *(6,7)*. Fast axonal transport is mediated by the motor-driven movement of vesicular structures along microtubules. By studying the interaction between α-synuclein and brain vesicles we discovered that the Ala30Pro mutation inhibits the interaction between mutant a-synuclein and brain vesicles *(6)*. Hypothetically, this inhibitory effect could perturb the fast axonal transport of α-synuclein thus increasing its concentration in the cell body where it may aggregate into Lewy bodies. The technique described in this chapter is modified from Brown & Rose *(8)* and allows the study of interactions between a-synuclein and brain vesicles and therefore the functional effects of pathogenic point mutations or deletions of specific domains. Information on the following points can be found in Jensen et al. *(6,9)* and references therein: (1) Mutagenesis, expression, and purification of recombinant human α-synucleins and (2) methodology for performing sodium dodecyl sulfate (SDS) gel electrophoresis and electroblotting.

From: *Methods in Molecular Medicine, vol. 62: Parkinson's Disease: Methods and Protocols*
Edited by: M. M. Mouradian © Humana Press Inc., Totowa, NJ

2. Materials

2.1. Biotinylation

1. Biotin-*N*-hydroxysuccinimide (Sigma).
2. Dimethylformamide.
3. 0.1 *M* $NaHCO_3$, pH 8.0.
4. 0.1 *M* Tris-HCl, pH 7.4.
5. Dialysis tubing (Spectrapor 7, cutoff 3500 kDa, Spectrum).

2.2. Preparation of Crude Rat Brain Vesicles

1. One adult rat brain hemisphere.
2. Dounce homogenizer (5 mL).
3. Homogenization buffer: 5 m*M* dithioerythreitol, 2 m*M* EDTA, 9% (w/v) sucrose, 25 m*M* 2-[N-morphoplino]ethanesulfonic acid (MES), pH 7.0 added proteinase inhibitor cocktail (Complete, Boehringer Mannheim).

2.3. Vesicle Flotation Assay for Binding of Biotin-α-Synuclein to Brain Vesicles

For a discussion on the virtues of the flotation assay, *see* **Note 1**.

1. Biotinylated wild-type and mutant α-synuclein.
2. Rotating tube holder or rocking table.
3. 75% (w/v) sucrose, 5 m*M* dithioerythreitol, 2 m*M* EDTA, 25 m*M* MES, pH 7.0. Heat the solution to dissolve the sucrose.
4. 5 m*M* dithioerythreitol, 2 m*M* EDTA, 25 m*M* MES, pH 7.0.
5. Peristaltic pump.
6. SW40 or other swinging rotor for an ultracentrifuge.
7. 10% Triton X-100.
8. Trichloroacetic acid.
9. Acetone (*see* **Note 2**).
10. 1X loading buffer: 20 m*M* Tris-HCl, pH 6.8, 20% glycerol, 2% SDS, 20 m*M* dithioerythreitol, bromophenol blue.
11. Nitrocellulose or other suited blotting membrane.
12. Horseradish peroxidase-conjugated streptavidin (Boehringer Mannheim).

3. Methods

All procedures are carried out at 4°C unless stated otherwise.

3.1. Biotinylation of α-Synuclein Peptides

1. A 5 m*M* stock solution of biotin-*N*-hydroxysuccinimide is made in dimethylformamide. This solution can be stored for years at –20°C.
2. α-Synuclein (1 mg/mL) is dialysed against 0.1 *M* $NaHCO_3$, pH 8.0.
3. Mix 1 mL α-synuclein and 120 µL biotin-*N*-hydroxysuccinimide and incubate for 1 h. Add 120 µL Tris-HCl, pH 7.4 and dialyze extensively against phosphate-

buffered saline (PBS) after 1 h. Supplement the biotin-α-synuclein to 50% glycerol (v/v) and store at –20°C in aliquots. Measure the protein concentration (Bio-Rad Protein Assay). The efficiency of the biotinylation reaction and comparison between different batches are assessed by determining the minimal amount of biotin-α-synuclein and its mutants that could be detected by dot-blot analysis using horseradish peroxidase-conjugated streptavidin (Boehringer Mannheim) followed by enhanced chemiluminescence (ECL; Amersham). This comparison must be performed carefully when the biotinylated peptides have to be compared subsequently with respect to binding efficiencies. Large differences in the efficiency of biotinylation would lead to large differences in peptide concentrations despite equal biotin-mediated signals.

3.2. Preparation of Crude Rat Brain Vesicles

1. An adult rat is killed by cervical dislocation, the skull is opened with scissors, and the brain is taken out by a thin spatula and placed in ice-cold isotonic saline. One-half of the cerebral hemisphere is homogenized in 2.5 mL homogenization buffer with 10 strokes. The homogenate is centrifuged at 560*g* (2500 rpm) in a cooled tabletop centrifuge to remove nuclei and large debris, and the remaining vesicles are isolated by ultracentrifugation at 100,000*g* for 1 h. The pellet is resuspended in 2.5 mL homogenization buffer and designated crude rat brain vesicles. The vesicles are used for binding assays within 24 h.

3.3. Biotin-α-Synuclein/Brain Vesicle Binding Assay

1. Dilute 60 μL crude brain vesicles with 40 μL homogenization buffer and incubate with 0.5 μg biotin-α-synuclein with approximately 5 μL of the stock solution for 2 h in an Eppendorf-like 1.5-mL centrifuge tube. Perform the incubation on a rotation mixer and make sure there is a small air bubble in the incubate to ensure mixing during the incubation.
2. Add 240 μL of 75% sucrose buffer to the incubate (final concentration 55%), mix gently and place the mixture in the bottom of a tube for the swing rotor. Place a 48–17% sucrose gradient above the vesicles and spin the gradient at 150,000*g* (50,000 rpm) for 16 h. The gradient is made by mixing the MES buffer with 75% sucrose buffer to prepare the 48 and 17% solutions. We recommend the SW40 rotor and a gradient of 3000 μL.
3. Stop the centrifuge without using the brake. A white band is visible approximately in the middle of the gradient when using a vesicle concentration as indicated. Label nine tubes and place 40 μL Triton X-100 in each. Collect nine fractions of 375 μL into the numbered tubes and vortex. Transfer 200 μL to new tubes and freeze the remaining for further analysis (such as sucrose concentration, protein content, repeated analysis, etc.). Precipitate the protein in the 200 μL sample by 50 μL of 50% trichloroacetic acid, vortex and spin 20,000*g* (15,000 rpm) in a cooled tabletop centrifuge. Wash the precipitate with 2X acetone. Dissolve the final precipitate in 1X loading buffer and heat to 95°C for 3 min. Adjust the pH with 0.5 *M* Tris-HCl, pH 7.4, if the loading buffer turns yellow. Spin the

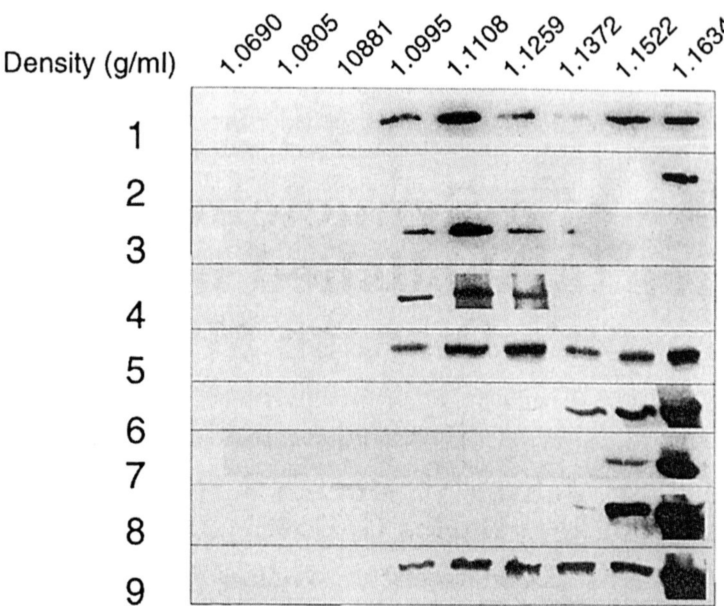

Fig. 1. Binding of α-synuclein proteins to rat brain vesicles. Adult rat brain extract was fractionated into postnuclear supernatant, cytosol, and vesicles. Binding of α-synuclein to vesicles was measured in a flotation assay. The gradient was divided into nine separate fractions (ranging in density from 1.0690 to 1.1634 g/mL), and α-synuclein was visualized in each fraction. Endogenous rat α-synuclein was measured in the postnuclear fraction (1), the cytosol (2), and the crude vesicle fraction (3). Endogenous rat SNAP25 was measured in the crude vesicle fraction as a marker for synaptic vesicles (4). Binding of biotinylated human α-synuclein proteins to crude vesicles was measured in fractions 5–9: wild-type α-synuclein (5); α-synuclein (30–140) (6); α-synuclein (55–140) (7); A30P α-synuclein (8); and A53T α-synuclein (9). Similar results were obtained in four separate experiments. The data show the flotation of vesicle-associated proteins to light fractions (approximately 1.1108 g/mL) in contrast to unbound proteins remaining in the dense bottom fraction (1.1522–1.1634 g/mL). (Reproduced with permission from **ref. *6***.)

samples at 20,000*g* (15,000 rpm) for 5 min to remove insoluble material and resolve the supernatant on a 10–20% gradient SDS polyacrylamide gel. Transfer the proteins from the gel onto a nitrocellulose membrane in an electroblotting apparatus, and block the membrane in 2% skimmed milk, 0.05% Tween-40, 150 m*M* NaCl, 25 m*M* Tris-HCl, pH 7.4. The distribution of various proteins in the sucrose gradient is visualized by horseradish peroxidase-conjugated reagents followed by enhanced chemiluminescence, as follows: (1) Biotinylated α-synuclein is probed by horse radish peroxidase conjugated streptavidin (**Fig. 1**, panels 5–9); (2) endogenous rat α-synuclein is probed by an anti-α-synuclein antibody

(**Fig. 1**, panel 3); and (3) other vesicle-associated proteins, e.g., synaptophysin, are probed by their respective specific antibodies (**Fig. 1**, panel 4). The same blot can be probed with different antibodies provided the molecular weights differ sufficiently. Otherwise the first set of antibodies must be stripped from the membrane by 200 m*M* glycine, pH 2.5, before the second set of antibodies is applied. The horseradish peroxidase-conjugated streptavidin bound to the biotinylated α-synuclein can be stripped off by 8 *M* urea, 200 m*M* glycine, pH 2.5.

4. Notes

1. The flotation technique for determinating binding of proteins to vesicles is elaborate compared with a simple assay based on pelleting of the membrane fraction. However, the flotation assay has some advantages that make it superior in some instances. First, the population of tracer binding vesicles is characterized in terms of its density. Second, by placing the sample in the bottom of the centrifuge tube, all aggregated tracer stays in the bottom fraction. The sedimentation assay would be the method of choice when a large number of variables is tested for their influence on vesicle binding, especially when the interaction has been demonstrated first by the flotation assay.
2. We precipitate the samples isolated from the gradient by trichloroacetic acid followed by acetone washing to remove sucrose and lipid as these substances negatively affect the subsequent gel electrophoresis. This labor-consuming procedure may not be required if only a very small volume is needed for analysis due to high activity of the tracer. Then the sample may be mixed directly with loading buffer for electrophoretic analysis. This must be determined for each experiment.

References

1. Polymeropoulos, M. H., Lavedan, C., Leroy, E., Ide, S. E., Dehejia, A., Dutra, A., et al. (1997) Mutation in the alpha-synuclein gene identified in families with Parkinson's disease. *Science* **276,** 2045–2047.
2. Kruger, R., Kuhn, W., Muller, T., Woitalla, D., Graeber, M., Kosel, S., et al. (1998) Ala30Pro mutation in the gene encoding alpha-synuclein in Parkinson's disease. *Nat. Genet.* **18,** 106–108.
3. Spillantini, M. G., Schmidt, M. L., Lee, V. M., Trojanowski, J. Q., Jakes, R., and Goedert, M. (1997) Alpha-synuclein in Lewy bodies. *Nature* **388,** 839–840.
4. Conway, K. A., Harper, J. D., and Lansbury, P. T. (1998) Accelerated in vitro fibril formation by a mutant alpha-synuclein linked to early-onset Parkinson disease. *Nat. Med.* **11,** 1318–1320.
5. El-Agnaf, O. M., Jakes, R., Curran, M. D., and Wallace, A. (1998) Effects of the mutations Ala30 to Pro and Ala53 to Thr on the physical and morphological properties of alpha-synuclein protein implicated in Parkinson's disease. *FEBS Lett.* **440,** 67–70.
6. Jensen, P. H., Nielsen, M. S., Jakes, R., Dotti, C. G., and Goedert, R. (1998) Binding of a-synuclein to brain vesicles is abolished by familial Parkinson's disease mutation. *J. Biol. Chem.* **273,** 26,292–26,294.

7. Jensen, P. H., Li, J.-Y., Dahlström, A., and Dotti, C. G. (1999) Axonal transport of synucleins are mediated by all rate components. Eur. *J. Neurosci.* **11,** 3369–3376.
8. Brown, D. A. and Rose, J. K. (1992) Sorting of GPI-anchored proteins to glycolipid-enriched membrane subdomains during transport to the apical cell surface. *Cell* **68,** 533–544.
9. Jensen, P. H., Højrup, P., Hager, H., Nielsen, M. S., Jacobsen, L., Olesen, O. F., et al. (1997) Binding of Ab to α- and β-synucleins: identification of segments in α-synuclein/NAC precursor that bind Aβ and NAC. *Biochem. J.* **323,** 539–546.

6

Molecular Biology of Dopamine-Induced Apoptosis

Possible Implications for Parkinson's Disease

Ilan Ziv, Anat Shirvan, Daniel Offen, Ari Barzilai, and Eldad Melamed

1. Introduction

The causes for the highly selective loss of dopaminergic neurons in the substantia nigra pars compacta in Parkinson's disease (PD) are still unknown. However, a major advance has been recently made with the introduction of the concept of apoptosis as the route leading this specific neuronal population to degeneration. Apoptosis, or programmed cell death (PCD), is an active, controlled program inherent in every living cell. Upon receiving certain signals, cells that are destined to die undergo a highly characteristic process of "suicide." This process consists of massive biochemical and morphological alterations, including cell shrinkage, loss of cell-to-cell contacts, blebbing of cell membranes, cytoskeletal rearrangements, and DNA condensation and fragmentation. It culminates in cell conversion to membrane-bound particles (apoptotic bodies) that are ready to be digested by neighboring macrophages ***(1–3)***.

Apoptosis plays a major role in the nervous system throughout life. During central nervous system (CNS) development, apoptosis is a major tool in the final construction of the highly organized neuronal networks, i.e., over 50% of original embryonal neural cells, which are either defective or form imperfect synapses, are eliminated by this death process ***(4,5)***. Apoptosis allows this strict selection in an organized and "clean" manner, without untoward spillage of intracellular substances and enzymes that may be harmful to neighboring cells.

The significance of apoptosis control in determining the fate of neuronal cells is further emphasized by the irreversible exit of neuronal cells from the cell cycle at the stage of terminal differentiation, as well as the lack of mature neuronal cell division shortly after birth ***(6)***. Thus, neuronal tissue homeostasis

From: *Methods in Molecular Medicine, vol. 62: Parkinson's Disease: Methods and Protocols*
Edited by: M. M. Mouradian © Humana Press Inc., Totowa, NJ

is determined, to a large extent, by the function and integrity of the intracellular "restraints" of the inherent apoptotic death program. Failure of these control systems of apoptosis may therefore lead to "inappropriate" activation of self-demise of neuronal cells, causing neuronal loss that does not serve the organism, but rather leads to clinical neurologic dysfunction ***(5,7)***.

Numerous lines of evidence in recent years have substantiated the concept that inappropriate apoptosis does play an important role in neurodegeneration in general and in the pathogenesis of PD in particular ***(8)***. Morphologic considerations support this possibility. The histopathology of PD is consistent with a protracted process of loss of individual neurons (calculated to be no more than several nigral cells per day), with cell elimination by neighboring macrophages or microglia. Some of the remaining neurons appear shrunken with their nuclei condensed ***(9)***. There is also evidence for degeneration of the neuronal axonal network. These features are highly suggestive of an apoptotic process. These data are supported by several studies that directly demonstrated with terminal deoxynucleotidyl transferase-mediated dUTP-biotin end labeling (TUNEL) histochemical staining the presence of neuronal apoptosis within postmortem nigral tissues from PD patients ***(10,11)***.

These considerations mark the threshold of activation of the apoptotic death process as a possible critical scenario of events, in which PD pathogenesis may be determined. A novel line of PD research is, therefore, aimed at examining two key possibilities for the mystery of PD etiology and pathogenesis: (1) is there a specific defect in the apoptosis control mechanisms in the nigral neurons of PD patients? and (2) is there an excessive challenge for the normal apoptosis control apparatus within PD nigrostriatal neurons?

This approach calls for evaluation of relations between apoptosis and morphologic and biochemic features, unique to the nigrostriatal neurons that are destined to degenerate in PD. Our research demonstrates that dopamine can constitute such a common denominator. Dopamine, the endogenous neurotransmitter, is synthesized and stored within the nigrostriatal neurons. Its concentration within the cell bodies of these neurons is estimated to be 0.1–1.0 m*M*, while its levels within the neuronal terminals may reach 10 m*M* ***(12,13)***. Its auto- and enzymatic oxidation creates neuromelanin, the pigment hallmark of the substantia nigra. The first clue that drew our attention to the possible role of this neurotransmitter in apoptosis came from an entirely different field, namely, melanoma research. Wick et al. described a substantial anticancer effect of DA, and showed that it is toxic to melanoma cells both in vitro and in vivo and is synergistic to the effect of irradiation ***(14,15)***. This clue was strengthened by the emerging concept of apoptosis as the mode of activity of many anticancer drugs ***(16)***. We therefore hypothesized that dopamine may act as an inducer of apoptosis in postmitotic neuronal cells.

1.1. Features of Dopamine-Induced Apoptosis in Neuronal Cells

The model we used was cultured, postmitotic, chick sympathetic neurons. Cells were exposed to dopamine at the above-described physiologic concentration range (0.1–0.5 m*M*), for 24 h. We found dopamine to be toxic to the cultured neuronal cells, with a lethal dose for 50% of cells (LD_{50}) of 0.1 m*M* ***(17,18)***. The process of DA-induced cell death was highly characteristic of apoptosis: cell bodies manifested severe shrinkage, chromatin condensation, and subsequent DNA fragmentation. Scanning electron microscopic studies revealed massive blebbing of cell membranes, with the ultimate conversion of the cell to clusters of membrane-bound particles, i.e., apoptotic bodies. Massive alterations in the axonal network were observed, with thinning, blebbing, and multifocal neurite disruption. Importantly, a characteristic apoptosis commitment point (ACP) could be determined. ACP is the time point beyond which apoptotisis can no longer be halted by removal of the triggering stimulus, marking the initiation of the irreversible execution phase of the death program. ACP for dopamine-induced apoptosis was found to be 5–6 h in our models.

Comparative studies in other cell types revealed that this effect of DA was not cell type specific, as we had observed it in other postmitotic cultured neuronal cells (e.g., mouse cerebellar granule cells), neuronal-like cell line (PC-12 cell), and nonneuronal cells (e.g., mouse thymocytes) ***(19,20)***. We also examined a possible apoptosis-triggering effect of other monoaminergic neurotransmitters, epinephrine (EN), norepinephrine (NE), and serotonin (SR). We found that induction of apoptosis is common to all these monoamines ***(20)***. Levodopa, the current cornerstone of pharmacological treatment of PD, was also found to be a potent apoptosis-inducing agent ***(21)***. A grading of relative potency of these agents was observed, with dopamine and levodopa being the most potent, followed by EN and NE; SR manifested significantly less toxic activity. Interestingly, this grading is in accordance with the relative involvement of the corresponding neuronal systems in PD, characterized by a most extensive degeneration of the nigrostriatal dopaminergic pathway, moderate involvement of the noradrenergic neurons of the locus ceruleus neurons, and less attrition in the serotonergic raphe nuclei. In yet another set of experiments, we showed that synthetic neuromelanin, the product of in vitro autooxidation and polymerization of DA, is also a potent inducer of neuronal apoptosis ***(22)***.

Collectively, these findings indicate that dopamine and related substances should be considered among the activators of the intrinsic cellular suicide program within the parkinsonian nigra. A nonreceptor-mediated process was suggested, since several cell types in which the proapoptotic effect of dopamine was found are devoid of receptors for this neurotransmitter. This prompted us to search for alternative pathways through which dopamine may exert its effect.

We found that oxygen free radical species (ROS) play an important causative role: dopamine-induced apoptosis could be effectively inhibited by cotreatment with several antioxidants ***(23)***. Interestingly, not all antioxidants were equally effective: thiol-containing antioxidants such as dithiothreitol (DTT) or *N*-acetylcysteine were found to be the most potent. By contrast, other antioxidants, namely, vitamins E and C were found to be less active. The thiol group, a common denominator among the active antioxidants, pointed at the glutathione system as a possible important intrinsic protective mechanism against the lethal effect of dopamine. Indeed, we found a strong inverse correlation between the levels of reduced glutathione, and the vulnerability of the cells to the death process induced by the neurotransmitter. The role of ROS in dopamine-induced apoptosis found in our studies is in accordance with the currently well-accepted important role of oxidative stress, both as a trigger and as a mediator of the intrinsic death program ***(24)***.

1.2. Molecular Basis of Dopamine-Induced Apoptosis

1.2.1. Genotoxicity

The role of DNA damage in the cascade of dopamine-induced cell death was first noted in the context of the anticancer effect of the neurotransmitter. Dopamine has been shown to cause DNA strand breaks and base modifications ***(25)***. Wick ***(15)*** also found that dopamine inhibited several enzymatic pathways that are operative in DNA repair processes, such as DNA polymerase, ribonucleotide reductase, and thymidylate synthase. DNA damage is known to be one of the major triggers of apoptosis, thus exemplifying the important role of the death program in eliminating defective, potentially hazardous cells. The cascade of events leading from DNA damage to apoptosis is currently the subject of intense research efforts. The enormous nucleotide consumption during the cellular effort to repair widespread DNA damage, coupled with increases in cellular free calcium and activation of poly (ADP-ribose) polymerase are regarded as important factors in this process ***(18)***.

Recent focus has been placed on the possible role of protooncogenes and tumor suppressor genes such as p53 in genotoxicity-triggered apoptosis. p53 is a tumor suppressor gene, active in the crucial cellular "decision point" where the fate of the cell in response to DNA damage is determined, either DNA repair or death by apoptosis ***(26)***. Malfunction of the p53 system has been found to be an important factor in the pathogenesis of numerous tumors. The possible role of genotoxicity in dopamine-induced apoptosis prompted us to examine whether p53 has a role in the death process induced by the neurotransmitter. Using cultured postmitotic cerebellar neurons, we found that dopamine causes marked DNA damage, which is temporally related to marked increases in phosphorylated (activated) p53 levels and also to the apoptosis commitment point. We also found that inhibition of p53 activity, using a temperature-sensitive mutant in leukemia LTR-6 cells, can dramatically attenuate dopamine toxicity. The p53 system and possibly other similar systems therefore play an important role in dopamine-induced apoptosis ***(27)***.

1.2.2. Abortive Reactivation of Cell-Cycle Associated Events

One of the approaches that we undertook to elucidate the molecular events underlying dopamine-induced apoptosis in postmitotic neurons was screening via the differential display method. This method allowed a comprehensive delineation of the alterations of gene expression during the death process, following exposure of the cells to dopamine. One of the striking findings was the marked induction of cell cycle-related genes during the early phases of the death process induced by the neurotransmitter. Marked increases in expression of the cell cycle-specific genes cyclin B1 and proliferating cell nuclear antigen were found. Interestingly, this upregulation of gene expression was observed early in the death process and was found to be cyclic, occurring in at least two waves. Whereas the first wave of cell cycle changes occurred prior to the death commitment point, the second wave coincided with it. Importantly, the temporal profile of the observed changes in gene expression did not match the profile of the events that occur during a normal cell cycle. Also, concomitant alterations in other important cell cycle regulators, i.e., cyclin D1 and cyclin-dependent kinases were not observed, and no active DNA synthesis was detected ***(28)***. These findings possibly unravel an exciting and rather unfortunate path undertaken by the postmitotic neuronal cells upon exposure to the apoptosis-triggering stimulus of dopamine. These terminally differentiated neurons, therefore, try to reenter the cell cycle upon exposure to the apoptotic signal, perhaps in an attempt to save themselves from death. However, this attempt is incomplete, unsynchronized, and unsuccessful. Since cell cycle impairment is considered among the most powerful apoptotic stimuli, it is conceivable that this defective attempt of the neuron to reenter the division cycle is readily detected by powerful cellular cell cycle control mechanisms as a severe cellular derangement, leading to activation of the "suicide" program.

1.2.3. Reactivation of Developmental Processes: The Collapsin Story

One of the hallmarks of neuronal apoptosis is attrition of the neuronal axonal network. The molecular mechanisms underlying these alterations are largely enigmatic. Our differential display screening of the molecular events that take place during the process of dopamine-induced apoptosis yielded the unexpected detection of upregulation of the collapsin system ***(29)***. This protein system is part of the axonal guidance apparatus active during CNS development. The collapsin family of proteins constitutes repulsive cue signals, which act to inhibit axonal growth in aberrant directions. Activity of this system beyond the embryonic stage, and especially during a cellular death process, is surprising. Further exploration of this field indeed led to the emergence of an important role of collapsin in dopamine-induced apoptosis. We found that the temporal profile of collapsin upregulation matches the kinetics of the death process. We also found this upregulation to be neuron specific. By exposing cultured postmitotic neurons to a small peptide corresponding to a conserved domain of the collapsin protein which includes the putative active site (the SEMA domain), we have been able to induce apoptosis. Furthermore, we have been able to inhibit dopamine-induced neuronal death dramatically using antibodies raised against the putative active site of collapsin.

Thus, during neuronal apoptosis, cells appear to reactivate and utilize systems that normally function exclusively during development. Specifically, the collapsin system seems to be a powerful tool, mediating axonal collapse during the apoptotic process. Our studies also suggest that this neuritic collapse may act as part of a vicious cycle, augmenting and accelerating the death process.

1.2.4. Induction of Stress-Associated Genes

Several stress-associated genes have been found to be upregulated during dopamine-induced apoptosis. These include, among others, HSP60, found in our differential display screening. Recently, dopamine-triggered apoptosis has been shown to be mediated, at least in part, through activation of the c-jun N-terminal kinase (JNK) ***(30)***. This activation includes increases in JNK activity as well as increased levels and phosphorylation of c-Jun. The functional role of this activation has also been shown as transient expression of a dominant negative mutant of SEK1, an upstream kinase of JNK, which prevented both JNK activation and dopamine-induced apoptosis. The JNK system, therefore, acts as a signaling pathway in the death process induced by this neurotransmitter. The inhibitory effect of the antioxidants *N*-acetylcysteine and catalase on JNK activation and subsequent apoptosis further suggests that this pathway acts downstream to dopamine-induced ROS formation.

1.2.5. Role of the Bcl-2 System

The Bcl-2 family is a group of proteins that act as a major control system of apoptosis. It consists of several structurally related proteins, of which several function as potent inhibitors of the death program (e.g., Bcl-2, Bclx-L); others function as inducers of apoptosis (e.g., Bax, Bak). Several of these proteins are strategically localized to the outer mitochondrial membrane. They can act as multifunctional proteins, e.g., they are capable of forming pores within the mitochondrial membrane, and they govern mitochondrial permeability transition, an opening of mega channels that plays an important role in the apoptotic cascade. In addition, members of the Bcl-2 family serve as docking proteins, regulating cytosolic levels of several downstream mediators of apoptosis ***(31)***. We found that overexpression of Bcl-2 in PC-12 cells effectively inhibited dopamine toxicity ***(32)***. In accordance with these results, we found that neuronal cells from Bcl-2-deficient mice are more susceptible to dopamine-induced apoptosis ***(33)***. These results demonstrate the strategic role of the Bcl-2 system in regulation of the cellular response to the apoptosis-triggering effect of the endogenous neurotransmitter.

1.3. Dopamine-Induced Apoptosis: Possible Significance for the Pathogenesis of Parkinson's Disease

The intensive research in the field of dopamine-induced apoptosis shows that dopamine should be considered among the neurotransmitters that may act as two-edged swords: although it plays an indispensable role in neuronal signal transduction, it also carries a significant toxic potential if not handled properly. The immediate analogy is to the excitotoxicity of glutamate and its analogs, which have recently been the focus of intensive research yielding significant clinical applications. Although both glutamate and dopamine can act as triggers of neuronal apoptosis, glutamate toxicity is primarily based on receptor activation, whereas dopamine toxicity probably utilizes different pathways mediated, at least in part, by ROS and genotoxicity.

Our studies also point to the "hostile" environment that prevails within and around the nigrostriatal neurons. By producing and storing dopamine, these neurons have to relentlessly face powerful apoptosis-triggering forces. As postmitotic cells, these neurons cannot rely on proliferation as a compensatory mechanism for maintenance of tissue homeostasis. Their longevity, expected to last throughout the life span of the organism, therefore depends solely on the continuous integrity and competence of the cellular systems that normally control and regulate the inherent death program and prevent the cells from being exposed to the toxicity of their transmitter. There are many ways by which nigrostriatal neurons may protect themselves from their own potentially injurious neurotransmitter. Among others, these include dopamine reuptake channels and vesiculation, antioxidant substances (e.g., glutathione, superoxide dismutase), trophic factors, the Bcl-2 system and the presence of surrounding glia. Although obviously dopamine cannot be claimed to be the cause of PD, it is now more conceivable to add this neurotransmitter to the array of factors that constantly challenge the apoptosis control systems within the nigrostriatal neuron, which collectively may render this specific neuronal population more vulnerable to degeneration. This could happen if one or more of the natural defense systems against dopamine toxicity fail, with the consequent exposure of neurons to the unchecked attack of dopamine.

The apoptotic threshold may, therefore be the "battlefield" where cell fate is determined by the interplay between apoptosis-triggering stimuli and the integrity of the cellular apoptosis-control systems. Exciting advances in apoptosis research have resulted in the translation of this once hypothetical notion to several well-characterized biologic systems that govern the cellular activation of apoptosis. These advances have revolutionized the approach to the pathogenesis of numerous neurologic disorders including PD. Neuronal cell death in PD should no longer be regarded as a passive process, but rather as an active cascade, which is controlled, at least in part, by intrinsic cellular systems. Research and modulation of these systems may hold promise for novel therapeutic strategies for the inhibition of neuronal loss in this common and progressive degenerative disorder. This potential is well exemplified by the Bcl-2 system.

In an effort to understand the molecular events associated with neuronal degeneration, we have focused on the early stages of the death process triggered by dopamine in cultured neuronal cells. To detect genes whose expression is selectively changed in response to dopamine treatment, we used the differential display method, which is capable of detecting differences in the mRNA repertoire between cell populations ***(34,35)***. This nonhypothesis-bound approach can be applied to different cultured neuronal cells, allowing the isolation of several dopamine-responsive genes, i.e., genes undergoing either up- or downregulation in response to dopamine exposure.

To focus on genes that may participate in modulating the early stages of the dopamine-induced apoptosis, the commitment point to the death process (ACP) was determined prior to application of the differential display technique. Thus, comparison was made between the repertoire of mRNA expressed in cultured cells undergoing dopamine-induced apoptosis and nonapoptotic cells. ACP was defined as the time point following dopamine administration from which neurons could not be rescued upon removal of dopamine. RNA for the differential display reactions was collected from apoptotic cultures at time points that were just prior to or soon after the ACP, as well as from control nonapoptotic cultures.

As a model system, we describe the use and application of the method to cultured chick sympathetic neurons. The method is composed of several steps that are described herein.

2. Materials

2.1. Preparation of Neuronal Cultures

1. Fertilized eggs (d 9).
2. DCCM-1: Serum-free medium, Biological Industries, Israel.
3. Chick embryo extract: Final concentration 2%.

4. Horse serum: Heat inactivated, final concentration 0.5%.
5. Fluorodeoxyuridine: Final concentration 20 µg/mL.
6. Uridine: Final concentration 50 µg/mL.
7. Glutamate.
8. Penicillin, streptomycin, and amphothericin B.
9. Nerve growth factor: Final concentration 10 ng/mL.
10. Poly-L lysine-coated plates.

2.2. Treatments and Measurement of Cell Viability

1. Dopamine (3-hydroxytyramine-hydrochloride, #CH8502, Sigma, St. Louis, MO).
2. Trypan blue (Biological Industries).
3. Alamar blue (Alamar Bioscience, CA).

2.3. RNA Preparation

1. Triazol kit (BRL Life Technologies, Gaithersburg, MD).
2. Diethylpyrocarbonated (DEPC)-treated water.
3. DNase I (BRL).
4. Agarose gel (1.5%).
5. Ethidium bromide.
6. RNase inhibitor (BRL).

2.4. Differential Display Reactions

1. Primers for the 3' end: Four sets of primers are used, poly dT12CA, poly dT12GA, poly dT12CG, and poly dT12AG.
2. Primers for the PCR step: Arbitrary primers of 10 nucleotides.
3. dNTP (Promega).
4. Taq DNA polymerase (Promega).
5. DNA sequencing apparatus.
6. Acrylamide gels (6%).
7. Fluorescent labels for proper orientation (Stratagene, La Jolla, CA).

2.5. Cloning and Sequencing Procedures

1. 4% agarose gels (1% SeaKem and 3% NuSieve).
2. Conventional DNA size markers.
3. MERmaid kit (Biolab, La Jolla, CA).
4. GETsorb kit (Genomed, NC).
5. Qiaquick kit (Qiagene, Hilden, Germany).
6. pGEM-T vector for cloning (Promega).
7. Bacterial growth plates of Luria-Bertani culture medium (LB) containing 100 g/mL ampicillin, 80 µg/mL 5-bromo-4-chloro-3-indolyl-β-D-galactoside (X-Gal), and 0.5 m*M* isopropylthio-β-D-galactoside (IPTG).
8. Qiagen plasmid preparation kit.
9. Sequenase II kit (Amersham Life Sciences, Cleveland, OH).
10. pUCM13 forward or reverse sequencing primers.

2.6. Northern Blot Analysis

1. 1% agarose, 2.2 *M* formaldehyde in 1X 3-(*N*-morpholino)propane sulfonic acid (MOPS) buffer, pH 7.0.
2. Qiagen nylon membrane.
3. Ultraviolet crosslinker.
4. Rediprime kit (Amersham) for preparation of labeled probe.
5. Washing solution: 0.1X standard sodium citrate (SSC), 0.1% sodium dodecyl sulfate (SDS).
6. Soft Laser scanning densitometer (Biomed Instruments, Fullerton, CA) and/or 202D video-based gel documentation system (Dinco and Rhenium, Israel).
7. Oligonucleotide of 18S rRNA, kinased.
8. T4 polynucleotide kinase (New England Biolabs).
9. A probe of glyceraldehyde 6-phosphate dehydrogenase (GAPDH).

3. Methods

3.1. Preparation of Neuronal Cultures and Treatment with Dopamine

1. Dissect paravertebral sympathetic ganglia at embryonic d 9 (E-9) ***(36)***.
2. Collect ganglions into L-15 medium (Biological Industries), and spin for 1 min at 150*g*. Wash twice in phosphate-buffered saline (PBS).
3. Incubate in the presence of trypsin: 25% in EDTA for 30 min at 37°C.
4. Collect cells and triturate in the above medium.
5. Spin cells at 150*g* for 5 min and resuspend in DCCM-1 medium, containing 2% chick embryo extract, 0.5% horse serum, 20 µg/mL fluorodeoxyuridine, and 50 µg/mL uridine (to kill non-neuronal cells); 2 mm each of glutamine, penicillin, streptomycin, and amphothericin B and 10 ng/mL nerve growth factor (NGF).
6. Plate the cells in 24 poly-L-lysine-coated wells (4×10^5 cells/well), or 35-mm tissue culture plates (10^6/cells) (Corning).
7. Grow cells in serum free medium DCCM-1 supplemented as in **step 5** above.

3.1.1. Treatments

1. Dissolve dopamine directly in the proper culture medium (*see* **Note 1**).
2. Treat sympathetic neurons (d 4–5 in culture, in the presence of NGF) for different time points with 300 µ*M* dopamine (determined earlier as the most potent concentration following detailed dose response studies ***(17,20)***.
3. Perform dopamine treatment in serum-free medium in the presence of NGF (10 ng/mL). Maintain plates in identical conditions but without exposure to dopamine to serve as controls.
4. Determine neuronal viability by Trypan blue exclusion assay and count live cells with a hemocytometer ***(20)***.
5. Alternatively, determine neuronal viability by use of Alamar blue reagent, which is a fluorescent -3-(4,5-dimethylthiazol-2-yl)-2,5-diphenyltetrazolium bromide (MTT) based reagent. Measure fluorescence with excitation at 570 nm and absorbance at 600 nm (*see* **Note 2**).

3.2. Determination of the Death Commitment Point

1. Treat neurons with 300 μ*M* dopamine.
2. At different time points following dopamine exposure (1–24 h), wash out the drug and replace with fresh medium without dopamine. Similar sets of untreated cells serve as controls.
3. Twenty-four hours after DA administration, monitor cell survival by Alamar blue (*see* **Note 3**).

3.3. RNA Preparation

1. Prepare total RNA from 10^6 sympathetic neurons using the Triazol kit.
2. Remove chromosomal DNA contamination by DNase I treatment (10 U/reaction).
3. Stop the reaction by EDTA and extract RNA with phenol/chloroform.
4. Dissolve RNA in DEPC-treated water and determine its concentration by absorbance at 260 nm.
5. Electrophorese RNA samples in 1.5% agarose gel and stain with ethidium bromide to assess concentration and integrity.
6. Store RNA at –70°C.

3.4. Differential Display Reactions

1. Use 50–100 ng of total RNA in each reverse transcription (RT) reaction, in a volume of 20 μL. Reactions are carried out essentially as described ***(34,35)***.
2. Use 3' end primers at a concentration of 2.5 μ*M*, and dNTP at 20 μ*M*. Each reaction employs one of the following primers: poly dT12CA, poly dT12GA, poly dT12CG, or poly dT12AG.
3. Incubate the mixture at 42°C for 90 min, and at 95°C for an additional 5 min, and then store in aliquots at –70°C. Perform control reactions in the absence of enzyme (*see* **Note 4**).

3.5. PCR Amplification

1. Use 2 μL of each RT reaction as a template for polymerase chain reaction (PCR), in a total volume of 20 μL. Carry out these reactions in triplicates.
2. Reactions are performed according to Liang et al. ***(34)*** and Bauer et al. ***(35)***, except that a single arbitrary primer of 10 mer is used, and therefore both ends of the amplified molecules are tagged with the same arbitrary primer. Under these conditions, selection of the mRNA population representing only coding regions can be achieved.
3. In a final volume of 20 μL combine: 1 μL of the primer (final concentration of 2.5 μ*M*); dNTP (final concentration of 20 μ*M*); 1 μL ^{35}S-dATP; $MgCl_2$ (concentration of 1.25 m*M*); 1 μL of *Taq* polymerase, and 2 μL of the appropriate 10X buffer.
4. Perform the PCR reaction under conditions appropriate for the specific primers. An example for conditions used is as follows: initial denaturation step of 1 min at 94°C, followed by 40 cycles of 30 s at 94°C; 1 min at 42°C; and 30 s at 72°C; and a 5 min incubation at 72°C. Store at 4°C.

5. Electrophorese the reaction mix in 6% denaturing sequencing gel within 24 h (*see* **Note 5**).

3.6. Rescue of Differentially-Expressed Bands

1. Pick cDNA bands that consistently show different expression patterns for further characterization.
2. To ensure precise orientation between the X-ray film and the dried gel, use fluorescent markers from Stratagene.
3. Cut out bands from the gel through the film and reexpose the gel to X-ray film to ensure that the appropriate band has been excised.
4. Extract DNA from the gel piece with 30 μL of water for 60 min at room temperature.
5. Take the aqueous phase immediately for reamplification. The conditions of the first 20 cycles are the same as in the differential display reaction.
6. Change primer and dNTP concentrations to 10 and 100 μ*M*, respectively.
7. Amplify for an additional 20 cycles.

3.7. Cloning and Sequencing of Bands of Interest

1. Recover reamplified cDNA bands from 4% agarose gels using either the MERmaid kit or the GETsorb kit.
2. Purify extracted DNA further by the Qiaquick kit and clone into the pGEM-T vector.
3. Prepare plasmid DNA using the Qiagen plasmid kit.
4. Sequence the insert using sequenase II and M13 forward or reverse primers.
5. Analyze the sequences using the National Center for Biotechnology Information GeneBank database (BLASTN algorithm) or the GeneBank and EMBL databases with the Fasta program (GCG Software, Madison WI).

3.8. Northern Blot Analysis

1. Use Northern blot analysis to verify the validity of the differential display reactions, in order to follow the regulation of mRNA of specific genes that were identified as up- or downregulated. Use total RNA prepared from dopamine-treated or untreated cells for Northern blot.
2. Load 5–10 μg of RNA corresponding to 10^6 cells in 1% agarose gel, 2.2 *M* formaldehyde in 1X MOPS buffer.
3. After electrophoresis, blot the gels onto Qiagen nylon membrane and crosslink with ultraviolet light.
4. Prepare probes by random priming using a Rediprime kit.
5. Wash blots at room temperature with 0.1X SSC, 0.1% SDS and expose to X-ray film.
6. For RNA quantification, assess intensity of bands by both soft Laser scanning densitometer and/or a video-based gel documentation system.
7. As a control for gel loading and transfer, strip membranes from radioisotope, and rehybridize with an 18S ribosomal RNA oligonucleotide, kinased according to Sambrook et al. *(37)*: Use 500 ng of oligonucleotide in a volume of 5 μL, add 3 μL buffer, 10 μL [λ-^{32}P]-ATP, 11 μL sterile water, and 1 μL polynucleotide kinase

enzyme. Incubate for 30 min at 37°C, and purify with a G-25 column. Add to hybridization buffer.

8. Normalize RNA quantities in each lane against rRNA levels. As an internal control, test the expression of GAPDH by rehybridizating the same blot with a probe of rat GAPDH, consisting of a 1500-bp fragment of its coding region *(28)*.

4. Notes

1. Dopamine is light sensitive and tends to lose activity easily even if stored under proper conditions (probably due to humidity and/or changes in temperature). Therefore, it is advisable to purchase several bottles with the smallest amount and store them unopened.
2. A similar approach can be applied to different apoptotic triggers or different neuronal cell types.
3. Determination of the commitment point should be specific to the trigger and the neuronal cell type.
4. To validate the reproducibility of altered expression, rescreen three different RNA preparations by identical differential display protocols.
5. To confirm reproducibility of the amplification for selected bands, each reaction is repeated at least three times with different preparations of RNA.

References

1. Thompson, C. B. (1995). Apoptosis in the pathogenesis and treatment of disease. *Science* **267,** 1456–1462.
2. Steller, H. (1995) Mechanisms and genes of cellular suicide. *Science* **267,** 1445–1449.
3. Searle, J, Kerr, J. F., and Bishop, C. J. (1982) Necrosis and apoptosis, distinct modes of cell death with fundamentally different significance. *Ann. Pathol.* **17,** 229–259.
4. Burek, M. J. and Oppenheim, R. W. (1996) Programmed cell death in the developing nervous system. *Brain Pathol.* **6,** 427–446.
5. Bredesen, D. E. (1995) Neural apoptosis. *Ann. Neurol.* **38,** 839–851.
6. Hayes, T. E., Valtz, N. L. M., and McKay R. D. G. (1991) Downregulation of CDC2 upon terminal differentiation of neurons. *New Biol.* **3.** 259–269.
7. Cotman, C. W. and Anderson, A. J. (1995) A potential role for apoptosis in neurodegeneration and Alzheimer's disease. *Cell. Mol. Neurobiol.* **10,** 19–45.
8. Ziv, I. and Melamed, E. (1998) Role of apoptosis in the pathogenesis of Parkinson's disease; a novel therapeutic opportunity? *Mov. Disord.* **13,** 865–870.
9. Ma, S. Y., Rinne, J. O., Collan, Y., Royata, M., and Rinne, U. K. (1996) A quantitative morphometrical study of neuron degeneration in the substantia nigra in Parkinson's disease. *J. Neurol. Sci.* **140,** 40–45.
10. Mochizuki, H., Mori, H., and Mizuno, Y. (1997) Apoptosis in neuro-degenerative disorders. *J. Neural Transm. 50,* 125–140.
11. Anglade, P., Vyas, S., and Javoy-Agid, F. (1995) Apoptotic degeneration of nigral dopaminergic neurons in Parkinson's disease. *Soc. Neurosci. Abst.* **21,** 1250.
12. Johnson, G. (1971) Quatitation of fluorescence of biogenic monoamines. *Prog. Hystochem. Cytochem.* **2,** 299–344.

13. Michel, P. P. and Hefti, F. (1990) Toxicity of 6-hydroxydopamine and dopamine for dopaminergic neurons in culture. *J. Neurosci. Res.* **26,** 428–435.
14. Wick, M. M. (1978) Dopamine: a novel antitumor agent active against B-16 melanoma in vivo. *J. Invest. Dermatol.* **71,** 163,164.
15. Wick, M. M. (1989) Levodopa/dopamine analogs as inhibitors of DNA synthesis in human melanoma cells. *J. Invest. Dermatol.* **92,** 329S–331S.
16. Eastman, A. (1990) Activation of programmed cell death by anticancer agents: cisplatin as a model system. *Cancer Cells* **2,** 275–280.
17. Ziv, I., Melamed, E., Nardi, N., Luria, D., Achiron, A., Offen, D., and Barzilai, A. (1994) Dopamine induces apoptosis-like cell death in cultured chick sympathetic neurons - a possible novel pathogenetic mechanism in Parkinson's disease. *Neurosci. Lett.* **170,** 136–140.
18. Ziv, I., Barzilai, A., Offen, D., Nardi, N., and Melamed, E. (1997) Nigrostiatal neuronal death in Parkinson's disease - a passive or an active genetically-controlled process? *J. Neural. Transm.* **49,** 69–76.
19. Offen, D., Ziv, I., Gordin, S., Barzilai, A., Malik, Z., and Melamed, E. (1995) Dopamine-induced programmed-cell-death in mouse thymocytes. *Biochim. Biophys. Acta* **1268,** 171–177.
20. Zilkha-Falb, R., Ziv, I., Nardi, N., Offen, D., Melamed, E., and Barzilai, A. (1997) Monoamine-induced apoptotic neuronal cell death. *Cell. Mol. Neurobiol.* **17,** 101–118.
21. Ziv, I., Zilkha-Falb, R., Offen, D., Shirvan, A., Barzilai, A., and Melamed, E. (1997) Levodopa induces apoptosis in cultured neuronal cells- a possible accelerator of nigrostriatal degeneration in Parkinson's disease? *Mov. Disord.* **12,** 17–23.
22. Offen, D., Ziv, I., Barzilai, A., Gordin, S., Glater, E., Hochman, A., and Melamed, E. (1997) Dopamine-melanin induces apoptosis in PC12 cells: possible implications for the etiology of Parkinson's disease. *Neurochem. Int.* **31,** 207–216.
23. Offen, D., Ziv, I., Sternin, H., Melamed, E., and Hochman, A. (1996) Prevention of dopamine-induced cell death by thiol antioxidants: possible implications for treatment of Parkinson's disease. *Exp. Neurol.* **141,** 32–39.
24. Payne, C. M., Bernstein, C., and Bernstein, H. (1995) Apoptosis overview, empahsizing the role of oxidative stress, DNA damage and signal transduction pathways. *Leuk. Lymph.* **19,** 43–93.
25. Moldeus, P., Nordenskjold, M., and Bolcsfoldi, G. (1983) Genetic toxicity of dopamine. *Mut. Res.* **124,** 9–23.
26. Yonich-Rouach, E., Grunwald, D., Wilder, S., Kimchi, A., May, E., and Oren, M. (1993) p53-mediated cell death: relationship to cell cycle control. *Mol. Cell. Biol.* **13,** 1415–1423.
27. Daily, D., Barzilai, A., Offen, D., Melamed, E., and Ziv, I. (1999) The involvement of p53 in dopamine-induced apoptosis of cerebellar granule neurons and leukemic cells over-expressing p53. *Cell. Mol. Neurobiol.* **2,** 261–276.
28. Shirvan, A., Ziv, I., Machlin, T., Zilkha-Falb, R., Melamed, E., and Barzilai, A. (1997) Two waves of cyclin B and proliferating cell nuclear antigen expression during dopamine-triggered neuronal apoptosis. *J. Neurochem.* **69,** 539–549.

29. Shirvan, A., Ziv, I., Fleminger, G., Machlin, T., Brudo, I., Melamed, E., and Barzilai, A. (1999) Semaphorins as mediators of neuronal apoptosis. *J. Neurochem.* **73,** 961–971.
30. Luo, Y., Umegaki, H., Wang X., Abe, R., and Roth, G. S. (1998). Dopamine induces apoptosis through an oxidation-involved SAPK/JNK activation pathway. *J. Biol. Chem.* **273,** 3756–3764.
31. Reed, J. C. (1997) Double identity for proteins of the Bcl-2 family. *Nature* **387,** 773–776.
32. Offen, D., Ziv, I., Panet, H., Wasserman, L., Stein, R., Melamed, E., and Barzilai, A. (1997) Dopamine-induced apoptosis is inhibited in PC-12 cells expressing Bcl-2. *Cell. Mol. Neurobiol.* **17,** 289–304.
33. Hochman, A., Sternin, H., Gorodin, S., Korsmeyer, S., Ziv, I., Melamed, E., and Offen, D. (1998) Enhanced oxidative stress and altered antioxidants in brains of Bcl-2-deficient mice. *J. Neurochem.* **71,** 741–748.
34. Liang P. and Pardee A. B. (1992) Differential display of eukaryotic messenger RNA by means of the polymerase chain reaction. *Science* **257,** 967–971.
35. Bauer D., Muller H., Reich J., Riedel H., Ahrenkiel V., Warthop I., and Strauss M. (1993) Identification of differentially expressed mRNA species by improved display technique (DDRT-PCR). *Nucleic Acid Res.* **21,** 4272–4280.
36. Greene L. A. (1977) Quantitative in vitro studies on the nerve growth factor (NGF) requirements for neurons. 1. Sympathetic neurons. *Dev. Biol.* **58,** 96–105.
37. Sambrook J., Fritsch E. F., and Maniatis T. (1989) *Molecular Cloning: A Laboratory Manual.* Cold Spring Harbor Laboratory Press, Cold Spring Harbor, NY.

7

Animal Models of Induced Apoptotic Death in the Substantia Nigra

Tinmarla F. Oo and Robert E. Burke

1. Introduction

Apoptosis is a form of cell death in which genetically regulated programs intrinsic to the cell bring about its own demise. In recent years, there has been a tremendous growth of interest in apoptosis as a mechanism of disease in a wide range of human disorders including the neurodegenerative diseases, such as Parkinson's disease (PD) *(1)*. This growth of interest has spawned an extraordinary number of recent discoveries about the molecular basis of apoptosis. It is important to emphasize, however, that much of this new knowledge has been attained in the study of relatively simple systems, such as invertebrate models or mammalian nonneural cell culture systems. Less is known about these mechanisms in neural cells, and much of what is known is based on studies of peripheral neural cells (such as sympathetic ganglia and PC12 cells) in tissue culture. Much less is known about central neurons; in particular, we know little about the regulation of apoptotic death in central neurons in living animals. It is especially important to try to identify the mechanisms of cell death in central neurons of known phenotype, particularly those implicated in human neurodegenerative disease, such as the dopamine neurons in PD. The purpose of the models we have developed of induced apoptosis in dopamine neurons of the substantia nigra (SN) is to try to translate what is being learned about the molecular mechanisms of apoptosis in simpler systems to these neurons.

Thus far, our studies of these models have shown, as would be expected, that there are important major parallels between the regulators of cell death in dopamine neurons and those identified in many simple mammalian cells. Nevertheless, a continued detailed analysis of these regulators in dopamine neu-

From: *Methods in Molecular Medicine, vol. 62: Parkinson's Disease: Methods and Protocols*
Edited by: M. M. Mouradian © Humana Press Inc., Totowa, NJ

rons is important, because there are now many precedents for differences in the mechanisms of apoptosis between different cell phenotypes, and even within a phenotype, depending on the nature of the death stimulus. Greene and his colleagues have shown that within postmitotic sympathetic ganglion neurons, the particular mechanisms of apoptosis differ when death is induced by trophic factor withdrawal, oxidative stress, and DNA damage *(2)*.

The models we describe in this chapter are developmental models. We have shown that during normal development, a natural cell death event with the morphology of apoptosis occurs within the dopamine neurons of the SN *(3,4)*. It would be predicted by classic neurotrophic theory that the magnitude of this death event would be regulated by early target interactions *(5,6)*, and we have shown that this is the case; destruction either of the striatal target with the excitotoxin quinolinic acid (QA) *(7)* or of intrastriatal dopamine terminals with the neurotoxin 6-hydroxydopamine (6-OHDA) *(8)* results in an approximately tenfold increase in the number of apoptotic profiles in the SN pars compacta (SNpc) (**Fig. 1**). In both of these models, apoptotic death has been identified within phenotypically defined dopamine neurons, and the apoptotic nature of the death process has been confirmed by ultrastructural and end-labeling (TUNEL) criteria.

The question arises as to whether developmental models of apoptosis are likely to be relevant to the cell death processes of adult-onset, neurodegenerative disorders, such as PD. At the core of the hypothesis that apoptosis may underlie adult-onset neurodegenerative disease is the concept that the genetic programs mediating apoptosis, which are normally active during development, become abnormally reactivated in the adult. Thus the study of mechanisms of apoptosis in a particular neuronal phenotype during development is entirely germane to the hypothesis that apoptosis may play a role in adult neurodegenerative disorders. Under no circumstance of neuron death in the adult brain (where apoptosis has been postulated to play a role) has it been proposed that an adult mechanism of apoptosis may be separate and distinct from those occurring in the developmental setting. On the contrary, it has been assumed that these processes are highly related, if not identical, and this assumption has led to numerous important discoveries of the mechanisms of apoptosis across species and developmental ages.

Horvitz and his colleagues made the assumption that the regulation of *developmental* cell death in the nematode *Chaemorhabditis elegans* is related to the regulation of apoptosis in other biologic contexts; this led to important insights into the functional role of Bcl-2 as a negative regulator of apoptosis, and to the discovery of the caspases *(9)*. Indeed, most of what we now know about the molecular basis of apoptosis derives from studies of developmental models. Such models include nerve growth factor (NGF) withdrawal from neonatal

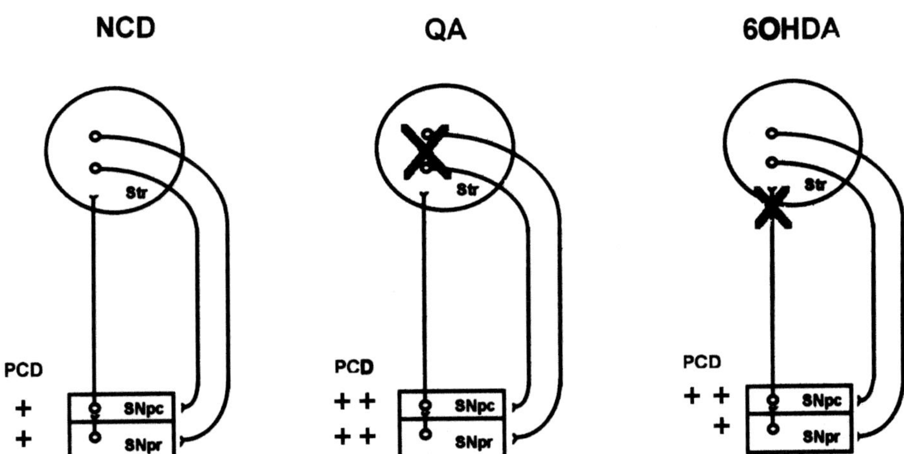

Fig. 1. Three paradigms of programmed cell death (PCD) in SN. A natural cell death event (NCD) with the morphology of apoptosis occurs in the SNpc *(3,4)* and SN pars reticulata (SNpr) (unpublished observations). This cell death event can be induced approximately tenfold by a developmental striatal axon-sparing lesion with QA *(7)*. In this model, there is induction of death in both the SNpc and SNpr. The morphology of cell death in this model is also apoptotic and appears identical to that observed in natural cell death. A cell death event can also be induced in SNpc by developmental destruction of dopaminergic terminals with 6-OHDA *(8)*.

sympathetic ganglia in culture, characterized by Johnson and coworkers ***(10)*** and others; withdrawal of serum from premitotic PC12 cells, or NGF withdrawal from postmitotic PC12 cells, characterized by Greene and collegues ***(11)*** and others ***(12)***; withdrawal of serum and potassium from postnatal cerebellar neurons ***(13)***; naturally occurring developmental cell death in motorneurons in chick, studied extensively by Oppenheim ***(14)*** and others; developmental degeneration of intersegmental muscles in hawkmoth, characterized by Schwartz and colleagues ***(15)***; and normal cell death in *Drosophila,* studied by Steller and others ***(16)***. We therefore propose that the study of the mechanisms of apoptosis in living dopamine neurons during development will provide useful knowledge about its regulation in other contexts, including that of disease in the adult brain.

We have used these models primarily to study the molecular correlates of apoptosis within dopamine neurons at a cellular level, using anatomic techniques ***(17–19)***. They also can be used for a regional analysis of the biochemical correlates of cell death. The striatal lesion model, induced by QA injection (**Fig. 2**), induces an increase in apoptotic death in SN that peaks by 24 h post

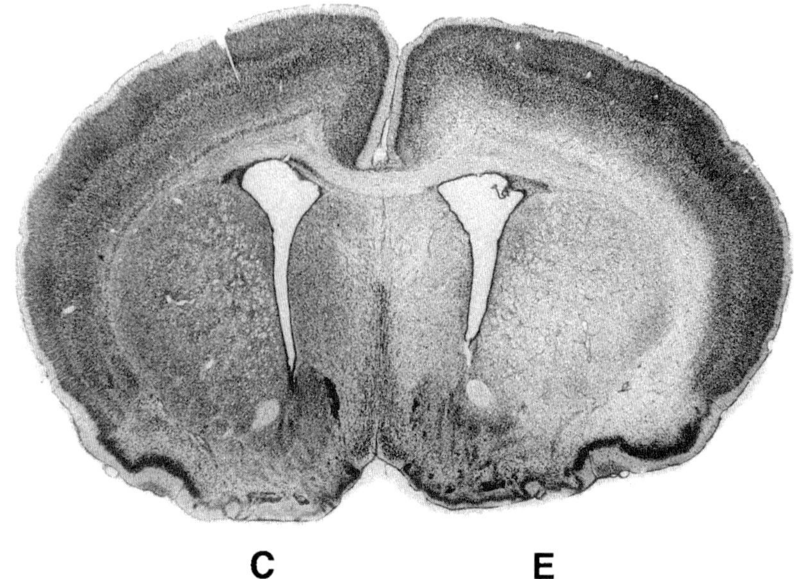

Fig. 2. Nissl stain of a coronal section of the striatum on postlesion d 2 following intrastriatal injection of QA on PND 14. Neuron loss is indicated by regions of pallor. It can be seen that there is pallor throughout the striatum on the experimental (E) side. Note that the lesion, while predominantly within the striatum, is not restricted to it, as there is also some pallor in the overlying cortex and in the adjacent medial septal area. C, control side.

lesion and abates by 96 h *(7)*. The intrastriatal 6-OHDA injection model results in a complete loss of dopaminergic terminals in the striatum (**Fig. 3A**), with complete preservation of intrinsic striatal neurons (**Fig. 3B**). In this model, induced death in the SN is delayed in its onset, beginning on the third postlesion day, and is more protracted in its course, continuing until postlesion d 10 *(8)*. This particular model is more selective for dopamine neurons, which, for some research questions, is an advantage. On the other hand, it is more destructive than the QA model; very few dopamine neurons survive. For this reason, the QA model may be more useful if one wishes to examine compensatory responses in surviving dopamine neurons.

2. Materials

2.1. Striatal Lesion with Quinolinic Acid

1. QA (Sigma , St. Louis, MO) is stored under desiccation at –20°C.
2. The vehicle for the QA injection is phosphate-buffered saline (PBS) 0.1 *M* (pH 7.1)/0.9% NaCl.

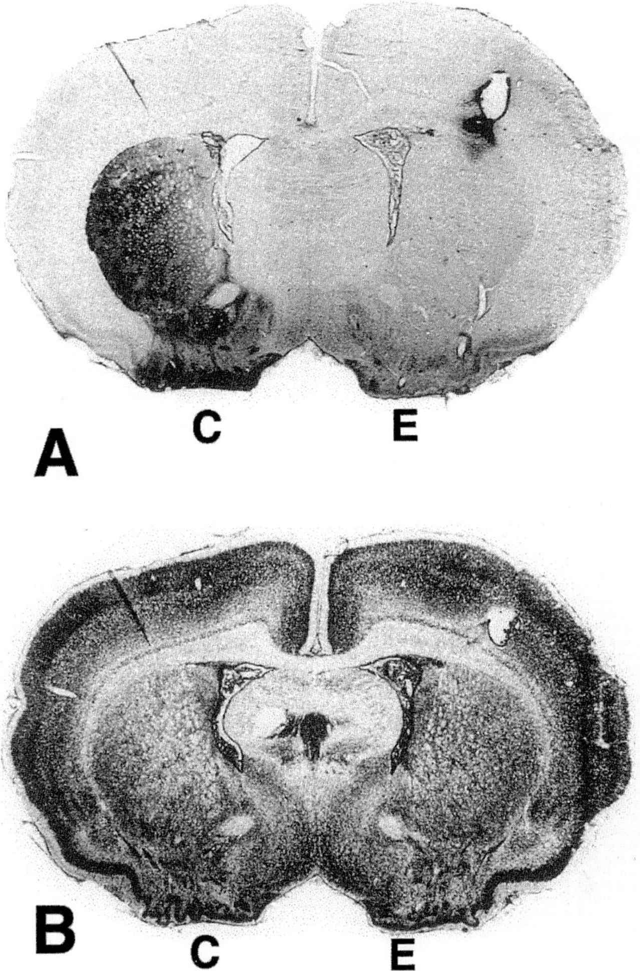

Fig. 3. Coronal sections of the striatum following intrastriatal injection of 6-OHDA. **(A)** Tyrosine hydroxylase (TH) immunostaining to demonstrate dopaminergic fibers within the striatum. Normal TH-positive fiber staining appears black, with an increasing medial-to-lateral gradient on the control (C) side. On the experimental (E) side, the striatum is devoid of staining. **(B)** Nissl stain demonstrating that there is no loss of intrinsic striatal neurons on the E side following the 6-OHDA lesion.

3. Anesthesia is induced by hypothermia alone (*see* **Note 1a**).
4. The intrastriatal QA infusion is performed with a CMA 100 microinfusion pump (Carnegie Medicin, Stockholm, Sweden).
5. Blue tubing connectors, fluorinated ethylene propylene (FEP) tubing, a cannula clip, and 500-µL syringes (Bioanalytical Systems, West Lafayette, IN).

6. A 28-gage cannula (Plastic One Products, Roanoke, VA). We cut the cannulae down to a 4-mm length in our lab. The cannula is held by the clip mounted on the arm of a David-Kopf stereotaxic apparatus and connected to the syringe using FEP tubing with blue tubing connectors.
7. A Dremel hand-held drill is used to make a skull burr hole.
8. After surgery, animals recover in a Thermo Care small animal incubator (Harvard Apparatus).

2.2 Dopaminergic Terminal Lesion with 6-OHDA

1. 6-OHDA-HBr (Regis, Morton Grove, IL), stored under nitrogen in a desiccator at –20°C.
2. L- ascorbic acid (Sigma), stored at room temperature.
3. Desmethylimipramine hydrochloride (DMI; Sigma), stored at 4°C.

2.3. Substantia Nigra Microdissection for Molecular and Biochemical Studies

1. A mouse brain matrix (30 g, coronal; Harvard Apparatus).
2. Large and small scissors and blunt and hooked forceps (Harvard Apparatus).
3. Petri dishes, spatula, razor blades, and sterile cryogenic vials (Nalgene; Fisher Scientific).

3. Methods

3.1. QA Injection

1. Timed pregnant rats (Sprague-Dawley; Charles River, Wilmington, MA) (*see* **Note 1**). We order multiple pregnancy females, i.e., multiparous females. These animals are more likely than nulliparous females to have larger litters and to nurse successfully.
2. Inspect the cage in the afternoon of each day; day of birth is defined as postnatal day (PND) 1.
3. Bring the pups into the lab on the day of the experiment and keep them at 33°C in the small animal incubator, separated from the dam. PND 7 pups are used for molecular and biochemical studies; PND 14 pups are used for anatomic studies for greater ease of tissue processing (*see* **Note 2**).
4. To prepare QA for injection, add 80.2 mg for each 1 mL of cold 0.1 *M* PBS and keep on ice. Add 70 μL of 10 *N* NaOH and mix thoroughly to dissolve the QA. Check pH with pH paper (range 6.0–8.0). Then, add 10 μL of 1 *N* NaOH stepwise to achieve pH 6.8. This solution, 480 m*M*, is stable for 3 d at 4°C.
5. Weigh each pup and anesthetize with hypothermia.
6. Load the 500-μL syringe with the QA solution and flush the tubing and cannula before the injection.
7. Place the anesthetized pup in the prone position on a ceramic plate, which has been stored at –20°C. Hypothermia provides additional anesthesia.
8. On the plate, support the chin with four glass microscope slides. It is essential to keep the chin level on glass slides to provide a correct and reproducible dorsal-ventral angle between the neck and the snout.

9. Place the pup and chilled plate on a Plexiglas stage.
10. Under a dissecting microscope, expose the skull by a midline incision, and drill a burr hole at 3.0 mm lateral to the left of bregma on the coronal suture.
11. Then move the Plexiglas stage onto the base platform of the stereotaxic apparatus toward the cannula holder.
12. Position the 28-gage cannula directly above the burr hole.
13. Pierce the dura with a needle and then insert the cannula, 4.0 mm vertically, into the striatum using the Kopf vertical adjustment knob.
14. Infuse QA at a rate of 0.50 μL/min for 2 min.
15. Slowly withdraw the cannula 2 min after the end of the infusion.
16. Suture the scalp with silk 5-0.
17. Inject PBS as a vehicle control.
18. We allow pups to recover in the small animal incubator at 33°C for 4 h, but the precise temperature should be determined empirically for each lab (*see* **Note 3**).
19. While animals are in the incubator, record their progress and behavior. As animals recover from anesthesia, they initially will rotate *away* from the side of the QA lesion. Eventually, rotational behavior stops, and animals will show normal motor and nursing behavior.
20. At the end of 4 h, return pups to the dams until the assigned postlesion day.

3.2. 6-OHDA Unilateral Injection

1. For the DMI injection, prepare 2.5 mg of DMI in 1 mL cold 0.9% NaCl.
2. Weigh the pups and treat them with 25 mg/kg DMI, subcutaneous interscapular injection, 30 min before 6-OHDA lesion (*see* **Note 4**).
3. In a test tube wrapped in aluminum foil, dissolve 15 mg 6-OHDA in 1 mL cold 0.9% (w/v) NaCl containing 0.02% (w/v) ascorbic acid (*see* **Note 5**). The solution must be clear. Any sign of brownish discoloration indicates that the 6-OHDA has oxidized, and it cannot be used.
4. Draw 500 μL of the solution into a syringe wrapped in foil and store the remaining volume on ice (*see* **Note 6**).
5. Flush the tubing and the cannula with fresh 6-OHDA before the injection.
6. Anesthetize the pup by inducing hypothermia.
7. Place the pup in the prone position on a chilled plate on a Plexiglas stage, with its chin resting on four glass slides as described above.
8. Under a dissecting microscope, expose the skull by a midline incision; drill a burr hole at 3.0 mm lateral to the left of bregma on the coronal suture.
9. The Plexiglas stage is moved onto the base platform of the stereotaxic apparatus toward the cannula holder, where a 28-gage cannula is inserted 4.0 mm vertically into the striatum as described above.
10. Infuse the 6-OHDA at a rate of 0.25 μL/min for 4 min.
11. Slowly withdraw the cannula 2 min after the end of the infusion.
12. Suture the scalp with Silk 5-0.
13. Flush the cannula and tubing before continuing onto another pup. Inject saline/ 0.02% ascorbate as vehicle control.

14. Allow the pups to recover in the small animal incubator for 4 h, and record their progress and behavior.
15. At the end of 4 h, return pups to the dams until the assigned postlesion day.

3.3. Substantia Nigra Microdissection for Molecular and Biochemical Studies

1. On the assigned postlesion day, using large scissors, remove the head of the rat pup.
2. Using scissors and forceps, remove the brain and place it into chilled 0.9% NaCl for approx 10 s.
3. Using the forceps, place the brain ventral surface down on a Petri dish on ice and remove the region caudal to the colliculi.
4. Again, with hooked forceps, place the brain into the mouse brain matrix with the ventral surface upward.
5. Mark both sides of each razor, to indicate the experimental side and avoid any possibility of left/right confusion.
6. With the ventral surface up, the left (experimental) side of the brain is on your right; thus mark the right side of each razor blade with an "E." Rest one razor blade in the third posterior slot. Rest a second razor in posterior slot 5. The blades should be just anterior (#5) and just posterior (#3) to the midbrain.
7. Push the blades into the brain at the same time.
8. Using a spatula, remove areas of the brain anterior and posterior to the razor blades.
9. Remove the blade in slot 5.
10. Using the spatula, pull the dorsal region of the brain from the edge of the block onto the second blade.
11. Remove the razor supporting the brain section from slot 3, and place the section on a Petri dish, *keeping the same orientation.*
12. Using forceps, dissect away and discard the cortices and mamillary body.
13. Using the razor blade, make a horizontal cut just below the cerebral aqueduct and discard the dorsal half of the section.
14. Then, with a vertical cut, split the remaining section in half. The portion on your left will be the right (control) side of the brain (*see* **Fig. 4**). The portion on your right will be the left (experimental) side.
15. Place each SN piece into appropriately labeled vials on dry ice. Each SN will weigh about 20 mg. The SNs can be stored at –80°C for 6 mo.

4. Notes

1. Although timed pregnant animals are somewhat more expensive than nontimed ones, we have found that the predictability of timed pregnancies, and the improved efficiency of planning experiments, make them well worth the additional expense.

1a. In our publications on these models, we specify that we use Metofane (Schering-Pough) for induction of anesthesia. However, Metofane is no longer available in the United States. For this reason we now anesthetize with hypothermia alone. Hypothermia provides a very effective, lasting anesthesia and is compatible with induction of both the QA and the 6OHDA models.

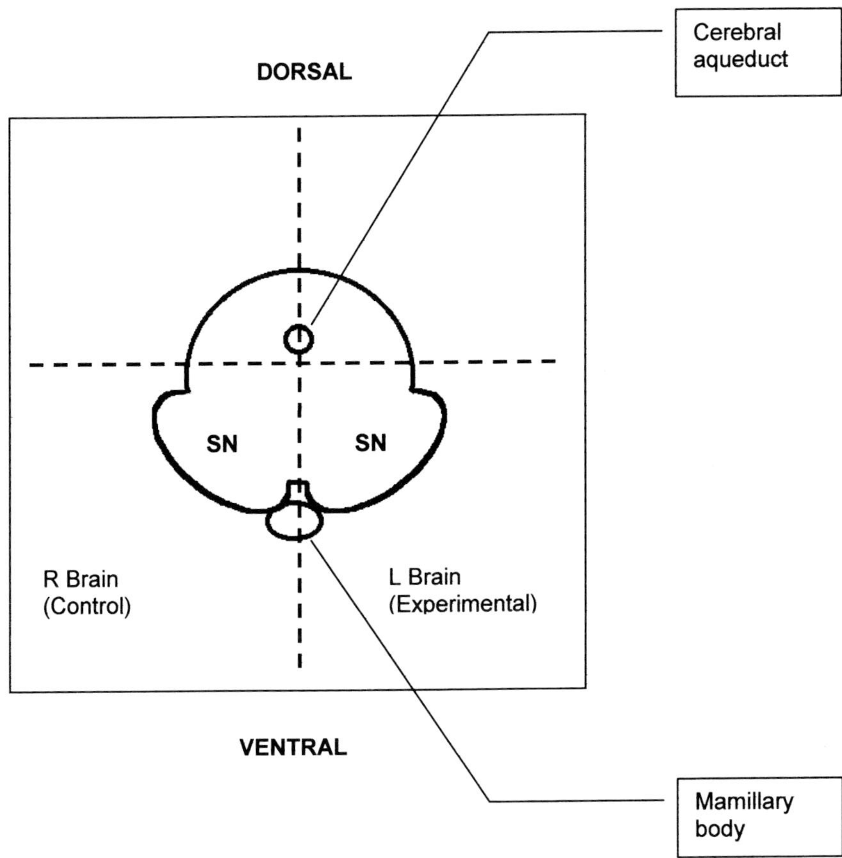

Fig. 4. Schematic of the mesencephalon demonstrating landmarks for substrantia nigra (SN) microdissection. The schematic depicts a 2.0-mm-thick section lying anterior surface up. The overlying cortex is not shown. We remove the mamillary body with forceps. We then cut the section horizontally (dotted line) just below the aqueduct and discard the dorsal piece. The ventral piece is then cut vertically (dotted line) in the midsagittal line to separate the left and right SN. Note that the "SN" piece contains not only SN, but also an overlying region of the central mesencephalon.

2. We have previously shown that the magnitude, distribution and morphology of cell death in SN is identical between PND 7 and PND 14 ***(20)***.
3. In our experience, a major potential source of variability in the striatal QA lesion model is the postoperative temperature of the animals. It has been demonstrated that body temperature does influence the magnitude of lesions made by excitotoxins ***(21)***. For this reason, we would suggest that any investigator who uses the striatal QA lesion model should, in their own lab, investigate the influence of different postoperative temperatures on the extent of the striatal lesion.

Although the striatum lies at a considerable distance from the SN, it is possible, if postoperative temperature is too high, for the QA injection actually to cause direct damage to the SN, leading to misleading results.

4. 6-OHDA, a light-sensitive compound, oxidizes easily at room temperature. Prepare 6-OHDA 15 min before the injection.
5. Note that NaCl must be used to dissolve 6-OHDA; in PBS it oxidizes immediately.
6. In our experience, 6-OHDA solution is stable for 1 h at room temperature. After this time, replenish the working solution to avoid injecting oxidized solution.

Reference

1. Stefanis, L., Burke, R. E., and Greene, L. A. (1997) Apoptosis in neurodegenerative disorders. *Curr. Opin. Neurol.* **10,** 299–305.
2. Park, D. S., Morris, E. J., Stefanis, L., et al. (1998) Multiple pathways of neuronal death induced by DNA-damaging agents, NGF deprivation, and oxidative stress. *J. Neurosci.* **18,** 830–840.
3. Janec, E. and Burke, R. E. (1993) Naturally occurring cell death during postnatal development of the substantia nigra of the rat. *Mol. Cell. Neurosci.* **4,** 30–35.
4. Oo, T. F. and Burke, R. E. (1997) The time course of developmental cell death in phenotypically defined dopaminergic neurons of the substantia nigra. *Dev. Brain. Res.* **98,** 191–196.
5. Barde, Y. A. (1989) Trophic factors and neuronal survival. *Neuron* **2,** 1525–1534.
6. Clarke, P. G. H. (1985) Neuronal death in the development of the vertebrate nervous system. *Trends Neurosci.* **8,** 345–349.
7. Macaya, A., Munell, F., Gubits, R. M., and Burke, R. E. (1994) Apoptosis in substantia nigra following developmental striatal excitotoxic injury. *Proc. Natl. Acad. Sci. USA.* **91,** 8117–8121.
8. Marti, M. J., James, C. J., Oo, T. F., Kelly, W. J., and Burke, R. E. (1997) Early developmental destruction of terminals in the striatal target induces apoptosis in dopamine neurons of the substantia nigra. *J. Neurosci.* **17,** 2030–2039.
9. Ellis, R. E., Yuan, J., and Horvitz, H. R. (1991) Mechanisms and functions of cell death. *Ann. Rev. Cell Biol.* **7,** 663–698.
10. Johnson, E. M. and Deckwerth, T. L. (1993) Molecular mechanisms of developmental neuronal death. *Ann. Rev. Neurosci.* **16,** 31–46.
11. Park, D. S., Stefanis, L., Yan, C. Y. I., Farinelli, S. E., and Greene, L. A. (1996) Ordering the cell-death pathway—differential-effects of Bc12, an interleukin-1-converting enzyme family protease inhibitor, and other survival agents on jnk activation in serum nerve growth factor-deprived PC12 cells. *J. Biol. Chem.* **271,** 21,898–21,905.
12. Pittman, R. N., Wang, S. L., Dibenedetto, A. J., and Mills, J. C. (1993) A system for characterizing cellular and molecular events in programmed neuronal cell death. *J. Neurosci.* **13,** 3669–3680.
13. Armstrong, R. C., Aja, T. J., Hoang, K. D., et al. (1997) Activation of the CED3/ICE-related protease CPP32 in cerebellar granule neurons undergoing apoptosis but not necrosis. *J. Neurosci.* **17,** 553–562.

14. Oppenheim, R. W. (1991) Cell death during development of the nervous system. *Ann. Rev. Neurosci.* **14,** 453–501.
15. Schwartz, L. M., Myer, A., Kosz, L., Engelstein, M., and Maier ,C. (1990) Activation of polyubiquitin gene expression during developmentally programmed cell death. *Neuron* **5,** 411–419.
16. White, K., Grether, M. E., Abrams, J. M., Young, L., Farrell, K., and Steller, H. (1994) Genetic control of programmed cell death in Drosophila. *Science* **264,** 677–683.
17. Henchcliffe, C. and Burke, R. E. (1997) Increased expression of cyclin-dependent kinase 5 in induced apoptotic neuron death in rat substantia nigra. *Neurosci, Lett.* **230,** 41–44.
18. Oo, T. F., Henchcliffe, C., James, D., and Burke, R. E. (1999) Expression of c-fos, c-jun, and c-jun N-terminal kinase (JNK) in a developmental model of induced apoptotic death in neurons of the substantia nigra. *J. Neurochem.* **72,** 557–564.
19. Jeon, B. S., Kholodilov, N. G., Oo, T. F., et al. (1999) Activation of caspase-3 in developmental models of programmed cell death in neurons of the substantia nigra. *J. Neurochem,* **73,** 322–333.
20. Kelly, W. J. and Burke, R. E. (1996) Apoptotic neuron death in rat substantia nigra induced by striatal excitotoxic injury is developmentally dependent. *Neurosci. Lett.* **220,** 85–88.
21. McDonald, J. W., Chen, C. K., Trescher, W. H., and Johnston, M. V. (1991) The severity of excitotoxic brain injury is dependent on brain temperature in immature rat. *Neurosci. Lett.* **126,** 83–86.

8

Apoptotic Morphology in Phenotypically Defined Dopaminergic Neurons of the Substantia Nigra

Tinmarla F. Oo and Robert E. Burke

1. Introduction

In the preceding chapter we described three paradigms by which we have studied programmed cell death in the substantia nigra (SN) of living animals: natural cell death and death induced either by developmental injury to the target striatum or by dopamine terminal destruction with the neurotoxin 6-hydroxydopamine (6-OHDA). In each of these paradigms, in order to relate experimental investigations specifically to dopamine neurons, the dopaminergic phenotype must be identified in conjunction with the demonstration of apoptotic morphology. This identification is essential, because apoptosis has been recognized in diverse neuronal populations and in glia *(1)*.

The principal method we have used is immunoperoxidase staining for tyrosine hydroxylase (TH), followed by counterstaining with thionin to demonstrate characteristic rounded, intensely basophilic chromatin clumps within the nucleus (**Fig. 1**). TH is the rate-limiting enzyme for catecholamine biosynthesis, and immunoperoxidase staining for TH has been widely used to demonstrate catecholaminergic neurons. Within the SN, the only catecholamine neurons present are dopaminergic, so TH immunostaining within this structure is generally accepted as evidence of the dopaminergic phenotype.

We have frequently used thionin counterstain to identify apoptotic chromatin clumps *(2–5)*. The specificity and sensitivity of this technique are important issues. With regard to specificity, particular morphologic features must be identified in order to consider a basophilic structure an apoptotic chromatin clump. The sturucture must (1) be round in shape; and (2) have distinctly bounded edges; (3) be intensely and (4) *uniformly* basophilic (i.e., its staining cannot be

From: *Methods in Molecular Medicine, vol. 62: Parkinson's Disease: Methods and Protocols*
Edited by: M. M. Mouradian © Humana Press Inc., Totowa, NJ

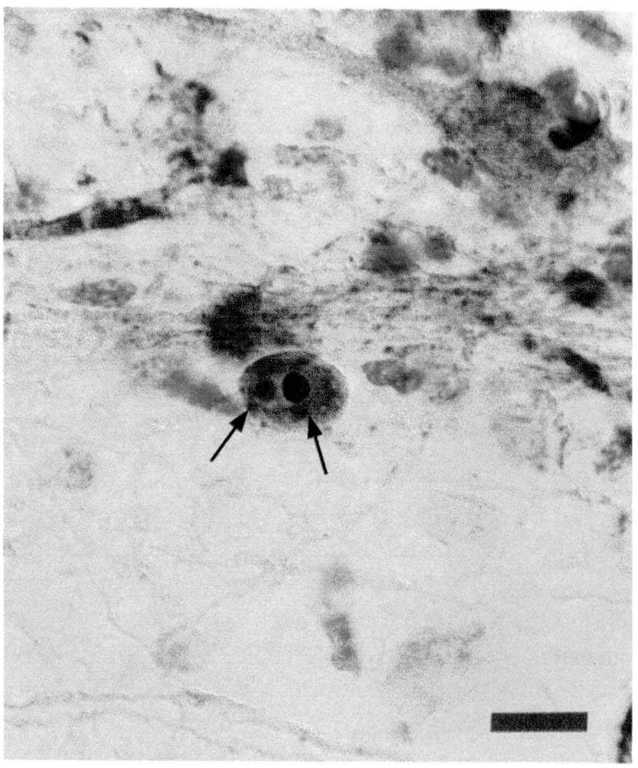

Fig. 1. An example of a brown, peroxidase-stained TH-positive neuron in the SNpc with apoptotic nuclear chromatin clumps (black arrows) demonstrated by thionin counterstain. Scale bar, 10 µm. (Reproduced with permission from **ref. *5***.)

mottled or heterogeneous); (5) it must be 2–4 µm in size; and (6) be located within a cellular profile, generally the nucleus. Not all basophilic clumps within the nucleus are apoptotic chromatin. For example, in the mouse brain, small, irregular, and heterogeneous basophilic clumps are frequently seen within neuronal nuclei due to heterochromatin ***(6)***.

Within a given model of apoptotic cell death, it is important not only to use these specific morphologic criteria, but also to demonstrate that profiles so identified at the light microscopic level are, in fact, apoptotic by ultrastructural analysis. We have shown that this is the case for both the target-injury ***(3)*** and 6-OHDA models (unpublished data). There are numerous precedents in the neuroscience literature for chromatin clumps to be identified on the basis of staining with basic dyes (thionin, cresyl violet, or toluidine blue), using the aforementioned morphologic criteria, and then to be demonstrated as apoptotic upon ultrastructural analysis ***(7–10)***. In view of such demonstrations, the use of basic dyes and observations at the light microscopic level by many investigators to identify and quantify apoptotic profiles in tissue sections seems justified ***(11–14)***.

The question arises of whether the technique of terminal deoxynucleotidyl transferase (TdT)-mediated dUTP nick end labeling (TUNEL) ***(15)***, which labels free 3'-ends in genomic DNA generated by endonuclease activity during apoptosis, is more specific than identification of apoptotic chromatin by basic dyes. In our assessment, this technique provides useful supplementary information to identify apoptosis, but it is not necessarily more specific than the basic dyes, when the morphologic criteria outlined above are used. There are now many demonstrations that TUNEL labeling can be false positive ***(16,17)***; it can label free 3'-ends in necrotic profiles as well as apoptotic ones. To avoid false positives with TUNEL labeling, it is essential to visualize not only a positive reaction product (i.e., chromogen deposition), but also apoptotic morphology (i.e., chromatin clumps). In our experience, in tissue sections, one of the best ways to achieve the latter is to perform a thionin counterstain ***(4,5)***. Cellular profiles so labeled satisfy both morphologic and histochemical (TUNEL) criteria for apoptosis. Thus, the usefulness of TUNEL as a specific indicator of apoptosis is, in the final analysis, dependent on demonstration of apoptotic chromatin clumps using a basic dye, or some other nuclear dye.

In our assessment, the use of basic dyes is also more sensitive than TUNEL labeling. In order for TUNEL labeling to be successful, tissue sections must be digested with proteases, such as proteinase K ***(15)***, or pepsin ***(18)***. This step must be done to allow access of either TdT or DNA polymerase ***(18)*** to nuclear genomic DNA. If this digestion step is not performed, the labeling procedure will not succeed. Thus, TUNEL depends on adequate penetration of macromolecular reagents. This is not the case for the staining of tissue sections with basic dyes, which are small, diffusable molecules. In our experience, when we perform TUNEL labeling successfully with adequate digestion, and then counterstain the sections with thionin, we frequently observe apoptotic profiles clearly defined by basophilic chromatin clumps that are TUNEL negative. Since these profiles have been confirmed in our models as apoptotic by ultrastructural criteria, we can only assume that they are false negative for TUNEL labeling, possibly because reagents have not adequately penetrated. Therefore, we prefer the use of a thionin counterstain to demonstrate apoptosis in phenotypically defined dopamine neurons. This method has been used successfully ***(19)***.

Although we prefer to use basic dyes to stain apoptotic chromatin clumps in tissue sections, other options exist. Other investigators have successfully used fluorescent dyes, such as acridine orange ***(19,20)*** or propidium iodide ***(14,21)***. Theoretically, such fluorescent nuclear dyes could be used in conjunction with fluorescent labeling of TH to identify apoptotic morphology within dopamine neurons. To our knowledge, there has been no direct comparison for sensitivity of fluorescent dyes with basic dyes. We have preferred the latter, in conjunction with the immunoperoxidase technique for TH, using diaminobenzidine as the chromogen, because these two labels are permanent and do not bleach. The sections are, therefore, easily viewed repeatedly by independent observers, and a high-quality image can still be photographed after multiple observations. On the other hand, an advantage of fluorescent double-labeling is that it is compatible with confocal laser imaging [e.g., see Waters et al. ***(20)*** and Tatton and Kish ***(19)***].

In our models of induced cell death, there are generally a sufficient number of TH-positive apoptotic profiles to make studies of time-course and the effects of pharmacologic interventions feasible. However, in the setting of natural cell death, the number of apoptotic TH-positive profiles is low *(22)*, making studies of negative regulation of cell death quite difficult. We have noted that only a small number of apoptotic profiles within the SN pars compacta (SNpc) are TH positive, and although it is possible that these profiles derive from nondopaminergic cells, we also have considered the possibility that they may represent nuclear remnants for which it is no longer possible to demonstrate the neuronal phenotype based on cytoplasmic markers. Such a possibility is supported by the general observation that, as a cell undergoes apoptosis, the cytoplasm is lost through a progressive process of cell membrane blebbing and then budding to form apoptotic bodies. We have shown within the SNpc that many apoptotic profiles have, by ultrastructural analysis, only a thin remaining rim of cytoplasm *(3)*. For such profiles, it is not possible to identify the original phenotype based on cytoplasmic markers. In addition, it is known that neuronal markers are downregulated during apoptosis *(23)*. For this additional reason, it may be difficult, if not impossible, to demonstrate by immunohistochemistry the original phenotype of the dying cell.

Based on these considerations, we have proposed that it may be useful to quantify not only TH-positive profiles within the SNpc (i.e., profiles meeting criteria for the dopaminergic phenotype at the *cellular* level), but also profiles that meet criteria for being within the SNpc at the *regional* level. In practice, we have defined apoptotic profiles as meeting regional criteria if they are within 15 μm of two TH-positive neurons (**Fig. 2**). We have shown that numbers of profiles meeting such regional criteria show a precise correlation with numbers of TH-positive profiles in terms of their time-course of expression during development and their magnitude ($r = 0.94$) *(22)*. We have concluded that profiles meeting regional criteria are likely to derive from dopamine neurons, and we quantify the numbers of these profiles, as well as profiles meeting cellular criteria for TH positivity, in some of our studies.

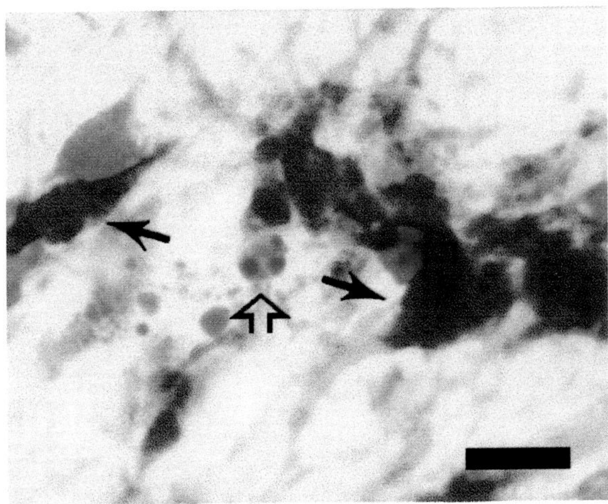

Fig. 2. An apoptotic profile within the SNpc by regional criteria. The profile (open arrow) contains three basophilic chromatin clumps and is within 15 µm of two TH-positive neurons, indicated by solid arrows. Scale bar = 10 µm. (Reproduced with permission from **ref.** *22*.)

2. Materials

2.1. Intracardiac Perfusion

1. Sodium chloride.
2. Sodium phosphate, monobasic (monohydrate; cat. no. S369) and dibasic (anhydrous; cat. no. S374; Fisher Scientific).
3. Sucrose (Fisher Scientific).
4. 0.2 *M* phosphate buffer (PB): 10.9 g Na_2HPO_4 and 3.1 g NaH_2PO_4 in 500 mL water.
5. Paraformaldehyde (Sigma, St. Louis, MO), stored at 4°C.
6. Large and small scissors and blunt and hooked forceps (Harvard Apparatus).

2.2. Tissue Sectioning

1. Sucrose.
2. 2-Methylbutane.
3. 22-mm square and 22 × 50-mm coverslips (Fisher Scientific).
4. Tissue-Tek OCT embedding compound (VWR Scientific Products).
5. Cryostat chucks and knife (Hacker Instruments, Fairfield, NJ).
6. Red sable brushes for transferring tissue sections (Ted Pella, Redding, CA).

2.3. TH Immunostaining

1. Mouse monoclonal anti-TH antibody (Boehringer Mannheim, Indianapolis, IN), stored at –20°C.

2. Biotinylated horse anti-mouse IgG (Vector, Burlingame, CA, catalog no. BA-2001.), stored at 4°C.
3. Normal horse serum (Vector), stored at 4°C.
4. Avidin-biotinylated horseradish peroxidase complex (ABC kit; Vector), stored at 4°C.
5. Diaminobenzidine (DAB) tetrahydrochloride dihydrate (Aldrich, Milwaukee, WI). We aliquot DAB as 50 mg in tubes and store at 4°C.
6. Glucose oxidase: 250,000 U (Sigma).
7. D(+) Glucose (Sigma).
8. Ammonium chloride (Sigma).
9. Trizma hydrochloride (Sigma).
10. Trizma base (Sigma).
11. Gelatin (Sigma).
12. Corning flat-bottomed tissue culture wells, glass scintillation vials, and Nalgene filter cups (0.2 µm; Fisher Scientific).

2.4. Thionin Counterstaining

1. The thionin solutions are prepared in advance and kept at room temperature.
2. Thionin: to prepare thionin stock solution, boil 1 g thionin in 100 mL water and then filter.
3. To prepare the buffer solution for thionin, add 7 g sodium acetate and 2 mL glacial acetic acid to 1 L of water.
4. Sodium acetate.
5. Ether.
6. Chloroform: Prepare the chloroform solution as 480 mL chloroform mixed with 60 mL ether and 60 mL of 95% (w/v) ethanol.
7. Formaldehyde: 39% (w/v).
8. Glacial acetic acid: To prepare formalin acetic acid solution, add 1 mL glacial acetic acid and 1 mL 39% formaldehyde to 1 L of water.
9. Butanol.
10. Histologic grade xylenes.
11. Permount. **Items 1–9** are purchased from Fisher Scientific and stored at room temperature.
12. Tissue-Tek staining outfit (Baxter, Edison, NJ).

3. Methods

3.1. Perfusion Fixation

1. To prepare the fixative (*see* **Note 1**), add 40 g paraformaldehyde to 450 mL nanopure water that is heated to 60°C.
2. Add 2.0 mL 1 *N* NaOH to dissolve paraformaldehyde.
3. Adjust the volume to 500 mL. This solution, 8% paraformaldehyde, is added to 500 mL of 0.2 *M* PB to yield 4% paraformaldehyde in 0.1 *M* PB (pH 7.1).
4. Store solution at 4°C.
5. On the assigned postlesion day, weigh the pup and place in a beaker containing gauze pads soaked in metofane for 4 min or halothane for 2 min.

6. Before preparing the animal for fixation, make certain that anesthesia is adequate by performing a tail pinch. There should be no evidence of a pain response (vocalization, withdrawal). Place the animal supine on a wetable surface near or over a sink.
7. To minimize exposure to paraformaldehyde vapor, keep water flowing in the sink as the fixative solution drains.
8. Using forceps and scissors, perform a thoracic dissection to expose the heart.
9. Using hooked forceps, clear the pericardium and insert a 20-gauge needle into the apex of the left ventricle of the heart; cut the auricle of the right atrium to allow drainage.
10. Perfused the rat intracardially with ice-cold 0.9% (w/v) NaCl for 5 min followed by cold 4% paraformaldehyde in 0.1 *M* PB for 10 min by gravity. The bottle of fixative should be 3.5 ft above the rat.
11. After fixation, carefully remove the brain and place it ventral surface down on a glass Petri dish lid, top up.
12. With a razor, make a cut between the colliculi and the cerebellum and discard the hindbrain.
13. Turn over the brain, ventral side up, and make a cut anterior to the hypothalamus.
14. Discard the anterior piece.
15. Postfix the remaining brain block in a glass scintillation vial containing 4% paraformaldehyde in 0.1 *M* PB for 1 wk at 4°C.
16. Place the brain in a cryoprotectant, 30% (w/v) sucrose in 4% paraformaldehyde in 0.1 *M* PB, for 2 d at 4°C.

3.2. Freezing and Sectioning

1. To freeze the brain, chill a beaker containing 2-methylbutane in powdered dry ice for 20 min.
2. To test the temperature of 2-methylbutane, apply OCT compound to a 22-mm square glass coverslip and lower it into the beaker (*see* **Note 2**).
3. Next, apply the OCT to a new coverslip and place the brain with the anterior surface down in the OCT; hold the coverslip with forceps and slowly lower it into the 2-methylbutane for 10 s (*see* **Note 3**).
4. Hold the brain on dry ice.
5. Apply fresh OCT to a cryostat chuck and attach the frozen brain with the anterior surface down in the OCT.
6. Cover immediately with fine, powdered dry ice.
7. Allow the brain and the cryostat knife to equilibrate in the cryostat for 30 min at –20°C before sectioning.
8. Mark the control side with a needle puncture made into the dorsal midbrain.
9. Section the brain at 20 μm from the posterior to the anterior planes encompassing the SN (Paxinos-Watson planes 2.7, 3.2, 3.7, 4.2).
10. Collect sections into cold PBS (0.1 *M* at pH 7.1).

3.3. TH Immunostaining

1. To prepare mouse monoclonal anti-tyrosine hydroxylase antibody, dissolve 40 μg of the lyophilized TH antibody in 1.0 mL nanopure water. Store the antibody as 25-μL aliquots at –80°C; it is stable for up to 2 yr in our experience.

2. For the secondary antibody, reconstitute 0.5 mg biotinylated horse antimouse IgG in 1.0 mL nanopure water and store at 4°C.
3. Process the sections for TH immunostaining by the free-floating method.
4. Rinse the sections twice in 0.1 *M* phosphate-buffered saline (PBS) for 15 min at 4°C.
5. Then incubate the sections overnight in the mouse monoclonal anti-TH antibody at 1:40 dilution in 10% normal horse serum in PBS at 4°C.
6. Rinse the sections twice in PBS with shaking for 15 min.
7. Incubate overnight in biotinylated horse anti-mouse IgG at 1:50 in 10% normal horse serum in PBS at 4°C.
8. Rinse the sections again twice in PBS with shaking for 15 min at room temperature.
9. Incubate with biotinylated horseradish peroxidase complex (ABC kit) at 1:600 in PBS for 1 h.
10. Rinse in PBS.
11. Prepare the DAB solution as 50 mg DAB added to 100 mL 0.1 *M* Tris buffer and then stir.
12. For the DAB reaction, dissolve 30 mg or 250,000 U glucose oxidase in 10 mL 0.1 *M* Tris buffer and store as 300-μL aliquots at –20°C. Aliquot ammonium chloride as 40 mg/0.2 mL Tris-HCl and D(+) glucose at 200 mg/0.8 mL. Store both at –20°C (*see* **Note 4**).
13. Add an aliquot each of ammonium chloride, glucose oxidase, and D(+) glucose to the DAB solution and then filter (Nalgene 0.2 μm) by vacuum before use.
14. Incubate the sections in DAB for about 10 min at room temperature with shaking.
15. During the incubation, choose sections at random and visualize under a dissecting microscope to achieve optimal staining. Look for brown chromogen deposition and monitor for any increase in background staining.
16. After DAB incubation, rinse the sections three times in Tris buffer and mount onto gelatin-coated slides.
17. Dry overnight at room temperature.
18. Sub the slides previously in 9 g gelatin in 1.5 L of water heated at 60°C for 10 min.
19. Dry at room temperature before use.

3.4. Thionin Counterstaining

1. For preparing thionin working solution, mix 45 mL of the thionin stock solution with 455 mL buffer solution.
2. For thionin staining, immerse the sections on the subbed slides at the times indicated for each solution in **Table 1**. According to the thickness of the sections, some adjustments may need to be made, based on empiric trials, for the time in the thionin working solution (**step 10**) and the decolorization in formalin/acetic acid (**step 13**).
3. After the thionin staining, coverslip the slides with Permount.
4. Study the slides under the microscope (*see* **Note 5**).

Table 1
Thionin Counterstain Procedure

Step	Solution	Time (min)
1.	95% (v/v) ethanol	20
2.	Chloroform solution	10
3.	95% ethanol	2
4.	100% ethanol	2
5.	Xylene	5
6.	100% ethanol	5
7.	95% ethanol	2
8.	95% ethanol	2
9.	Nanopure H_2O	2
10.	Thionin working solution	7
11.	Nanopure H_2O	2
12.	Nanopure H_2O	2
13.	Formalin acetic acid solution	10 s
14.	Nanopure H_2O	2
15.	Nanopure H_2O	2
16.	95% ethanol	2
17.	95% ethanol	2
18.	100% butanol	2
19.	Cedarwood oil	5
20.	Xylene	5
21.	Xylene	5
22.	Xylene	5

4. Notes

1. The preparation of the fixative solution *must* be performed in a hood. Exposure of the eyes and face to heated paraformaldehyde can cause serious injury.
2. The OCT must freeze instantly. If the 2-methylbutane is not cold enough, the brain will freeze too slowly, causing freezing artifacts.
3. Do not keep the brain in 2-methylbutane for more than 10 s, because it will develop cracks.
4. We prefer to generate a fresh, continuous supply of H_2O_2 by the glucose oxidase reaction. In our experience, stored, refrigerated H_2O_2 solutions inevitably deteriorate, at variable rates, resulting in occasional, unpredictable failures of the DAB-peroxidase chromogen reaction.
5. Once TH-positive apoptotic profiles have been identified, the next goal is to quantify them in tissue sections, which can be an arduous task. It is beyond the scope of this chapter to discuss current methods of counting cellular profiles in tissue sections, or to review some of the controversies. For these aspects there are excellent recent reviews ***(25–27)***. Briefly, many reports have effectively made

the case that unbiased stereologic methods should be used to avoid double-counting errors when counting geometrically complex neuronal profiles, which are relatively large in relation to section thickness *(25,26)*. Such procedures avoid some of the assumptions or profile geometry and orientation made by earlier methods, such as the Abercrombie correction *(28)*, which assumed that profiles are uniform and spherical. However, a number of considerations suggest that traditional methods of counting are likely to provide reasonable estimates of the numbers of apoptotic profiles within tissue sections. First, the criterion structure for counting (an ensemble of chromatin clumps surrounded by a nucleus) is small (about 5 µm) in relation to section thickness for immunohistochemistry (20–60 µm), thus minimizing double-counting error. Second, apoptotic profiles tend to be spherical in shape, as assumed by traditional methods. Third, apoptotic profiles are rarely split by the microtome blade in paraffin *(14)* and frozen *(22)* sections, thus minimizing the split profiles that result in double-counting errors. Based on these considerations, we and others *(14)* have proposed that, for apoptotic profiles, traditional methods of counting are likely to be acceptable.

Whatever method one chooses for counting apoptotic profiles, two technical points must be borne in mind. First, when counting TH-positive profiles in thick sections, it is important to realize that an apoptotic profile may be superimposed on a TH-positive neuron in the section. It is therefore essential to use a high-power (100×) oil-immersion objective to examine the profile by focusing up and down to make sure that the apoptotic chromatin clumps are in the same plane of focus as the chromogen reaction product in the cytoplasm. Second, apoptotic chromatin clumps must be contained in a cellular profile to qualify for counting as an "apoptotic profile." Not infrequently, apoptotic chromatin clumps can be observed lying free in the extracellular space. Since more than one such clump could arise from a single apoptotic cellular profile, such "free" chromatin clumps should not be counted.

Acknowledgments

This work was supported by NIH NINDS grant NS26836 (REB), The Parkinson's Disease Foundation, The Lowenstein Foundation, and The Smart Family Foundation.

References

1. Oppenheim, R. W. (1991) Cell death during development of the nervous system. *Ann. Rev. Neurosci.* **14,** 453–501.
2. Janec, E. and Burke, R. E. (1993) Naturally occurring cell death during postnatal development of the substantia nigra of the rat. *Mol. Cell Neurosci.* **4,** 30–35.
3. Macaya, A., Munell, F., Gubits, R. M., and Burke, R. E. (1994) Apoptosis in substantia nigra following developmental striatal excitotoxic injury. *Proc. Natl. Acad. Sci. USA* **91,** 8117–8121.
4. Oo, T. F., Henchcliffe, C., and Burke, R. E. (1995) Apoptosis in substantia nigra following developmental hypoxic-ischemic injury. *Neuroscience* **69,** 893–901.

5. Marti, M. J., James, C. J., Oo, T. F., Kelly, W. J., and Burke, R. E. (1997) Early developmental destruction of terminals in the striatal target induces apoptosis in dopamine neurons of the substantia nigra. *J. Neurosci.* **17,** 2030–2039.
6. Moser, F. G., Dorman, B. P., and Ruddle, F. H. (1975) Mouse-human heterocaryon analysis with a 33 258 Hoechst-Giemsa technique. *J. Cell. Biol.* **66,** 676–680.
7. Cunningham, T. J., Mohler, I. M., and Giordano, D. L. (1982) Naturally occurring neuron death in the ganglion cell layer of the neonatal rat: Morphology and evidence for regional correspondence with neuron death in superior colliculus. *Dev. Brain Res.* **2,** 203–215.
8. Ferrer, I., Bernet, E., Soriano, E., del Rio, T., and Fonseca, M. (1990) Naturally occurring cell death in the cerebral cortex of the rat and removal of dead cells by transitory phagocytes. *Neuroscience* **39,** 451–458.
9. Ferrer, I. (1992) The effect of cycloheximide on natural and X-ray-induced cell death in the developing cerebral cortex. *Brain Res.* **588,** 351–357.
10. Sloviter, R. S., Dean, E., and Neubort, S. (1993) Electron microscopic analysis of adrenalectomy induced hippocampal granule cell degeneration in the rat: apoptosis in the adult central nervous system. *J. Comp. Neurol.* **330,** 337–351.
11. Williams, R. W. and Rakic, P. (1988) Elimination of neurons from the rhesus monkey's lateral geniculate nucleus during development. *J. Comp. Neurol.* **272,** 424–436.
12. Gould, E., Woolley, C. S., and Mcewen, B. S. (1991) Naturally occurring cell death in the developing dentate gyrus of the rat. *J. Comp. Neurol.* **304,** 408–418.
13. Sengelaub, D. R. and Finlay, B. L. (1982) Cell death in the mammalian visual system during normal development : I. Retinal ganglion cells. *J. Comp. Neurol.* **204,** 311–317.
14. Clarke, P. G. H. and Oppenheim, R. W. (1995) Neuron death in vertebrate development: *In vivo* methods, in *Methods in Cell Biology: Cell Death* (Schwartz L. M. and Osborne B. A., eds.), Academic Press, New York, pp. 277–321.
15. Gavrieli, Y., Sherman, Y., and Ben-Sasson, S. A. (1992) Identification of programmed cell death in situ via specific labeling of nuclear DNA fragmentation. *J. Cell. Biol.* **119,** 493–501.
16. Grasl-Kraupp, B., Ruttkay-Nedecky, B., Koudelka, H., Bukowska, K., Bursch, W., and Schulte-Hermann, R. (1995) *In situ* detection of fragmented DNA (TUNEL assay) fails to discriminate among apoptosis, necrosis, and autolytic cell death: A cautionary note. *Hepatology* **21,** 1465–1468.
17. Ishimaru, M. J., Ikonomidou, C., Tenkova, T. I., et al. (1999) Distinguishing excitotoxic from apoptotic neurodegeneration in the developing rat brain. *J. Comp. Neurol.* **408,** 461–476.
18. Wijsman, J. H., Jonker, R. R., Keijzer, R., van de Velde, C. J. H., Cornelisse, C. J., and van Dierendonck, J.-H. (1993) A new method to detect apoptosis in paraffin sections: in situ end-labeling of fragmented DNA. *J. Histo. Cytochem.* **41,** 7–13.
19. Tatton, N. A. and Kish, S. J. (1997) In situ detection of apoptotic nuclei in the substantia nigra compacta of 1-methyl-4-phenyl-1,2,3,6-tetrahydropyridine-treated mice using terminal deoxynucleotidyl transferase labelling and acridine orange. *Neuroscience* **77,** 1037–1048.

20. Waters, C. M., Moser, W., Walkinshaw, G., and Mitchell, I. J. (1994) Death of neurons in the neonatal rodent and primate globus- pallidus occurs by a mechanism of apoptosis. *Neuroscience* **63,** 881–894.
21. Tompkins, M. M., Basgall, E. J., Zamrini, E., and Hill, W. D. (1997) Apoptotic-like changes in Lewy-body-associated disorders and normal aging in substantia nigral neurons. *Am. J. Path.* **150,** 119–131.
22. Oo, T. F. and Burke, R. E. (1997) The time course of developmental cell death in phenotypically defined dopaminergic neurons of the substantia nigra. *Dev. Brain Res.* **98,** 191–196.
23. Freeman, R. S., Estus, S., and Johnson, E. M. (1994) Analysis of cell cycle related gene expression in postmitotic neurons selective induction of cyclin D1 during programmed cell death. *Neuron* **12,** 343–355.
24. Lundquist, I. and Josefsson, J. O. (1971) Sensitive method for determination of peroxidase activity in tissue by means of coupled oxidation reaction. *Anal. Biochem.* **41,** 567–577.
25. Saper, C. B. (1996) Any way you cut it: A new journal policy for the use of unbiased counting methods. *J. Comp. Neurol.* **364,** 5.
26. Coggeshall, R. E. and Lekan, H. A. (1996) Methods for determining numbers of cells and synapses: A case for more uniform standards of review. *J. Comp. Neurol.* **364,** 6–15.
27. Guillery, R. W. and Herrup, K. (1997) Quantification without pontification: choosing a method for counting objects in sectioned tissues. *J. Comp. Neurol.* **386,** 2–7.
28. Abercrombie, M. (1946) Estimation of nuclear populations from microtome sections. *Anat. Rec.* **94,** 239–247.

9

The Role of Nitric Oxide in Parkinson's Disease

Serge Przedborski and Ted M. Dawson

1. Introduction

Neurodegenerative disorders are adult-onset disabling neurologic conditions such as Parkinson's disease (PD) in which specific subsets of brain neurons are dying. Without exception, the frequency of these disorders is increasing dramatically as the proportion of elderly in our society grows. The search for efficacious therapies, if not to prevent, at least to slow down or halt the progression of these diseases, is of major public health importance. However, this goal can only be achieved through a better understanding of the causes and mechanisms by which neurons die in these degenerative disorders. We review here the question of nitric oxide (NO), a small and ubiquitous molecule believed to be a pivotal element in the cascade of deleterious events underlying neurodegeneration in PD. Since NO synthases (NOS) are the only known enzymes that produce NO, in this chapter particular attention is paid to the anatomic distribution and catalytic activity of these enzymes in the brain. We also provide several experimental protocols commonly used for quantitative and qualitative studies of NOS.

1.1. Nitric Oxide

NO has emerged as a protean biologic effector molecule that acts as an intercellular messenger molecule in the nervous system, regulating vascular tone and blood pressure, and controlling platelet activation, and when synthesized in high amounts by activated macrophages, it is an antimicrobial and antitumor molecule. Although NO is a gas in its native state, in most biologic systems it acts as a dissolved nonelectrolyte. The only exception is in the lung and in paranasal sinus air, where it is present in the gaseous phase. NO is synthesized by one of the three distinct NOS isoforms isolated to date. Depending

From: *Methods in Molecular Medicine, vol. 62: Parkinson's Disease: Methods and Protocols*
Edited by: M. M. Mouradian © Humana Press Inc., Totowa, NJ

on the site of production, the amount of NO produced, and the targets within the local environment, NO can have many diverse functions. The identification of NO as a neurotransmitter has refined our conventional understanding of how neurons communicate, since, in contrast to classical neurotransmitters, NO is not stored in synaptic vesicles, is not released by exocytosis, and does not mediate its actions by binding to cell surface receptors. In the nervous system, NO has a dual role as a physiologic messenger and as a mediator of lethal processes in a variety of neurodegenerative disorders and toxic insults to the nervous system.

1.2. Parkinson's Disease

The cardinal clinical features of PD include tremor, stiffness, and slowness of movement, all of which are attributed to the dramatic loss of dopaminergic neurons in the substantia nigra pars compacta (SNpc) ***(1)***. Its prevalence has been estimated at approx 1,000,000 in North America, with approx 50,000 newly affected individuals each year ***(1)***. The most potent treatment for PD remains the administration of a precursor of dopamine, L-dopa, which, by replenishing the brain with dopamine, alleviates almost all PD symptoms. However, chronic administration of L-dopa often causes motor and psychiatric side effects that may be as debilitating as PD itself ***(2)***. Furthermore, there is no supportive evidence that L-dopa therapy impedes the progressive death of SNpc dopaminergic neurons. Therefore, without undermining the importance of L-dopa therapy in PD, it remains essential to elucidate the cascade of events that underlie the neurodegenerative process. To this end and in light of the rarity of available postmortem brain samples from PD patients, many investigators, including ourselves, have focused their research efforts on experimental models of PD such as the one produced by the parkinsonian toxin l-methyl-4-phenyl-1,2,3,6-tetrahydropyridine (MPTP). Consequently, most of the currently available data regarding NO in PD derive from studies carried out in the MPTP model and not in PD *per se*.

1.3. The MPTP Model of Parkinson's Disease

MPTP is a byproduct of the chemical synthesis of a meperidine analog with potent heroin-like effects. MPTP can induce a parkinsonian syndrome in humans almost indistinguishable from PD ***(3)***. It was recognized as a neurotoxin in early 1982, when several young drug addicts mysteriously developed a syndrome similar to PD after the intravenous use of street preparations of meperidine analogs contaminated with MPTP ***(4)***. Since the discovery that MPTP causes parkinsonism in human and nonhuman primates as well as in various other mammalian species, it has been used extensively as a model of PD ***(3,5,6)***. In human and nonhuman primates, MPTP produces an irreversible and severe parkinsonian syndrome that replicates almost all the PD features including tremor, rigidity, slowness of movement, postural instability, and even freezing. The responses to traditional antiparkinsonian therapies are virtually identical to those seen in PD, as are the complications of such therapies. However, in PD the neurodegenerative process is believed to occur over several years, whereas MPTP produces a clinical condition consistent with "end-stage PD" in a few days ***(7)***. Except for a few cases ***(8a)***, no human pathologic material has been available. Thus, the comparison between PD and the MPTP model is largely limited to nonhuman primates ***(9)***.

According to neuropathologic data, MPTP administration causes damage to the dopaminergic pathways identical to that seen in PD ***(10)***, with a resemblance that goes beyond the degeneration of SNpc dopaminergic neurons. Like PD, MPTP causes greater loss of dopaminergic neurons in the SNpc than in the ventral tegmental area ***(11,12)*** and greater degeneration of dopaminergic nerve terminals in the putamen than in the caudate nucleus ***(13)***. On the other hand, two typical neuropathologic features of PD have, until now, been lacking in the MPTP model. First, except for the SNpc, the other pigmented nuclei such as the locus coeruleus have been spared, according to most published reports. Second, the eosinophilic intraneuronal inclusions, called Lewy bodies, so characteristic of PD have thus far not been convincingly observed in MPTP-induced parkinsonism ***(8a,9)***. Also worth noting is the fact that postmortem brain samples from PD patients ***(14)*** show a selective defect in the same mitochondrial electron transport chain complex that is affected by MPTP ***(15,16)***. Abnormalities in parameters of oxidative stress in postmortem PD brain tissue suggest that this disease is caused by an overproduction of free radicals ***(17)***, the same highly reactive tissue-damaging species that are suspected of being involved in MPTP-induced dopaminergic toxicity in vivo ***(18–20)***. However, despite this impressive resemblance between PD and the MPTP model, MPTP has never been recovered from postmortem brain samples or body fluids of PD patients. Altogether, these findings are consistent with the hypothesis that MPTP does not cause PD but is an excellent experimental model. Accordingly, it can be speculated that elucidating MPTP molecular mechanism(s) should lead to important insights into the pathogenesis and treatment of PD.

1.3.1. Metabolism of MPTP

The metabolism of MPTP is a complex, multistep process ***(21)***. After its systemic administration, MPTP, which is highly lypophilic, rapidly crosses the blood-brain barrier. Once in the brain, the pro-toxin MPTP is metabolized to 1-methyl-4-phenyl-2,3-dihydropyridinium ($MPDP^+$) by the enzyme monoamine oxidase B (MAO-B) within nondopaminergic cells, and then (probably by spontaneous oxidation) to 1-methyl-4-phenylpyridinium (MPP^+), the active toxic compound. Thereafter, MPP^+ is released (by an unknown mechanism) in the extracellular space. Brain inflow of MPTP, together with its transformation into MPP^+, determines the amount of MPP^+ available to enter dopaminergic neurons. Extracellular MPP^+ is then taken up by plasma membrane dopamine transporters, for which it has high affinity *(22)*.

Alterations in many of these MPTP metabolic steps modify MPP^+ potency. For instance, blockade of MAO-B by pargyline and deprenyl *(23)* or of dopamine transporters by mazindol *(24)* prevents MPTP-induced dopaminergic toxicity. Striatal content of MPP^+ is linearly and positively correlated with the magnitude of dopaminergic damage *(25)*.

1.3.2. Mechanism of Action of MPTP

Once inside dopaminergic neurons, MPP^+ is concentrated by an active process within the mitochondria *(26)*, where it impairs mitochondrial respiration by inhibiting complex I of the electron transport chain *(27,28)* through its binding at or near the same site as the mitochondrial poison rotenone *(29,30)*. The inhibition of complex I impedes the flow of electrons along the mitochondrial electron transport chain, leading to a deficit in adenosine triphosphate (ATP) formation. It appears, however, that complex I activity should be reduced >70% to cause severe ATP depletion *(31)* and that, in contrast to in vitro paradigms, in vivo MPTP causes only a transient 20% reduction in mouse striatal and midbrain ATP levels *(32)*. These findings raise the question as to whether MPP^+-related ATP deficit can be the sole factor underlying MPTP-induced dopaminergic neuronal death. Another consequence of complex I inhibition by MPP^+ is an increased production of free radicals, especially of superoxide *(33–35)*. From the aforementioned findings, it may be speculated that the initiation of MPP^+'s deleterious cascade of events results from energy failure and oxidative stress, which individually may not be sufficient to kill cells, but in combination may well be lethal. A similar scenario of interplay among mitochondrial dysfunction, energy failure, and oxidative stress has been postulated for PD *(36)*.

The importance of MPP^+-related superoxide production in dopaminergic toxicity in vivo is demonstrated by the fact that transgenic mice with increased brain activity of copper/zinc superoxide dismutase (SOD1) are significantly more resistant to MPTP-induced dopaminergic toxicity than their wild-type littermates *(18)*. This finding strongly suggests that the superoxide radical plays a pivotal role in the MPTP neurotoxic process. However, superoxide is poorly reactive, and it is the general consensus that this radical does not cause serious direct injury *(37)*. Instead, superoxide is believed to exert many or most of its toxic effects through the generation of other reactive species such as the hydroxyl radical, whose oxidative properties can ultimately kill cells *(37)*. For instance, superoxide facilitates hydroxyl radical production by hydrogen per-

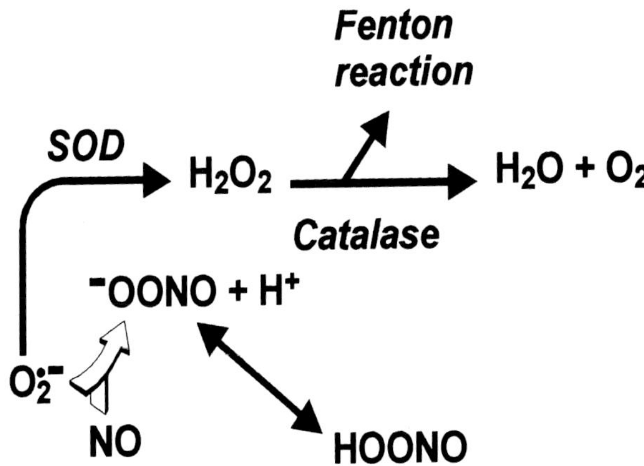

Fig. 1. Superoxide ($O_2^{\bullet -}$) can react with superoxide dismutase (SOD) to produce hydrogen peroxide (H_2O_2), which in turn can react with catalase to produce water and oxygen or enter the Fenton reaction. Alternatively, superoxide can also react with nitric oxide (NO) to produce peroxynitrite ($^{-}OONO$) and peroxynitrous acid (HOONO).

oxide and transitional metals such as iron (i.e., the Fenton reaction; **Fig. 1**) *(37)*. Although this reaction can readily take place in vitro, its occurrence in vivo is subordinate to such factors as low pH *(38)*. Despite this unfavorable pH constraint, MPTP does stimulate the formation of hydroxyl radicals *in vivo*, as evidenced by the increase in the hydroxyl radical-dependent conversion of salicylate into 2,3- and 2,5-dihydroxy-benzoates *(19)*.

Superoxide can also react with NO to produce peroxynitrite, another potent oxidant *(39)* (**Fig. 1**). At physiologic pH and in aqueous milieu, this reaction proceeds five times faster than the decomposition of superoxide by SOD *(40)* (see thick white arrow in **Fig. 1**). The intracellular concentration of SOD1 is estimated to be 10–40 μ*M* *(41)*. Thus, NO concentration has to be approximately 10 μ*M* for peroxynitrite formation to be competitive, which is not unrealistic as NO production at the cellular level is estimated at 1–10 μ*M* *(39)*. The situation is different, however, for superoxide, whose basal intracellular concentration is low *(42)*. Thus, under normal conditions, superoxide is limiting, and it is likely that minimal peroxynitrite formation occurs. Conversely, in pathologic conditions, should superoxide concentrations increase, as in response to MPTP administration, formation of appreciable amounts of peroxynitrite is expected. In light of this and of our previous work on superoxide *(18)*, we *(43)* and others *(19,20)* have assessed the role of NO in the MPTP neurotoxic process. These studies show that inhibition of NOS attenuates, in a dose-dependent fashion, MPTP-induced striatal dopaminergic loss in mice *(19,43)*. We also demonstrate that 7-nitroindazole (7-NI), a compound that inhibits NOS activity without significant cardiovascular effects in mice *(44)*, is profoundly neuroprotective against MPTP-induced SNpc dopaminergic neuronal death *(43)*. The protective effect of the NOS antagonist 7-NI against MPTP-induced striatal and SNpc dopaminergic damage was subsequently demonstrated in monkeys *(20)*.

1.4. Proposed Mechanism of MPTP Action

From the above findings, the following scheme can be proposed to explain both selectivity and dopaminergic toxicity (**Fig. 2**): MPTP is converted to MPP^+, which is transported into dopaminergic neurons via the dopamine transporter. MPP^+ inhibits enzymes in the mitochondrial electron transport chain, resulting in ATP deficit and increased "leakage" of superoxide from the respiratory chain. Superoxide cannot readily transverse cellular membranes and so remains in the cell and organelle in which it is produced. In contrast, NO is membrane permeable and diffuses into neighboring neurons. If the neighboring cell has elevated levels of superoxide, then there is an increased probability of superoxide reacting with NO to form peroxynitrite, which is highly reactive, damaging lipids, proteins, and DNA. In this scheme, it is the site of generation of superoxide that determines whether a cell will succumb to NO- and peroxynitrite-mediated deleterious effects. Since dopaminergic neurons selectively accumulate MPP^+, which in turn stimulates superoxide production, these neurons are selectively at risk.

1.4.1. Source of NO and NO Synthase

As summarized above, there is strong evidence that NO participates in the MPTP neurotoxic process. Because MPTP selectively kills dopaminergic neurons, it is expected that the deleterious cascade of events that underlie the neurodegeneration takes place inside dopaminergic neurons. As illustrated in **Fig. 2**, there are experimental arguments to indicate that superoxide concentration is indeed increased inside dopaminergic neurons by MPP^+. However, NO is produced by NOS, which thus far has not been identified inside dopaminergic neurons in rodents; although this needs to be confirmed, low levels of NOS might be present in dopaminergic neurons in humans *(45)*. In contrast to their lack of NOS, at least in rodents, dopaminergic structures are surrounded by NOS-containing fibers and cell bodies in the striatum, and, to a lesser extent, in the SNpc *(45,46)*. Because NO is uncharged and lypophilic *(47)*, it is able to travel away from its site of synthesis and inflict remote cellular damage without the need for any export mechanisms. It is suggested that NO, which is highly diffusible, can travel in random directions up to 150–300 μm during the 5–15 s that correspond to its estimated half-life in physiologic and aqueous conditions *(47)*. Although this modeling may depart from the actual in vivo

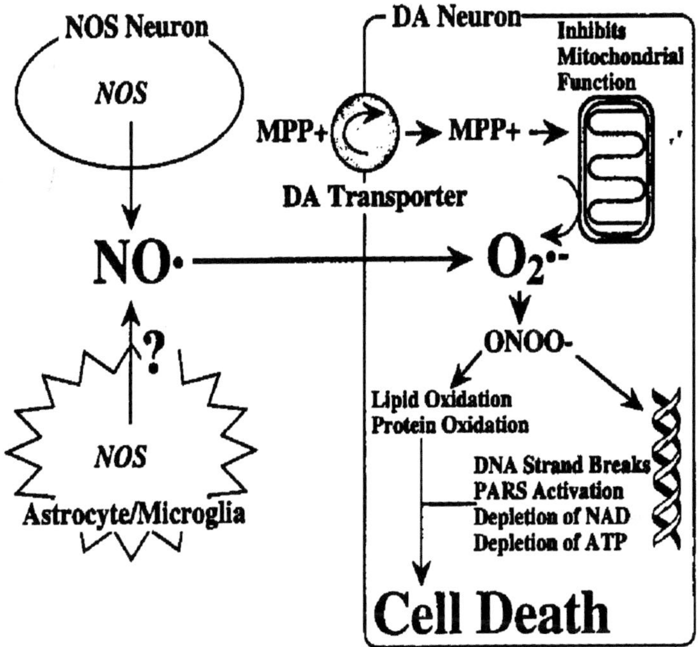

Fig. 2. Proposed scheme for selectivity of MPTP-induced dopaminergic neurotoxicity. DA, dopamine. (Reproduced with permission from **ref. *43***.)

situation encountered by a molecule of NO, it gives credence to the hypothesis that NO can cover a distance several times greater than the diameter of a cell. As shown in **Fig. 2**, we are thus speculating that the NO production involved in MPTP toxicity takes place in nondopaminergic cells present in the vicinity of dopaminergic structures.

Another question pertinent to the origin of NO in the MPTP model is which isoforms of NOS are primarily involved in this process? Nitric oxide is formed from arginine by NOS, which oxidizes the guanidino nitrogen of arginine, releasing NO and citrulline. To date, three distinct NOS isoenzymes have been purified and molecularly cloned (**Table 1**): neuronal NOS (nNOS, NOS I), inducible NOS (iNOS, NOS II), and endothelial NOS (eNOS, NOS III). These isoforms fall into two general categories on the basis of regulation of enzymatic activity. The first category comprises the constitutively expressed eNOS and nNOS isoforms, whose production of NO is Ca^{2+}/calmodulin dependent and is tightly controlled by mechanisms regulating intracellular Ca^{2+} levels. The second category comprises iNOS, which is not present constitutively (at least in most cells), but rather its mRNA transcription and translation are induced as part of an immune response in many cell types by endotoxin or

Table 1
Properties of NO Synthase Isoforms

First identified	Isoform	Name	Subcellular location	Denatured molecular mass	Regulation	Cofactors	No. amino acids	mRNA (kb)
Brain	I	Neuronal NOS (nNOS)	Soluble > particulate	160,000	Ca^{2+}/calmodulin	NADPH, FAD/FMN, tetrahydro-biopterin	1429 (rat)	10.5 (rat)
Macrophage	II	Inducible or macrophage NOS (iNOS)	Soluble > particulate	130,000	Inducible by cytokines, Ca^{2+} independent	Calmodulin, NADPH, FAD/FMN, tetrahydro-biopterin	1144 (mouse)	4.4–5.0 (mouse)
Endothelium	III	Endothelial NOS (eNOS)	Particulate > soluble	135,000	Ca^{2+}/calmodulin	NADPH, FAD/FMN, tetrahydro-biopterin	1203 (human)	4.3 (human)

inflammatory cytokines (e.g., γ-interferon, interleukin-1, or tumor necrosis factor). This inducible isoform contains calmodulin and is not regulated by intracellular changes in Ca^{2+} levels. Since all three isoforms of NOS have been identified in the brain, each of these can individually or in combination be involved in the production of NO used in MPTP neurotoxic process.

1.5. NOS Immunohistochemistry

There are at least two ways to explore the distribution of NOS proteins, by NOS immunohistochemistry or by nicotinamide adenine dinucleotide phosphate (NADPH)-diaphorase histochemistry; both approaches have advantages and disadvantages. However, rather than being exclusive, as we can see from the literature, both methods are often used within the same study.

1.5.1. Anti-NOS Antibodies

The main advantage of NOS immunohistochemistry over NADPH-diaphorase is that it allows the study of each NOS isoform separately. Anti-NOS antibodies directed against each NOS isoform are now commercially available; several of these, whether they are monoclonals or polyclonals, produce good results in immunohistochemistry as well as in Western blot.

The production of isoform-specific antibodies can be accomplished through a variety of approaches, including the production of monoclonal antibodies against purified protein, fusion protein, or synthesized peptides from the deduced amino acid sequence. Polyclonal antibodies directed against regions of the NOS isoforms with low homology can also be used to generate isoform-selective antibodies. Selection of peptides has been made easier by the development of computer programs that can assist in the design of peptides. Certain considerations are important to keep in mind. The peptide should be unique to your protein or at the very least have a low homology to the known isoforms. In addition, it should have a high antigenic index, and it is extremely helpful if it is water soluble. The methods, techniques, and theory behind the production of both monoclonal and polyclonal antibodies as well as the potential pitfalls that may arise in making antibodies are beyond the scope of this chapter and can be found in **ref. *48***.

1.5.2. Localization of NO Synthase Isoforms

Neuronal NOS is the predominant isoform of NOS in the brain. Its catalytic activity and protein are identifiable throughout the brain ***(45,49)***. Relevant to MPTP, nNOS is present in high density in the striatum within intrinsic medium-sized neurons colocalizing with somatostatin and neuropeptide Y ***(48)***. In the midbrain, nNOS is found in cholinergic neurons and within serotoninergic fibers ***(46,48)***. Thus, both by its abundance and its localization, nNOS appears to be an excellent candidate for producing NO following MPTP. This is in agreement with our demonstration that mutant mice deficient in nNOS ***(49)*** are partially protected against MPTP-induced striatal dopaminergic toxicity ***(43)***. The finding that mice are better protected by the NOS antagonist 7-NI than by the lack of nNOS expression suggests that nNOS is important but may not be the sole isoform of NOS involved in the MPTP neurotoxic process. Can it be iNOS?

In the normal brain, iNOS is not detectable ***(50)*** or is minimally expressed ***(51)***. However, under pathologic conditions, iNOS expression can significantly increase in activated astrocytes as well as in other cells such as microglia ***(52)***, invading macrophages, and even neurons ***(53)***. This was shown in the brain after kainic acid lesion ***(54)***, ischemic damage ***(55)***, and stab wounds ***(52)***. A similar scenario seems to exist in the MPTP model. Indeed, it appears that early in the course of MPTP-induced dopaminergic neuron degeneration there is an increase in striatal and midbrain iNOS activity (***55a***) consistent with the strong astrocytic and microglial reaction that occurs in these brain regions following MPTP administration ***(55a,56,57)***. Changes in iNOS activity are already substantial 24 h after MPTP administration, which precedes the peak of dopaminergic neurodegeneration. Therefore, NO derived from iNOS may play a substantial role in MPTP-induced dopaminergic neurodegeneration. Since iNOS is induced following MPTP, it may not play a significant role in the initiation of the MPTP toxic process, but instead may amplify its propagation by fueling injured dopaminergic neurons with increasing amounts of NO. This view is consistent with our recent report of attenuated MPTP-induced SNpc degeneration in iNOS knockout mice (***55a***).

eNOS is localized in the endothelium of blood vessels in the periphery and in the nervous system. Aside from endothelial cells, eNOS has also been localized in different discrete regions of the brain by autoradiography ***(58)*** and immunostaining ***(48)***. Although these studies report only low levels of eNOS in several brain regions, eNOS is particularly abundant in the hippocampus and in the olfactory bulb within neurons and neuropil. The presence of eNOS in the parenchyma, along with the fact that the brain is generously vascularized, makes it possible that eNOS contributes to the basal concentration of NO in the brain. As such, eNOS may have some importance in the MPTP neurotoxic process. Alternatively, its role in the vasculature ***(59)*** may be more significant for MPTP. As mentioned above, the striatal content of MPP^+, which is a determining factor in dopaminergic neurotoxicity, is tightly regulated by cerebral inflow of MPTP and outflow of MPP^+. Therefore, eNOS, by modulating blood vessel tone and thus cerebral perfusion, may alter the amount of blood-borne MPTP that gets into the brain and the kinetics of disappearance of MPP^+. Should the cause of PD be related to an endogenous or exogenous blood-borne toxin, eNOS may be a therapeutic target for this disease.

1.6. NADPH-Diaphorase Histochemistry

Under appropriate conditions of paraformaldehyde fixation, NADPH-diaphorase staining can be used to identify all NOS isoforms. For unknown reasons, NOS is resistant to paraformaldehyde fixation, whereas all other NADPH-dependent oxidative enzymes are inactivated by fixatives.

1.6.1. Localization of NADPH-Diaphorase

In the brain, the highest density of NADPH-diaphorase is evident in the cerebellum and in the olfactory bulb ***(60,61)***. The accessory olfactory bulb has even more prominent staining. Other areas of high-density staining include the pedunculopontine tegmental nucleus, the superior and inferior colliculi, the supraoptic nucleus, the islands of Calleja, the caudate-putamen, and the dentate gyrus of the hippocampus. In the cerebellum, NADPH-diaphorase occurs in glutaminergic granule cells as well as in γ-aminobutyric acid (GABA)-ergic basket cells. In the cerebral cortex, NADPH-diaphorase staining colocalizes with somatostatin, neuropeptide Y, and GABA. In the corpus striatum, NADPH-diaphorase neurons also stain for somatostatin and neuropeptide Y. In the pedunculopontine tegmental nucleus of the brain stem, NADPH-diaphorase neurons stain for choline acetyltransferase but do not stain for somatostatin and neuropeptide Y. Even though there does not seem to be a single neurotransmitter that colocalizes with NADPH-diaphorase, all NADPH-diaphorase neurons identified co-localize with NOS ***(62)***. NOS catalytic activity accounts for diaphorase staining because transfection of cultured human kidney 293 cells with nNOS cDNA produces cells that stain for both nNOS and NADPH-diaphorase ***(62)***.

NADPH-diaphorase has been localized to the endothelium of blood vessels in the periphery and in the nervous system. NADPH-diaphorase is also concentrated in the hippocampus and is evident in pyramidal cells of the CA1 region and in granule cells of the dentate gyrus. eNOS or a closely related isoform accounts for NADPH-diaphorase staining in this structure. Using high concentrations of glutaraldehyde fixatives, we found that NADPH-diaphorase staining provides robust staining of pyramidal cells of the CA1 region.

NADPH-diaphorase has also been identified in neutrophils, macrophages, microglia, and astrocytes.

1.7. NOS Catalytic Activity

In several studies, it is important to gather information about the actual enzymatic activity of NOS. This question arises consistently when, for example, one wishes to determine whether, in a pathologic condition such as PD, changes in NOS activity occur or how intense and lasting is the inhibition of NOS activity following administration of a NOS antagonist. Among the different methods available to assess NOS activity, the most reliable and straightforward is based on the conversion of [^{3}H]arginine into [^{3}H]citrulline (*see* **Subheading 3.**).

1.8. Peroxynitrite and Nitrotyrosine

Superoxide is produced by many biologic reactions, especially by mitochondrial respiration ***(37)***. It can be engaged in numerous reactions including the direct oxidation of biological molecules (e.g., cathechols) and the production of hydroxyl radicals (**Fig. 1**). Similarly, NO exerts many biologic effects that can be defined as direct (i.e., resulting from the reactions between NO and specific biologic molecules) or indirect (i.e., resulting from the reactions between reactive nitric oxide species [RNOS], which are derived from NO oxidation, and specific biologic targets) ***(41)***. Most, if not all, of the direct effects of NO appear to be related to biologic regulatory effects and not to neurotoxicity ***(41)***; although NO can directly affect mitochondrial respiration in vitro ***(63)***, the deleterious consequence of this effect remains to be determined in vivo. Conversely, the indirect actions of NO, which are mediated by RNOS such as nitrite (NO_2^-), nitrate (NO_3^-), and peroxynitrite and its protonated derivative peroxynitrous acid (N_2O_3H) are unquestionably deleterious ***(41)***; in aqueous conditions, RNOS such as NO^+ and NO^- react rapidly with water and thus are unlikely to be major participants in noxious reactions.

In light of the above, it appears that since they are weak oxidants, neither superoxide nor NO is believed to be sufficiently damaging by themselves to participate directly in the MPTP toxic process. In contrast, peroxynitrite fulfils the role of the toxic mediator between superoxide and NO. The versatility of peroxynitrite as an oxidant is impressive: it can react with antioxidants (e.g., ascorbate, glutathione), unsaturated fatty acid in lipids, amino acid residues (e.g., cysteine, methionine, and tyrosine), and purine bases (e.g., guanine) ***(64,65)***. By damaging DNA, peroxynitrite may stimulate the activity of poly(ADP-ribose) synthetase (PARP) ***(66)***, which in turn may exacerbate MPP^+-induced ATP depletion ***(66–68)***. One persistent fingerprint left by peroxynitrite is nitration of phenolic rings including tyrosine ***(69)***. As such, detection and quantification of nitrotyrosine is important indirect evidence that peroxynitrite is involved in a pathologic process. Aside from being a marker, tyrosine nitration may also be deleterious, as it can inactivate enzymes and receptors that depend on tyrosine residues for their activity ***(70,71)*** and prevent phosphorylation of tyrosine residues important for signal transduction ***(72,73)***.

This cascade of events appears quite relevant to the mode of action of MPTP, as we have demonstrated that, following MPTP administration to mice, both striatal and midbrain levels of nitrotyrosine in proteins increase in a time-dependent fashion and that tyrosine hydroxylase (TH), the rate-limiting enzyme in dopamine synthesis, becomes inactivated by tyrosine nitration ***(74)***. Nitrotyrosine has been successfully detected and quantified by different methods including high-performance liquid chromatography (HPLC), mass spectrometry, and immunobased assays ***(75)***. Although these are not described in detail, we discuss them briefly and emphasize some important practical aspects.

1.8.1. Quantification of Nitrotyrosine

Several HPLC-based methods with ultraviolet (UV) or fluorescent detection have been used to quantify and separate chlorotyrosine and nitrotyrosine from tyrosine and other tyrosine analogs ***(76,77)***. These techniques, however, like other UV or fluorescent detection-based methods, lack sensitivity. Two HPLC methods with electrodetection have recently been developed ***(76,77)***; as anticipated, they are significantly more sensitive and, thus, more appropriate to quantify the minute amounts of nitrotyrosine presumably present in the brain. However, there are some concerns about whether these HPLC methods are actually detecting tyrosine analogs such as nitrotyrosine or an artifact ***(78)***. Until this issue is resolved, it would be preferable to utilize a method that combines the possibility of quantifying tyrosine analogs such as isotope dilution gas chromatography combined with mass spectrometry (GC/MS) ***(79–82)***. Relevant to the existence of peroxynitrite in the MPTP model, it has been demonstrated that MPTP significantly increases striatal levels of *free nitrotyrosine* in mice ***(19)***. Although this finding provides major impetus to the implication of peroxynitrite in the MPTP model, one should be aware that the relationship between free and protein nitrotyrosine is unknown and that the physiopathologic role, if any, of free nitrotyrosine remains to be determined.

1.8.2. Visualization of Nitrotyrosine

Although the HPLC and GC/MS methods are highly sensitive, they do not provide information as to where at an anatomic or cellular level the changes in tyrosine nitration occur after MPTP administration. A similar issue was successfully addressed recently in spinal cord from amytrophic lateral sclerosis (ALS) patients ***(83)*** and in rejected transplanted kidney ***(84)*** in which levels of nitrotyrosine, determined by HPLC, were more than twofold higher in tissue extracts from these pathologic conditions compared with controls. In both situations, immunohistochemical analysis of nitrotyrosine revealed that conspicuous immunoreactivity was localized in spinal cord motor neurons ***(83)*** and in kidney tubular cells *(84)*. Both locations are pertinent to the pathological processes that underlie ALS and chronic kidney transplant rejection. These immunohistochemical studies were performed by using specific antinitrotyrosine antibodies. Both mouse monoclonal and rabbit polyclonal antinitrotyrosine antibodies *(85)* are now commercially available from Upstate Biotechnology (UBI, Lake Placid, NY). Both were raised against nitrated keyhole limpet hemocyanin (KLH) and specifically recognize peroxynitrite-modified proteins including KLH, bovine serum albumin (BSA), catalase, histone, lysozyme, actin, rat brain homogenate, and heart homogenate, but not the corresponding native proteins. Nitrotyrosine (0.3 m*M*) can completely block the monoclonal or the polyclonal antibody binding to nitrated BSA; however, in routine use, concentrations as high as 10 m*M* nitrotyrosine may be necessary to block antibody binding fully. In contrast, a 10 m*M* concentration of either tyrosine, aminotyrosine, chlorotyrosine, hydroxytyrosine, or phosphotyrosine has no effect on antibody binding to nitrated BSA. It is, however, recommended to verify the specificity of the antibodies by two sets of controls on each tissue sample to confirm the presence of nitrotyrosine as follows: (1) blockade with an excess of nitrotyrosine; and (2) reduction to aminotyrosine with a strong reducing agent such as dithionite. Surprisingly, to our knowledge, to date no published studies exist regarding the identification of nitrotyrosine immunostaining in the MPTP model or in PD.

1.8.3. Target Proteins of Tyrosine Nitration in Dopamine Neurons

Aside from their use for immunostaining, the antinitrotyrosine antibodies have been used for immunoprecipitating and immunoblotting of tyrosine nitrated proteins *(74,86)*. These techniques are the cornerstone methods used to identify manganese SOD (SOD2) as a specific target of tyrosine nitration in the rejected kidney transplant *(84)*. This method also enabled us to demonstrate that TH is a major target of tyrosine nitration following MPTP administration *(74)*. Both immunoblot and the immunoprecipitation using the antinitrotyrosine antibodies are straightforward *(74)* and require the same type of controls as described for immunostaining.

2. Materials

Unless specified, all reagents required for the assays referenced in this chapter can be obtained from standard commercial sources and preferentially should be of the highest purity. Some technical comments and detailed recipes for the preparation of the necessary buffers and reaction solutions are given.

1. Water quality is a key factor to the success and reproducibility of the assays described in this chapter. Pure water refers to both low ion content and no infectious agents such as bacteria, fungi, and algae. This type of high-quality water

can be obtained from a distilled or a deionized water station. It is also advisable to autoclave distilled or deionized water whenever possible.

Caution: Some enzymatic reactions (e.g., horseradish peroxidase) may be inhibited by deionized water and thus, unless mandatory, it is advisable to use high-quality distilled water.

2. 0.2 *M* phosphate buffer (PB), pH 7.4**:** Prepare the following two stock solutions:
   a. Stock solution A: 0.2 *M* NaH_2PO_4 (12 g NaH_2PO_4 in 500 mL H_2O, or 13.9 g of $NaH_2PO_4 \cdot H_2O$ in 500 mL H_2O).
   b. Stock solution B: 0.2 *M* Na_2HPO_4 (28.4 g Na_2HPO_4 in 1 L H_2O).

   To make 0.2 *M* PB at pH 7.4: mix 1 part of solution A with 4 parts of solution B (e.g., 100 mL of A + 400 mL of B). This stock solution can be used to prepare the fixative solution (*see* **step 4**) or be diluted with an equal volume of distilled water to provide 0.1 *M* PB.
3. Tris-buffered saline (TBS): 50 m*M* Tris-HCl, pH 7.2 and 1.5% NaCl. Store at room temperature.
4. Fixative solution (4% paraformaldehyde/0.1 *M* PB): Depolymerize 8% paraformaldehyde in distilled H_2O (8 g in 100 mL H_2O) by heating to 80°C for 30 min while stirring. Do not exceed 80°C. If paraformaldehyde boils, start over.

   Caution: Wear gloves and mask while weighing and preparing paraformaldehyde. The solution must be heated in a fume hood.
   a. Clear paraformaldehyde solution with 1–2 drops of 10 *M* NaOH. *Solution will turn from a turbid appearance to a clear solution.*
   b. Let solution cool to room temperature (RT), check volume, and replace any H_2O that may have evaporated.
   c. Add an equal volume of 0.2 *M* PB, pH 7.4, to make a final solution of 4% paraformaldehyde/0.1 *M* PB.
   d. Filter 4% paraformaldehyde/0.1 *M* PB solution through a 0.22-µm filter unit and use within 1 wk (older 4% paraformaldehyde/0.1 *M* PB solution may contain crystals of formalin, which may cause tissue artifacts).
5. NADPH staining solution: Prepare buffer solution and stain mix as follows:
   a. Buffer solution: 0.1 *M* Tris-HCl, pH 7.2, 0.2% Triton X-100, 0.02% NaN_3.
   b. Stain Mix: 1 m*M* β-NADPH reduced form (8.33 mg in 10 mL buffer solution), 0.2 m*M* nitroblue tetrazolium (NBT) (1.64 mg in 10 mL buffer solution). Dissolve β-NADPH and NBT in the buffer solution in separate tubes. β-NADPH is readily soluble in the buffer, but NBT may need to be sonicated for 10 min. Mix β-NADPH and NBT together in a 1:1 ratio and filter before application to cells. The final concentration of the stain mix should be 1 m*M* β-NADPH reduced form and 0.2 m*M* NBT. Since the two compounds are solubilized in separate tubes, each tube should contain a 2X concentration, so that when mixed together in a 1:1 ratio the final concentration is 1X. *The final staining mix should be filtered before use to prevent formation of dark blue precipitates.*
6. NOS enzymatic activity reaction mix: Prepare buffer solution and reaction mix as follows:
   a. Reaction buffer: 50 m*M* Tris-HCl, pH 7.4, 2.5 m*M* dithiothreitol (DTT; 3.8 mg/mL), 10 µ*M* tetrahydrobiopterin (BH_4; 3.1 mg/mL). *Although Tris-*

HCl can be kept at 4°C for an extended period, DTT and BH_4 must be added to Tris-HCl on the day of the assay.

b. NADPH solution (1.25 m*M*): Dissolve 5 mg of NADPH in 5 mL of reaction buffer. This tube must be protected from light and kept on ice.
c. $CaCl_2$ solution (28 m*M*): Dissolve 78 mg of $CaCl_2$ in 5 mL reaction buffer.
d. Radioactive solution: Mix 12.5 µL L-[2,3-^{3}H]arginine (specific activity: 36.8 Ci/mmol; Dupont-NEN, Boston, MA) with 1250 µL reaction buffer. This tube must be protected from light and kept on ice. *Ten microliters of this radioactive mix should produce 250,000–500,000 dpm.*
e. Stopping buffer: 20 m*M* HEPES, pH 5.5, 1 m*M* EDTA, and 1 m*M* EGTA.
f. Resin suspension: Wash 100 g Dowex AG50WX-8 (Pharmacia, Piscataway, NJ) resin (hydrogen form) with 200 mL 1 *N* NaOH to convert it from the hydrogen to the Na form. Gently stir the mixture for 15 min at RT, let the mix settle, then pour off the liquid, and repeat the NaOH wash two more times. Afterward, wash the resin several times with distilled water until the pH (use pH paper) of the resin suspension is between 7.0 and 8.0. Then decant and resuspend the resin with stopping buffer. *The prepared resin suspension can be kept for several weeks in a beaker covered with parafilm at 4°C.*

3. Methods

3.1. NOS Immunostaining Protocol

1. Anesthetize rats or mice with pentobarbital (35–45 mg/kg intraperitoneal injection) and perfuse them with cold saline followed by 4% paraformaldehyde/0.1 *M* PB containing 0.1% glutaraldehyde (250 mL for rats and 75 mL for mice).
2. Remove the brains and postfix tissues for 2 h in 4% paraformaldehyde/0.1 *M* PB.
3. Cryoprotect brains by immersing them in 20% (v/v) glycerol in PB. Alternatively, the brains can be cryoprotected in 30% (v/v) sucrose in PB by sequentially bathing the tissue in 10, 20, and 30% sucrose.
4. Permeabilize slide-mounted or free-floating tissue sections in TBS containing 0.4% Triton X-100 for 30 min at RT (*see* **Note 1**).
5. Block tissue sections for 1 h in TBS containing 4% normal goat serum (NGS), 0.2% Triton X-100, and 0.02% NaN_3 at RT.
6. Incubate sections overnight at 4°C in TBS containing 0.1% Triton X-100, 2% NGS, and 0.02% NaN_3 with the appropriate dilution of primary antibody.
7. Rinse tissue sections with TBS containing 1% NGS (3 X 10 min).
8. Incubate tissue sections with a biotinylated goat-anti-rabbit antibody (Vector) at a 1:200 dilution for 1 h at RT in TBS containing 1.5% NGS.
9. Rinse tissue sections 2 X 10 min in TBS containing 1% NGS and then 2 X 10 min in TBS.
10. Incubate tissue sections with an avidin-biotin-horseradish peroxidase complex (Vector Elite, Vector) at a 1:50 dilution in TBS for 1 h at RT.
11. Rinse tissue sections 3 X 10 min in TBS.
12. Develop color with a substrate solution consisting of 0.1% H_2O_2 and 0.5 mg/mL diaminobenzidine in TBS.
13. Rinse section with TBS.

14. Mount sections on gelatin-coated glass slides and allow to air dry prior to counterstaining (facultative) with thionin, which gives a light blue/purple color to the nucleus of all cells and to Nissl bodies of neurons.
15. Dehydrate the sections and coverslip using Permount (Fisher) (*see* **Note 2**).

3.2. NADPH-Diaphorase Histochemistry

1. Anesthetize rats or mice with pentobarbital, perfuse, and process brains as described for NOS immunohistochemistry (*see* **Subheading 3.1., steps 2–4**).
2. Incubate sections at 37°C in the NADPH-diaphorase staining mix.
3. Check staining at 30 min under a light microscope.
4. Let stain for 30–90 min. Cells that contain NOS should turn purple/dark blue.
5. Stop the reaction by rinsing the tissue sections (3 X 10 min) in cold TBS (*see* **Note 3**).
6. Mount sections on gelatin-coated glass slides.
7. If counterstaining is required, use any dye that produces a color other than blue/purple such as crystal green.
8. Dehydrate sections and coverslip using Permount (Fisher) (*see* **Note 2**).

3.3. NOS Catalytic Activity

3.3.1. Tissue Preparation

1. Sacrifice rats or mice by decapitation and quickly remove the brains.
2. Dissect out regions of interest such as striatum and cerebellum freehand on an ice-cold glass Petri dish *(87)*.
3. Immediately freeze the samples on dry ice and store at –80°C until analysed.

3.3.2. Radioenzymatic Assay

nNOS and eNOS catalytic activity are assayed by measuring Ca^{2+}-dependent activity; iNOS is assayed by measuring the Ca^{2+}-independent conversion of [^{3}H]arginine to [^{3}H]citrulline ***(49)***.

1. On the day of the assay, sonicate frozen tissue samples in 20 volumes (w/v) 50 m*M* Tris-HCl, pH 7.4, buffer containing 1 m*M* EDTA and 1 m*M* EGTA and keep on ice.
2. Add 25 μL of homogenate to the various reaction tubes, which should be placed on ice and prepared as described in **Table 2** (*see* **Note 4**).
3. Incubate tubes for 15 min at 25°C.
4. Terminate the reaction by the addition of 3 ml of cold stopping buffer.
5. Apply the total resulting volume progressively to a mini-column packed with 0.5–1.0 mL Dowex AG50WX-8 resin.
6. Quantify [^{3}H]citrulline by liquid scintillation counting of the eluate. For each experiment, the blank (background) is generated by omitting NADPH (*see* **Note 2**).

4. Notes

1. Although we use TBS, phosphate-buffered saline would give the same result in most instances. However, be aware that many enzymes, including horseradish

Table 2
Experimental Tubes (Duplicate) for NOS Activity Assay[a]

	Ca^{2+}-dependent activity		Ca^{2+}-independent activity		Blank	
	1	2	1	2	1	2
Tris buffer	0	0	10	10	90	90
Radioactive	10	10	10	10	10	10
$CaCl_2$	10	10	0	0	0	0
Homogenate	25	25	25	25	25	25
NADPH	80	80	80	80	0	0
Total volume	125	125	125	125	125	125

[a]All volumes are in µL. NADPH starts the reaction, so it should be added last.

peroxidase, can be inhibited by phosphate. Thus, unless required, TBS would be the preferred buffer.

2. In case of failure in any of the assays described above, do not dismiss the possibility that the culprit could be the water (e.g., inhibition caused by deionized water, infection), buffer (e.g., incorrect concentration or pH), and degradation or omission of the primary or secondary antibodies as well as key reagents such as NADPH.
3. For NADPH-diaphorase, be aware that when the solution turns pink/purple, the reaction should be stopped. Optimal NADPH-diaphorase staining is usually obtained prior to the solution turning pink/purple.
4. For NOS activity, if only nNOS activity is to be studied, then it is preferable to centrifuge the tissue homogenate (18,000*g*, 15 min, 4°C) and use 25 µL of the supernatant for the reaction since nNOS is a soluble enzyme.

Acknowledgment

S.P. is supported by NINDS grants R29 NS37345, RO1 NS38586, and P50 NS538370, the U.S. Department of Defense (DAMD 17-99-1-9474), The Parkinson's Disease Foundation, the Lowenstein Foundation, and the Smart Foundation. S.P. is also a recipient of the Cotzias Award from the American Parkinson Disease Association. T.M.D. is supported by NINDS grant P50 NS38377, the U.S. Army Medical Research and Material Command grant 98222087 and the Mitchell Family Foundation.

References

1. Fahn, S. and Przedborski, S. (2000) Parkinsonism in *Merritt's Neurology* (L. P. Rowland, ed.), Lippincott Williams & Wilkins, New York, pp. 679–693.
2. Fahn, S. (1989) Adverse effects of levodopa in Parkinson's disease, in *Handbook of Experimental Pharmacology*, vol. 8 (Calne, D. B., ed.), Springer-Verlag, Berlin, pp. 386–409.

3. Przedborski, S., Jackson-Lewis, V., Djaldetti, R., Liberatore, G., Vila, M., Vukosavic, S., and Almer, G. (2000). The parkinsonian toxin MPTP: action and mechanism. *Restor. Neurol. Neurosci.* **16,** 135–142.
4. Langston, J. W., Ballard, P., and Irwin, I. (1983) Chronic parkinsonism in humans due to a product of meperidine-analog synthesis. *Science* **219,** 979–980.
5. Heikkila, R. E., Sieber, B. A., Manzino, L., and Sonsalla, P. K. (1989) Some features of the nigrostriatal dopaminergic neurotoxin 1- methyl-4-phenyl-1,2,3,6-tetrahydropyridine (MPTP) in the mouse. *Mol. Chemic. Neuropathol.* **10,** 171–183.
6. Kopin, I. J. and Markey, S. P. (1988) MPTP toxicity: implication for research in Parkinson's disease. *Annu. Rev. Neurosci.* **11,** 81–96.
7. Langston, J. W. (1987) MPTP: the promise of a new neurotoxin, in *Movement Disorders 2* (Marsden, C. D. and Fahn, S., eds.), Butterworths, London, pp. 73–90.
8. Davis, G. C., Williams, A. C., Markey, S. P., Ebert, M. H., Caine, E. D., Reichert, C. M., and Kopin, I. J. (1979) Chronic parkinsonism secondary to intravenous injection of meperidine analogs. *Psychiatry Res.* **1,** 249–254.

8a. Langston, J. W., Forno, L. S., Tetrud, J., Reeves, A. G., Kaplan, J. A., and Karluk, D. (1999) Evidence of active nerve cell degeneration in the substantia nigra of humans years after 1-methyl-4-phenyl-1,2,3,6-tetrahydropyridine exposure. *Ann. Neurol.* **46,** 598–605.

9. Forno, L. S., DeLanney, L. E., Irwin, I., and Langston, J. W. (1993) Similarities and differences between MPTP-induced parkinsonism and Parkinson's disease: Neuropathologic considerations. *Adv. Neurol.* **60,** 600–608.
10. Agid, Y., Javoy-Agid, F., and Ruberg, M. (1987) Biochemistry of neurotransmitters in Parkinson's disease, in *Movement Disorders 2* (Marsden, C. D. and Fahn, S., eds.), Butterworths, London, pp. 166–230.
11. Seniuk, N. A., Tatton, W. G., and Greenwood, C. E. (1990) Dose-dependent destruction of the coeruleus-cortical and nigral- striatal projections by MPTP. *Brain Res.* **527,** 7–20.
12. Muthane, U., Ramsay, K. A., Jiang, H., Jackson-Lewis, V., Donaldson, D., Fernando, S., Ferreira, M., and Przedborski, S. (1994) Differences in nigral neuron number and sensitivity to 1-methyl- 4-phenyl-1,2,3,6-tetrahydropyridine in C57/bl and CD-1 mice. *Exp. Neurol.* **126,** 195–204.
13. Moratalla, R., Quinn, B., DeLanney, L. E., Irwin, I., Langston, J. W., and Graybiel, A. M. (1992) Differential vulnerability of primate caudate-putamen and striosome-matrix dopamine systems to the neurotoxic effects of 1- methyl-4-phenyl-1,2,3,6-tetrahydropyridine. *Proc. Natl. Acad. Sci. USA* **89,** 3859–3863.
14. DiMauro, S. (1993) Mitochondrial involvement in Parkinson's disease: The controversy continues. *Neurology* **43,** 2170–2172.
15. Nicklas, W. J., Yougster, S. K., Kindt, M. V., and Heikkila, R. E. (1987) MPTP, MPP+ and mitochondrial function. *Life Sci.* **40,** 721–729.
16. Gluck, M. R., Youngster, S. K., Ramsay, R. R., Singer, T. P., and Nicklas, W. J. (1994) Studies on the characterization of the inhibitory mechanism of 4'-alkylated 1-methyl-4-phenylpyridinium and phenylpyridine analogues in mitochondria and electron transport particles. *J. Neurochem.* **63,** 655–661.
17. Przedborski, S. and Jackson-Lewis, V. (1998) Experimental developments in movement disorders: update on proposed free radical mechanisms. *Curr. Opin. Neurol.* **11,** 335–339.

18. Przedborski, S., Kostic, V., Jackson-Lewis, V., Naini, A. B., Simonetti, S., Fahn, S., Carlson, E., Epstein, C. J., and Cadet, J. L. (1992) Transgenic mice with increased Cu/Zn-superoxide dismutase activity are resistant to N-methyl-4-phenyl-1,2,3,6-tetrahydropyridine-induced neurotoxicity. *J. Neurosci.* **12,** 1658–1667.
19. Schulz, J. B., Matthews, R. T., Muqit, M. M. K., Browne, S. E., and Beal, M. F. (1995) Inhibition of neuronal nitric oxide synthase by 7-nitroindazole protects against MPTP-induced neurotoxicity in mice. *J. Neurochem.* **64,** 936–939.
20. Hantraye, P., Brouillet, E., Ferrante, R., Palfi, S., Dolan, R., Matthews, R. T., and Beal, M. F. (1996) Inhibition of neuronal nitric oxide synthase prevents MPTP-induced parkinsonism in baboons. *Nature Med.* **2,** 1017–1021.
21. Przedborski, S. and Jackson-Lewis, V. (1998) Mechanisms of MPTP toxicity. *Mov. Disord.* **13 (Suppl 1),** 35–38.
22. Mayer, R. A., Kindt, M. V., and Heikkila, R. E. (1986) Prevention of the nigrostriatal toxicity of 1-methyl-4-phenyl-1,2,3,6-tetrahydropyridine by inhibitors of 3,4-dihydroxyphenylethylamine transport. *J. Neurochem.* **47,** 1073–1079.
23. Heikkila, R. E., Manzino, L., Cabbat, F. S., and Duvoisin, R. C. (1984) Protection against the dopaminergic neurotoxicity of 1-methyl-4-phenyl-1,2,3,6-tetrahydropyridine by monoamine oxidase inhibitors. *Nature* **311,** 467–469.
24. Javitch, J. A., D'Amato, R. J., Strittmatter, S. M., and Snyder, S. H. (1985) Parkinsonism-inducing neurotoxin, N-methyl-4-phenyl-1,2,3,6-tetrahydropyridine: uptake of the metabolite N-methyl-4-phenylpyridinium by dopamine neurons explain selective toxicity. *Proc. Natl. Acad. Sci. USA* **82,** 2173–2177.
25. Giovanni, A., Sieber, B. A., Heikkila, R. E., and Sonsalla, P. K. (1991) Correlation between the neostriatal content of the 1-methyl-4- phenylpyridinium species and dopaminergic neurotoxicity following 1-methyl-4-phenyl-1,2,3,6-tetrahydropyridine administration to several strains of mice. *J. Pharmacol. Exp. Ther.* **257,** 691–697.
26. Ramsay, R. R. and Singer, T. P. (1986) Energy-dependent uptake of N-methyl-4-phenylpyridinium, the neurotoxic metabolite of 1-methyl-4-phenyl-1,2,3,6-tetrahydropyridine, by mitochondria. *J. Biol. Chem.* **261,** 7585–7587.
27. Nicklas, W. J., Vyas, I., and Heikkila, R. E. (1985) Inhibition of NADH-linked oxidation in brain mitochondria by MPP+, a metabolite of the neurotoxin MPTP. *Life Sci.* **36,** 2503–2508.
28. Mizuno, Y., Sone, N., and Saitoh, T. (1987) Effects of 1-methyl-4-phenyl-1,2,3,6-tetrahydropyridine and 1-methyl-4-phenylpyridinium ion on activities of the enzymes in the electron transport system in mouse brain. *J. Neurochem.* **48,** 1787–1793.
29. Ramsay, R. R., Krueger, M. J., Youngster, S. K., Gluck, M. R., Casida, J. E., and Singer, T. P. (1991) Interaction of 1-methyl-4-phenylpyridinium ion (MPP^+) and its analogs with the rotenone/piericidin binding site of NADH dehydrogenase. *J. Neurochem.* **56,** 1184–1190.
30. Higgins, D. S., Jr. and Greenamyre, J. T. (1996) [^{3}H]dihydrorotenone binding to NADH: Ubiquinone reductase (Complex I) of the electron transport chain: An autoradiographic study. *J. Neurosci.* **16,** 3807–3816.
31. Davey, G. P. and Clark, J. B. (1996) Threshold effects and control of oxidative phosphorylation in nonsynaptic rat brain mitochondria. *J. Neurochem.* **66,** 1617–1624.

32. Chan, P., DeLanney, L. E., Irwin, I., Langston, J. W., and Di Monte, D. (1991) Rapid ATP loss caused by 1-methyl-4-phenyl-1,2,3,6- tetrahydropyridine in mouse brain. *J. Neurochem.* **57,** 348–351.
33. Rossetti, Z. L., Sotgiu, A., Sharp, D. E., Hadjiconstantinou, M., and Neff, M. (1988) 1-Methyl-4-phenyl-1,2,3,6-tetrahydropyridine (MPTP) and free radicals in vitro. *Biochem. Pharmacol.* **37,** 4573–4574.
34. Hasegawa, E., Takeshige, K., Oishi, T., Murai, Y., and Minakami, S. (1990) 1-Mehtyl-4-phenylpyridinium (MPP+) induces NADH-dependent superoxide formation and enhances NADH-dependent lipid peroxidation in bovine heart submitochondrial particles. *Biochem. Biophys. Res. Commun.* **170,** 1049–1055.
35. Cleeter, M. W., Cooper, J. M., and Schapira, A. H. (1992) Irreversible inhibition of mitochondrial complex I by 1-methyl-4-phenylpyridinium: evidence for free radical involvement. *J. Neurochem.* **58,** 786–789.
36. Beal, M. F. (1995) Aging, energy, and oxidative stress in neurodegenerative diseases. *Ann. Neurol.* **38,** 357–366.
37. Halliwell, B. and Gutteridge, J. M. (1991) *Free Radicals in Biology and Medicine*, Clarendon Press, Oxford.
38. Liochev, S. I. and Fridovich, I. (1994) The role of $O_2^{\bullet-}$ in the production of $HO^{\bullet-}$: In vitro and in vivo. *Free Radic. Biol. Med.* **16,** 29–33.
39. Beckman, J. S., Beckman, T. W., Chen, J., Marshall, P. A., and Freeman, B. A. (1990) Apparent hydroxyl radical production by peroxynitrite: implications for endothelial injury from nitric oxide and superoxide. *Proc. Natl. Acad. Sci. USA* **87,** 1620–1624.
40. Huie, R. E. and Padmaja, S. (1993) The reaction of NO with superoxide. *Free Radic. Res. Commun.* **18,** 195–199.
41. Wink, D. A., Matthews, R. T., Grisham, M. B., Mitchell, J. B., and Ford, P. C. (1996) Direct and indirect effects of nitric oxide in chemical reactions relevant to biology, in *Nitric Oxide. Part A. Source and Detection of NO; NO Synthase* (Packer, L., ed.), Academic Press, New York, pp. 12–31.
42. Beckman, J. S., Chen, J., Crow, J. P., and Ye, Y. Z. (1994) Reactions of nitric oxide, superoxide and peroxynitrite with superoxide dismutase in neurodegeneration. *Prog. Brain Res.* **103,** 371–380.
43. Przedborski, S., Jackson-Lewis, V., Yokoyama, R., Shibata, T., Dawson, V. L., and Dawson, T. M. (1996) Role of neuronal nitric oxide in MPTP (1-methyl-4-phenyl-1,2,3,6-tetrahydropyridine)-induced dopaminergic neurotoxicity. *Proc. Natl. Acad. Sci. USA* **93,** 4565–4571.
44. Moore, P. K., Wallace, P., Gaffen, Z., Hart, S. L., and Babbedge, R. C. (1993) Characterization of the novel nitric oxide synthase inhibitor 7-nitro indazole and related indazoles: antinociceptive and cardiovascular effects. *Br. J. Pharmacol.* **110,** 219–224.
45. Bredt, D. S., Glatt, C. E., Huang, P. L., Fotuhi, M., Dawson, T. M., and Snyder, S. H. (1991) Nitric oxide synthase protein and mRNA are discretely localized in neuronal populations of the mammalian CNS together with NADPH diaphorase. *Neuron* **7,** 615–624.
46. Leonard, C. S., Kerman, I., Blaha, G., Taveras, E., and Taylor, B. (1995) Interdigitation of nitric oxide synthase-, tyrosine hydroxylase-, and serotonin-contain-

ing neurons in and around the laterodorsal and pedunculopontine tegmental nuclei of the guinea pig. *J. Comp. Neurol.* **362,** 411–432.

47. Lancaster, Jr. J. R. (1996) Diffusion of free nitric oxide, in *Nitric Oxide. Source and Detection of NO; NO Synthase* (Packer, L., ed.), Academic Press, New York, pp. 31–50.
48. Dawson, T. M. and Dawson, V. L. (1996) Generation of isoform-specific antibodies to nitric oxide synthases, in *Nitric Oxide. Source and Detection of NO; NO Synthase* (Packer, L., ed.), Academic Press, New York, pp. 349–358.
49. Huang, P. L., Dawson, T. M., Bredt, D. S., Snyder, S. H., and Fishman, M. C. (1993) Targeted disruption of the neuronal nitric oxide synthase gene. *Cell* **75,** 1273–1285.
50. Lowenstein, C. J., Glatt, C. S., Bredt, D. S., and Snyder, S. H. (1992) Cloned and expressed macrophage nitric oxide synthase contrasts with the brain enzyme. *Proc. Natl. Acad. Sci. USA* **89,** 6711–6715.
51. Keilhoff, G., Seidel, B., Noack, H., Tischmeyer, W., Stanek, D., and Wolf, G. (1996) Patterns of nitric oxide synthase at the messenger RNA and protein levels during early rat brain development. *Neuroscience* **75,** 1193–1201.
52. Simmons, M. L. and Murphy, S. (1992) Induction of nitric oxide synthase in glial cells. *J. Neurochem.* **59,** 897–905.
53. Nathan, C. and Xie, Q. W. (1994) Regulation of biosynthesis of nitric oxide. *J. Biol. Chem.* **269,** 13,725–13,728.
54. Wallace, M. N. and Fredens, K. (1992) Activated astrocytes of the mouse hippocampus contain high levels of NADPH-diaphorase. *Neuroreport* **3,** 953–956.
55. Nakashima, M. N., Yamashita, K., Kataoka, Y., Yamashita, Y. S., and Niwa, M. (1995) Time course of nitric oxide synthase activity in neuronal, glial, and endothelial cells of rat striatum following focal cerebral ischemia. *Cell. Mol. Neurobiol.* **15,** 341–350.

55a. Liberatore, G. T., Jackson-Lewis, V. Vukosavic, S., Mandir, A. S., Vila, M., McAuliffe W. G. et al. (1999) Inducible nitric oxide synthase stimulates dopaminergic neurodegeneration in the MPTP model of Parkinson disease. *Nat. Med.* **5,** 1403–1409.

56. Francis, J. W., Von Visger, J., Markelonis, G. J., and Oh, T. H. (1995) Neuroglial responses to the dopaminergic neurotoxicant 1-methy-4-phenyl-1,2,3,6-tetrahydropyridine in mouse striatum. *Neurotoxicol. Teratol.* **17,** 7–12.
57. Czlonkowska, A., Kohutnicka, M., Kurkowska-Jastrzebska, I., and Czlonkowski, A. (1996) Microglial reaction in MPTP (1-methyl-4-phenyl-1,2,3,6-tetrahydropyridine) induced Parkinson's disease mice model. *Neurodegeneration* **5,** 137–143.
58. Hara, H., Waeber, C., Huang, P. L., Fujii, M., Fishman, M. C., and Moskowitz, M. A. (1996) Brain distribution of nitric oxide synthase in neuronal or endothelial nitric oxide synthase mutant mice using [^{3}H]L-N^{G}-nitro-arginine autoradiography. *Neuroscience* **75,** 881–890.
59. Dawson, T. M. and Dawson, V. L. (1996) Nitric oxide synthase: role as a transmitter/mediator in the brain and endocrine system. *Annu. Rev. Med.* **47,** 219–227.
60. Bredt, D. S., Hwang, P. M., and Snyder, S. H. (1990) Localization of nitric oxide synthase indicating a neural role for nitric oxide. *Nature* **347,** 768–770.

61. Hope, B. T., Michael, G. J., Knigge, K. M., and Vincent, S. R. (1991) Neuronal NADPH diaphorase is a nitric oxide synthase. *Proc. Natl. Acad. Sci. USA* **88,** 2811–2814.
62. Dawson, T. M., Bredt, D. S., Fotuhi, M., Hwang, P. M., and Snyder, S. H. (1991) Nitric oxide synthase and neuronal NADPH diaphorase are identical in brain and peripheral tissues. *Proc. Natl. Acad. Sci. USA* **88,** 7797–7801.
63. Bolaños, J. P., Almeida, A., Stewart, V., Peuchen, S., Land, J. M., Clark, J. B., and Heales, S. J. R. (1997) Nitric oxide-mediated mitochondrial damage in the brain: mechanisms and implications for neurodegenerative diseases. *J. Neurochem.* **68,** 2227–2240.
64. Beckman, J. S. (1994) Peroxynitrite versus hydroxyl radical: the role of nitric oxide in superoxide-dependent cerebral injury. *Ann. NY Acad. Sci.* **738,** 69–75.
65. Uppu, R. M., Squadrito, G. L., Cueto, R., and Pryor, W. A. (1996) Selecting the most appropriate synthesis of peroxynitrite, in *Nitric Oxide. Physiological and Pathological Processes* (Packer, L., ed.), Academic Press, New York, pp. 285–295.
66. Szabó, C., Zingarelli, B., O'Connor, M., and Salzman, A. L. (1996) DNA strand breakage, activation of poly(ADP-ribose) synthetase, and cellular energy depletion are involved in the cytotoxicity in macrophages and smooth muscle cells exposed to peroxynitrite. *Proc. Natl. Acad. Sci. USA* **93,** 1753–1758.
67. Zhang, J., Pieper, A., and Snyder, S. H. (1995) Poly(ADP-ribose) synthetase activation: an early indicator of neurotoxic DNA damage. *J. Neurochem.* **65,** 1411–1414.
68. Mandir, A. S., Przedborski, S., Jackson-Lewis, V., Wang, Z. Q., Simbulan-Rosenthal, M., Smulson, M. E., et al. (1999) Poly (ADP-ribose) polymerase activation mediates MPTP-induced parkinsonism. *Proc Natl Acad Sci USA* **96,** 5774–5779.
69. Ohshima, H., Friesen, M., Brouet, I., and Bartsch, H. (1990) Nitrotyrosine as a new marker for endogenous nitrosation and nitration of proteins. *Fd. Chem. Toxic.* **28,** 647–652.
70. Ischiropoulos, H., Zhu, L., Chen, J., Tsai, M., Martin, J. C., Smith, C. D., and Beckman, J. S. (1992) Peroxynitrite-mediated tyrosine nitration catalyzed by superoxide dismutase. *Arch. Biochem. Biophys.* **298,** 431–437.
71. Trotti, D., Rossi, D., Gjesdal, O., Levy, L. M., Racagni, G., Danbolt, N. C., and Volterra, A. (1996) Peroxynitrite inhibits glutamate transporter subtypes. *J. Biol. Chem.* **271,** 5976–5979.
72. Kong, C.-K., Yim, M. B., Stadtman, E. R., and Chock, P. B. (1996) Peroxynitrite disables the tyrosine phosphorylation regulatory mechanism: Lymphocyte-specific tyrosine kinase fails to phosphorylate nitrated cdc2(6-20)NH_2 peptide. *Proc. Natl. Acad. Sci. USA* **93,** 3377–3382.
73. Martin, B. L., Wu, D., Jakes, S., and Graves, D. J. (1990) Chemical influences on the specificity of tyrosine phosphorylation. *J. Biol. Chem.* **265,** 7108–7111.
74. Ara, J., Przedborski, S., Naini, A. B., Jackson-Lewis, V., Trifiletti, R. R., Horwitz, J., and Ischiropoulos, H. (1998) Inactivation of tyrosine hydroxylase by nitration following exposure to peroxynitrite and 1-methyl-4-phenyl-1,2,3,6-tetrahydropyridine (MPTP). *Proc. Natl. Acad. Sci. USA* **95,** 7659–7663.

75. Crow, J. P. and Ischiropoulos, H. (1996) Detection and quantification of nitrotyrosine residues in proteins: In vivo marker of peroxynitrite. *Methods Enzymol.* **269,** 185–194.
76. Crow, J. P. (1999) Measurement and significance of free and protein-bound 3-nitrotyrosine, 3-chlorotyrosine, and free 3-nitro-4-hydroxyphenylacetic acid in biologic samples: a high-performance liquid chromatography method using electrochemical detection. *Methods Enzymol.* **301,** 151–160.
77. Kettle, A. J. (1999) Detection of 3-chlorotyrosine in proteins exposed to neutrophil oxidants. *Methods Enzymol.* **300,** 111–120.
78. Kaur, H., Lyras, L., Jenner, P., and Halliwell, B. (1998) Artefacts in HPLC detection of 3-nitrotyrosine in human brain tissue. *J. Neurochem.* **70,** 2220–2223.
79. Leeuwenburgh, C., Hardy, M. M., Hazen, S. L., Wagner, P., Oh-ishi, S., Steinbrecher, U. P., and Heinecke, J. W. (1997) Reactive nitrogen intermediates promote low density lipoprotein oxidation in human atherosclerotic intima. *J. Biol. Chem.* **272,** 1433–1436.
80. Leeuwenburgh, C., Rasmussen, J. E., Hsu, F. F., Mueller, D. M., Pennathur, S., and Heinecke, J. W. (1997) Mass spectrometric quantification of markers for protein oxidation by tyrosyl radical, copper, and hydroxyl radical in low density lipoprotein isolated from human atherosclerotic plaques. *J. Biol. Chem.* **272,** 3520–3526.
81. Pennathur, S., Jackson-Lewis, V., Przedborski, S., and Heinecke, J. W. (1999) Mass spectrometric quantification of 3-nitrotyrosine, ortho-tyrosine, and o,o'-dityrosine in brain tissue of l-methyl-4-phenyl-1,2,3, 6- tetrahydropyridine-treated mice, a model of oxidative stress in Parkinson's disease. *J. Biol. Chem.* **274,** 34,621–34,628.
82. Heinecke, J. W., Hsu, F. F., Crowley, J. R., Hazen, S. L., Leeuwenburgh, C., Mueller, D. M., Rasmussen, J. E., and Turk, J. (1999) Detecting oxidative modification of biomolecules with isotope dilution mass spectrometry: sensitive and quantitative assays for oxidized amino acids in proteins and tissues. *Methods Enzymol.* **300,** 124–144.
83. Beal, M. F., Ferrante, R. J., Browne, S. E., Matthews, R. T., Kowall, N. W., and Brown, R. H., Jr. (1997) Increased 3-nitrotyrosine in both sporadic and familial amyotrophic lateral sclerosis. *Ann. Neurol.* **42,** 644–654.
84. McMillan-Crow, L. A., Crow, J. P., Kerby, J. D., Beckman, J. S., and Thompson, J. (1996) Nitration and inactivation of manganese superoxide dismutase in chronic rejection of human renal allografts. *Proc. Natl. Acad. Sci. USA* **93,** 11,853–11,858.
85. Beckman, J. S., Ye, Y. Z., Anderson, P. G., Chen, J., Accavitti, M. A., Tarpey, M. M., and White, C. R. (1994) Extensive nitration of protein tyrosines in human atherosclerosis detected by immunohistochemistry. *Biol. Chem. Hoppe Seyler* **375,** 81–88.
86. Ye, Y. Z., Strong, M., Huang, Z.-Q., and Beckman, J. S. (1996) Antibodies that recognize nitrotyrosine, in Nitric Oxide. Physiological and Pathological Processes (Packer, L., ed.), Acedemic Press, New York, pp. 201–209.
87. Reches, A., Wagner, H. R., Jiang, D., Jackson, V., and Fahn, S. (1982) The effect of chronic L-DOPA administration on supersensitive pre- and postsynaptic dopaminergic receptors in rat brain. *Life Sci.* **31,** 37–44.

10

Oxidative Stress Indices in Parkinson's Disease

Biochemical Determination

Moussa B. H. Youdim, Noam Drigues, and Silvia Mandel

1. Introduction

Parkinson's disease (PD) is associated with progressive degeneration of melanin-containing dopamine neuron cell bodies arising in the substantia nigra pars compacta (SNpc) and projecting terminals to the striatum. The disease is best characterized biochemically as a deficiency of striatal dopamine. The mechanism of neurodegeneration remains an enigma despite a large body of investigation and several hypotheses ***(1–5)***. In the past decade much has been learned about the chemical pathology of the disease. This progress has been helped by elucidation of the mechanism of the neurotoxic actions of 6-hydroxydopamine (6-OHDA) and *N*-methyl-4-phenyl-1,2,3,6-tetrahydropyridine (MPTP), which are used to induce animal models of this disease. Thus, the most valid current hypothesis concerning the pathogenesis of idiopathic PD is progressive oxidative stress (OS), which can generate excessive reactive oxygen species (ROS) selectively in the SNpc ***(1–9)***, and subsequent biochemical abnormalities (**Table 1**). In addition, the ROS scavenging system may also diminish, which would exaggerate the condition leading to accumulation of ROS. In PD, it is thought that both these events occur; **Table 1** gives a summary of the biochemical changes identified to date in the SNpc of PD patients. Iron, monoamine oxidase B (MAO-B), copper/zinc superoxide dismutase (Cu/Zn-SOD), and heme oxygenase (radical producing) are increased; reduced glutathione (GSH) and vitamin C (radical scavenging) are decreased. Whether OS is a primary or secondary event in PD has not been established, but when it does occur, OS can lead to a cascade of events resulting in the demise of the nigrostriatal dopaminergic neurons. One approach toward protection of such neurons is the use of radical scavengers or iron chelators as neuroprotective drugs ***(10)***.

From: *Methods in Molecular Medicine, vol. 62: Parkinson's Disease: Methods and Protocols*
Edited by: M. M. Mouradian © Humana Press Inc., Totowa, NJ

Table 1
Biochemical Alterations in Substantia Nigra of Parkinson's Disease Indicating Oxidative Stress

Elevated	Decreased
Iron (in microglia, astrocytes, oligodendrocytes, and melanized dopamine neurons and mitochondria)	GSH (GSSG unchanged); GSH/GSSG ratio decreased
Ferritin	Mitochondrial complex I
Mitochondrial monoamine oxidase B	Calcium binding protein (calbindin 28)
Lipofuscin	Transferrin and transferrin receptor
Ubiquitin	Vitamins E and C
Cu/Zn-superoxide dismutase	Copper
Cytotoxic cytokines (TNF-α, IL-1, IL-6)	
Inflammatory transcription factor NFκB	
Heme oxygenase-1	
Ratio of oxidized to reduced glutathione (GSSG/GSH)	
Nitric oxide	
Neuromelanin	

1.1. Iron and Parkinson's Disease

A significant increase of iron is observed in the SNpc of PD patients. This metal appears in reactive microglia, oligodendrocytes, astrocytes, and melanin-containing dopamine neurons, where it is bound to melanin (for review, *see* **ref. *11***). Whether the increased iron observed in the SNpc of parkinsonian brains as well as in the MPTP and 6-OHDA models has a primary or secondary role in the neurodegenerative process is not known. Nevertheless, reactive, free, and chelatable tissue iron has a major role in the production of the reactive hydroxyl radical, which can result in OS ***(12)***. This transitional-redox metal can be responsible for the initiation of membrane lipid peroxidation as a consequence of its interaction with available hydrogen peroxide by Fenton chemistry ***(12)***. Intranigral ***(13,14)***, but not intraventricular ***(15)***, injection of iron produces a relatively selective lesion of nigrostriatal dopamine neurons associated with motor deficit and chemical parkinsonism in rats. The biochemical events that may lead to this toxicity could be related to the well-established cytotoxic properties of iron. In the rodent models induced by iron, MPTP, and 6-OHDA, neuroprotection can be achieved by iron chelators (e.g., desferrioxamine), vitamin E, and lipoic acid ***(16–18)***. Indeed, activation of macrophages in the periphery has been directly linked to an iron-induced inflammatory process and gene regulation of nuclear factor κappa B (NFκB), interleukin (IL)-1β, IL-6, and tumor necrosis factor-α (TNF-α), an effect that is prevented by the prototype iron chelator desferrioxamine ***(19–22)***. Thus, the observed elevation of iron in the activated microglia and dopamine neurons of parkinsonian SNpc can act in concert to initiate OS via promotion of ROS such as superoxide, hydroxyl radical, and nitric oxide and activate the inflammatory transcription factor NFκB ***(23)***.

Much of what has been learnt about nigrostriatal dopaminergic neurodegeneration has come from studies of the mechanism of the neurotoxic actions of 6-OHDA and MPTP. 6-OHDA is a highly reactive substance that is readily auto-oxidized and oxidatively deaminated by MAO to give rise to hydrogen peroxide and ROS ***(24)***. Substantial evidence indicates that this neurotoxin exerts its neurodegenerative action via OS ***(25–27)*** and by being one of the most potent mitochondrial complex I inhibitors ***(25)***. The possibility that an endogenous substance similar to 6-OHDA or some other neurotoxin may be formed in the brain and be involved in the neurodegenerative process has been hypothesized on many occasions ***(28)***. More recently, a number of in vitro studies have clearly shown that dopamine in the presence of sufficient amounts of iron and hydrogen peroxide can be converted to 6-OHDA and 5-OHDA ***(29,30)***. Thus the excessive iron that accumulates in the SNpc of PD brains ***(5)***, together with the presence of dopamine and the absence of sufficient GSH, could act as an endogenous promoter of neurotoxicity and can theoretically give rise to 6-OHDA in the brain ***(28)***.

The identification of MPTP ***(31)***, its neurodegenerative-parkinsonian property in humans as well as in non-human primates ***(32)***, and the ability of the MAO-B inhibitor l-deprenyl (l-selegiline) to prevent its neurodegenerative action ***(33,34)***, strengthened this notion. However, MPTP is a synthetic man-made substance, and to date no such toxin has been identified in the environment or in brain. MPTP exerts dopaminergic neurotoxicity via its conversion to the reactive metabolite 1-methyl-4-phenylpyridine (MPP^+) by the enzyme MAO-B. MPP^+ initiates neurodegeneration via OS, sustained release and oxidation of dopamine, increased iron, generation of ROS, depletion of GSH, lipid peroxidation, and inhibition of mitochondrial complex I ***(35–39)***. However, the mitochondrial complex I inhibitory (Ki = 10 mM) ***(38)*** activity of MPP^+ is far less than that of 6-OHDA (Ki = 1.3 μM) ***(25)***. Furthermore, these neurotoxins induce an inflammatory process, which results in proliferation of reactive microglia, similar to what has been observed in PD ***(40)***.

The reactive microglia in the SNpc of PD are positive for HLA-DR ***(41,42)***. It is thought that the reactive microglia are responsible for induction of inflammatory damage resulting from their ability to generate substantial amounts of ROS ***(43)***. A similar inflammatory process is also seen in PD brains where several-fold increases in inflammatory cytotoxic cytokines (IL-1β, IL-2, IL-6, and TNF-α) are observed ***(43–47)***. 6-OHDA shares many of the biochemical events occurring in MPTP neurotoxicity and in idiopathic PD (**Table 1**). These include its ability to generate ROS and deplete GSH ***(24)***, release iron from ferritin in vitro and in SNpc of rats, mice, and monkeys ***(48–51)***, and, unlike MPTP, deplete mitochondrial adenosine triphosphate (ATP) ***(25,38,39)***.

Several studies have shown a selective and progressive increase in iron ***(1–6)*** with a concomitant loss of GSH content in the parkinsonian SNpc with advancing disease ***(5,6)***. Indeed, a link between cellular "iron overload" and depletion of GSH exists in other diseases (e.g., lung toxicity by paraquat, nephrotoxicity, cholestatic liver disease, Alzheimer's disease, ischemic heart and brain diseases) in which OS is reported to occur ***(52)***. Tissue GSH, a cofactor of glutathione peroxidase, is essential and responsible for the removal of hydrogen peroxide. In systemic organs, excess hydrogen peroxide is removed by mitochondrial catalase, peroxidase, and glutathione peroxidase. In the brain, on the other hand, the only major enzyme responsible for removal and disposition of hydrogen peroxide is glutathione peroxidase. In the presence of free tissue iron or low-molecular-weight iron complex (e.g., ATP-iron complex or iron citrate) and the absence of GSH, the highly reactive hydroxyl radical may be formed by the classical Fenton reaction from accumulated hydrogen peroxide, leading to lipid peroxidation ***(12)***. Thus, if hydrogen peroxide is overproduced and inadequately cleared in PD, OS may result. Indeed, our own extensive studies, supported by those from other laboratories on the biochemistry of the SN in PD, are compatible with neurochemical changes associated with OS ***(1–11)***, specifically in the pars compacta.

A closer examination of the chemical pathology of parkinsonian SNpc reveals the similarity to the neurotoxic events observed in the 6-OHDA, MPTP, and iron models of PD. These include exaggerated increase of iron in the microglia and dopamine neurons of SNpc ***(11)***, leading to the reported increase in dopamine turnover, hydroxyl radical generation, lipid peroxidation, dopamine depletion, inhibition of mitochondrial complex I, and nigrostriatal dopamine neuron loss associated with significant motor dysfunction.

1.2. Indices of Oxidative Stress

The cell generates ROS continuously. Such species are normally produced as a defense mechanism by the cell and are eventually scavenged. Under normal circumstances, a tight balance exists between their production and disposition. However, in certain diseases this balance is thought to shift in favor of ROS accumulation, leading to a state of OS, in which radicals attack the lipid bilayer of the cell membrane, resulting in lipid peroxidation. In addition, oxidation of proteins to carbonylated byproducts, oxidation of DNA, and depletion of cellular GSH occur. In the brain, hydrogen peroxide is disposed of by glutathione peroxidase. In the presence of its rate-limiting-cofactor, GSH, glutathione peroxidase converts hydrogen peroxide to water and oxygen. In this reaction, GSH is oxidized to GSSG (oxidized glutathione). In many instances in which OS occurs, as is the case in PD, the tissue concentration of GSH falls, whereas that of GSSG remains relatively constant. The decreased ratio of GSH/GSSG has also been used as an index of OS. There are several high-performance liquid chromatography (HPLC) methods for measuring the GSH/GSSG ratio ***(53)***.

For the identification and estimation of oxidative stress, it is essential to measure lipid peroxidation, protein oxidation and/or glutathione. For an excellent review on the subject of lipid peroxidation, its mechanism, and the thiobarbituric acid (TBA) test see Gutteridge and Halliwell ***(12)***. In this chapter, we describe methods to quantify three indices of oxidative stress, namely malondialdehyde, protein carbonyl and glutathione.

1.2.1. Malondialdehyde Determination by HPLC

Malondialdehyde (MDA) is a byproduct of membrane lipid peroxidation, and its measurement has been used as an index of ROS liberation and subsequent damage. MDA is found in biologic tissues in its free form as well as covalently bound to other molecules such as proteins and nucleic acids. Membrane lipid peroxidation is thought to be responsible for the demise of the cell. MDA has been used as an index of cell toxicity in a variety of diseases such as cancer, aging, nephrotoxicity, cholestatic liver disease, lung toxicity, neurodegenerative diseases such as PD, Alzheimer's disease, and multiple sclerosis. Its scrutiny in PD has aroused much interest, and one report, although not confirmed, suggests increased lipid peroxidation in the SN of PD brains ***(54)***.

Several procedures for the determination of MDA levels in biologic samples exist; many are based on the color reaction of MDA with TBA, which was originally reported in 1944 by Kohn and Liversedge ***(55)***. This is the classic and most widely employed method for the determination of MDA in tissue homogenates. The rationale for the TBA test is based on the reaction of MDA with TBA to form a pink complex. A sample is mixed at low pH with TBA and heated to form a chromogen that absorbs light at 532–546 nm and is fluorescent at 553 nm.

The method is excellent due to its high sensitivity; however the major setback is its very low specificity. The concept of TBA-reactive substances (TBARS) refers to the various molecules that react with TBA and form adducts, in addition to the $(TBA)_2$-MDA adduct ***(56)***. Furthermore, when using tissue homogenates, there is a real chance that other pigments will absorb light at the same wavelength. A major portion of MDA measured with this procedure is considered to be generated during the initial stage of acid-heating reaction ***(57)***. A major step forward was achieved in 1983 when Bird et al. integrated HPLC into the assay *(58)*. Since then, several HPLC methods have been developed that have the ability to differentiate between MDA-TBA adduct and other TBARS (*59*; for review *see* **ref.** ***12***). However, some methods use the HPLC technology to measure MDA levels without reaction with TBA *(60,61)*. Although simpler than ours, these methods yield very low levels of MDA because they detect only the free form. The method we describe here, adapted from the publication of Chirico *(62)*, uses the reaction of MDA with TBA and measures MDA levels after HPLC separation.

Indeed, Gutteridge and Halliwell *(12)* have suggested in their excellent review that separation and identification of volatile derivatives by gas chromatography (GC) and mass spectrometry (MS), respectively, will give a more precise information about the chemical nature of the compounds in question. They strongly suggest that measurement of MDA adducts by HPLC or GC and MS should be the method of choice as an index of lipid peroxidation analysis.

1.2.2. Determination of Protein Carbonyl

ROS generated in a variety of biologic systems have been implicated in the mechanism of aging and age-associated pathologies such as artherosclerosis, Alzheimer's diseases, and PD. In a recent study conducted in different brain areas of postmortem parkinsonian brains, an increase in protein oxidation specifically in the SNpc was reported *(63)*. Nucleic acids, proteins, and membrane lipids constitute important targets for oxidative modification. Among the various oxidative modifications of amino acid residues, carbonyl formation may be an early marker of protein oxidation *(64)*. Exposure of proteins to reactive oxygen species leads to the introduction of carbonyl groups into protein side chains, specifically into lysine, arginine, proline, or threonine *(64–66)*, resulting in alteration of the protein structure. The carbonyl assay was developed as a general assay for oxidative protein damage. Usually, the carbonyl groups in the protein side chains are derivatized to 2,4-dinitrophenylhydrazone (DNP-hydrazone), by reacting with 2,4-dinitrophenylhydrazine (DNPH), and measured spectrophotometrically *(67,68)*. In brain tissue, carbonyl levels vary over a wide range depending on which methodology is used. Lyras and coworkers *(69)* compared several techniques for determination of brain carbonyls. The authors concluded that reacting DNPH reagent with soluble proteins, before precipitation with trichloroacetic acid, and determining the protein levels in the final suspension and not in the initial homogenate, give more accurate results *(69)*, compared with those described by Reznick and Packer *(68)*.

We describe here a method based on derivatization of protein carbonyls to DNP-hydrazone, except the protein samples are separated by polyacrylamide gel electrophoresis, followed by Western blotting *(70,71)*, and analyzed for carbonyl content by immunoassay with anti-DNP antibodies. This is followed by exposure to a peroxidase-conjugated second antibody directed against the first antibody. The membrane is then treated with chemiluminescence reagents (luminol and enhancer) and subsequently exposed to X-ray film.

One of the major advantages of this technique is the possibility of identifying specific proteins that have undergone carbonyl modifications by peptide sequencing analysis of bands of interest *(71)*. Another advantage is that, semiquantitative assessment of protein carbonyls is possible by densitometric quantification of the relevant bands, relative to known DNP-labeled standards *(63)*. In addition, this method requires much lower protein amounts (10–20 µg) and has very high sensitivity, allowing detection of fentomoles of carbonyl residues.

1.2.3. Reduced and Oxidized Glutathione Levels

GSH, its oxidized form GSSG, and particularly the GSH/GSSG ratio are important indices for the level of oxidative stress to which a tissue is subjected. Numerous methods for measuring GSH and GSSG levels in biologic tissues are available, but most have disadvantages such as low sensitivity, mainly to GSSG, and require separate assays for GSH and GSSG (reviewed in **ref.** *72*). The most commonly used procedures, those of Reed et al. *(53)* and Fahey and Newton *(72)* measure derivatives of GSH. The first uses dinitrophenyl derivatives, and its sensitivity is too low for small tissue samples such as brain regions. The second procedure, which is very sensitive, uses bimane adducts after two steps of derivatization. High-performance liquid chromatography (HPLC) methods partially solve some of the problems. The first method for measuring thiols using HPLC was published in 1977 by Rabenstein and Saetre *(73)* and was adapted by Mefford and Adams for brain tissue *(74)*. Assays that measure specifically using HPLC and electrochemical detection are abundant. Most of the assays use sodium phosphate buffer at a low pH as the mobile phase. However, the specifications of the guard and analytical cells differ from one method to the other, probably because of different homogenization media and different detectors.

GSH and GSSG concentrations in brain homogenates are measured by colorimetric detection and seperated by HPLC. The method we use is that of Blum-Degan et al. *(75)* and Krien et al. *(76)*.

2. Materials

2.1. Malondialdehyde Determination

1. Standard solution: As a standard, use a 1,1,3,3-tetraethoxypropane (TEP) solution. Dilute the solution with double-distilled water (DDW) to a concentration of 0.045 µ*M* to 0.45 m*M* and store at 4°C until use.
2. Butylated hydroxytoluene (BHT) 0.2% (w/v): BHT is added as an antioxidant to prevent the sample from being oxidized during the assay *(77)*. Dissolve 0.2 g of BHT in 100 mL of absolute ethanol.

3. H_3PO_4 0.44 *M*: dissolve 4.31 g in 100 mL DDW.
4. TBA 0.6% (w/v): 0.6 g in 100 mL DDW, heated to 60°C to dissolve.
5. Mobile phase: 65% 50 m*M* KH_2PO_4-KOH at a pH of 7.0 and 35% absolute methanol.
6. Methanol/water, 80:20, for washing.
7. Sucrose 0.3 *M*.
8. A Spherisorb 5ODS2 (C_{18}) column (4.6 × 150 mm) with a Reverse Phase S_{10} ODS2 Guard Cart guard cell (30 × 14.6 mm).
9. HPLC apparatus, e.g., Waters Millipore fitted with a detector set at 532 nm. Set the flow rate at 0.8 mL/min.
10. Teflon-glass homogenizer.

2.2. Carbonyl Proteins

1. Derivatization solution: 10 m*M* DNPH in 2 *N* HCl.
2. Neutralization solution: 10 *N* NaOH.
3. Transfer buffer, for 1 L: 12.5 m*M* Tris base (1.45 g), 95 m*M* glycine (7.20 g), 20% methanol (200 mL). Bring to 1 L with dH_2O.
4. 10X Tris buffered saline (TBS), for 1 L: 200 m*M* Tris base (24.22 g), 1.5 *M* NaCl (85g). Bring to 1 L with dH_2O.
5. 1X TBS-T, for 1 L: 100 mL of 10X TBS, 0.5 mL of Tween 20 (0.05% final). Bring to 1 L with dH_2O.
6. Blocking solution, for 1 L: 100 mL TBS-T, 1% bovine serum albumin (BSA) (10 g). Bring to 1 L with dH_2O.
7. First anti-DNP antibody: Rabbit anti-dinitrophenyl (DNP) antibody from DAKO (V 0401).
8. Second antibody: Peroxidase-conjugated goat anti-rabbit antibody from Jackson Immuno Research (cat. no. 111-035-003).
9. 2X Laemmli gel loading buffer, 10 mL: 0.5 *M* Tris-HCl buffer, pH 6.8 (2.5 mL), 10% SDS (4 mL), glycerol (2 mL), 0.2% bromophenol blue solution (20 mg), bring to 10 mL with dH_2O. The buffer can be aliquoted and kept at room temperature. Add β-mercaptoethanol to a final concentration of 10% only at the time of the assay.
10. Chemiluminescent reagents: SuperSignal Substrate, Western Blotting (Luminol/ Enhancer Solution, Stable Peroxide Solution) supplied by Pierce, or equivalent.
11. Membranes: Optitran (supported nitrocellulose; supplied by Shleicher & Schuell) or Hybond ECL (pure nitrocellulose), supplied by Amersham, or an equivalent.

2.3. Glutathiones

1. 5% Metaphosphoric acid with 500 μ*M* (19.67 mg in total 100 mL) bis(3-amino-ethyl)-amine-N,N,N',N'',N'''-pentaacetic acid-Ca,^{3}Na (DTPA).
2. Mobile phase: 2.5 m*M* $NaH_2PO_4 \cdot 7HO$ (670.1 mg in 1 L DDW). Set the pH at 3.0 using phosphoric acid.
3. GSH and GSSG standards: Prepare a stock solution in 150 m*M* H_3PO_4 and dilute the standard freshly each time glutathiones are to be analyzed.
4. Detector: we use a Coulochem 5100A (ESA, Inc.).

5. Analytical cell (cat. no. 5011, ESA) set at E1 = 0.6 V and E2 = 0.9 V.
6. Column: Nucleosil C18 reversed-phase column. Flow set at 1 mL/min.

3. Methods

3.1. Malondialdehyde Determination

1. Homogenize brain tissue with a Teflon-glass homogenizer in 0.3 M sucrose to a 10% w/v suspension. Then centrifuge this preparation at 600*g* for 20 min. Carefully decant the supernatant and centrifuge at 25,000*g* for 45 min (*see* **Note 1**). Resuspend the precipitate, which contains mitochondrial nerve endings and membranes, in 0.3 *M* sucrose. Set the protein concentration for the sample at about 10 µg/mL.
2. Take 100 µL of the sample or standard solution and mix with 10 µL of BHT (*see* **Note 2**). React 600 µL of 0.44 M H_3PO_4 with the mixture and incubate for 10 min at room temperature. Add 200 µL of TBA, mix, and incubate at 90°C water for 45 min. Cool the mixture in ice water (*see* **Notes 3** and **4**).
3. Prepare two blanks, one with no reagent and the second with no sample. The first one will be used to zero the equipment and the second as a comparison for the samples, which will be subtracted by its value.
4. Inject 50 µL of the sample to the column.
5. A peak of the MDA-TBA adduct is eluted at a retention time of 4.8 min. Using the standard solution, confirm the identity of the peak and quantify the level of MDA adducts in the sample (*see* **Note 5**).
6. After running each sample, wash the column for 30 min with methanol/water. Replace the guard cell after 60 determinations.

3.2. Carboyl Protein

3.2.1. Derivatization

1. Homogenize tissue in 0.32 *M* sucrose in 0.05 *M* phosphate buffer, pH 7.4, containing a mix of protease inhibitors. We use the Complete™ (Boehringer Mannheim) protease inhibitors mix. Transfer 10 µL of a protein sample containing 15–20 µg of protein into a 1.5-mL microtube. Design a second tube as negative control and add another 10 µL of protein sample.
2. Denature by adding 1.76 µL of 20% SDS solution to both tubes to a final concentration of 3%.
3. Derivatize the samples by adding 10 µL DNPH solution. To the tube serving as negative control, add 10 µL of 2 *N* HCl instead of DNPH solution.
4. Incubate at room temperature for 15 min. Do not allow the reaction to continue for more than 30 min since a nonspecific reaction of nonoxidized proteins might occur.
5. Neutralize by adding 2 µL 10 *N* NaOH to both tubes. Check pH. It should be approx 7.0–7.4. If needed, add another 1 µL of NaOH and check again.
6. Add 20 µL of gel loading buffer to each tube. The samples are ready to load into polyacrylamide gel. Heating is not required. Use protein molecular weight standards already containing DNP residues as internal control for the procedure.

3.2.2. Western Blot

1. Subject samples to SDS-polyacrylamide gel electrophoresis (PAGE) (12% gel) and electroblot to nitrocellulose membrane according to standard procedures *(78)*.
2. Transfer the membrane to a plastic container a little bigger in size than the membrane so it can move freely during shaking incubations. Block nonspecific sites by incubating the membrane in blocking solution for 1 h with gentle shaking. The membrane should be completely covered with the solution while being shaken. Use about 0.4 mL for each cm^2 of membrane (*see* **Note 6**).
3. Decant the blocking solution. Dilute first antibody stock to 1:1000 in blocking solution just before use and add the solution, immersing the membrane completely. Incubate while shaking for 1 h at room temperature or overnight at 4°C. For assessing specificity of the resulting bands, a parallel membrane containing the same samples will not be exposed to primary antibody. This will allow detection of nonspecific binding of the secondary antibody.
4. Rinse the membranes twice with TBST and perform four washes with TBST x 1, 5 min each.
5. Dilute secondary antibody stock to 1:5000 in blocking solution and incubate the membrane for 1 h at room temperature with gentle shaking.
6. Wash the membrane as described in **step 4**.
7. Drain excess TBST from the membrane and incubate the blot with Super Signal Substrate Working Solution prepared by mixing equal parts of Luminol/Enhancer Solution and Stable Peroxide Solution prior to use. Make sure that the solution covers the membrane. Shake for 1–3 min.
8. Drain off excess reagent by holding the membrane from one corner and touching the opposite edge against a piece of Whatman #3 filter paper.
9. Place the membrane, protein side up, on a sheet of plastic wrap and cover with a second layer of plastic. Remove any air pockets. If there are any, you may lift up the plastic sheet and lay it again on the membrane surface. Leave about 2 cm of plastic wrap around the membrane to avoid leakage of excess reagent.
10. Place the membrane, protein side up, in a film cassette and place an autoradiography film on top of the membrane in a darkroom equipped with a red safe light (*see* **Note 7**).
11. Expose initially for 30 s and develop. The exposure time can be varied to achieve an optimal blot. The attached DNP in the standard mix allows you to visualize the proteins and facilitates selection of exposure times to distinguish between carbonyl-positive and -negative proteins. Only lanes containing proteins that have undergone oxidative modification and were derivatized will be labeled; no signal will be observed in the negative control (*see* **Notes 8–10**).

3.3. Glutathiones

1. Dissect the tissues on ice and place immediately in liquid nitrogen. If the homogenization is on a different day, store them at –70°C (*see* **Note 11**).

2. Homogenize the tissue in 150 m*M* orthophosphoric acid with 500 μ*M* bis (3-amino-ethyl)-amine-N,N,N',N'',N'''-pentaacetic acid-Ca (DTPA). Use a ratio of 19 μL for each mg of tissue (*see* **Note 12**).
3. Centrifuge the homogenate at 4°C for 5 min at 12,000*g* and filter the supernatant through molecular weight filter (5 kDa).
4. Inject a 20-μL aliquot of the filtrate into the HPLC system. If dilution is needed, use water. We dilute the filtrate 1:10.
5. Identify the peaks of GSH and GSSG by comparing the sample chromatogram with one of commercial standards (*see* **Note 13**). Calibrate the GSH levels by using various concentrations of GSH and GSSG. Use 1–20 n*M* GSH and 0.125–5 n*M* GSSG (*see* **Note 14**).
6. The retention time for GSH and GSSG is 7 and 16 min, respectively (*see* **Note 15**).

4. Notes

1. It is highly recommended that duplicates be used after the sample supernatant is obtained.
2. Although BHT is used as an antioxidant, one cannot fully prevent the decomposition of preoxidized lipids during the procedure, and the concomitant release of MDA.
3. When reacting with TBA, the pH of the sample must be below 3.0 for bound MDA to be released and adducts to form ***(79)***. Do not fix the pH lower than 1.5 because it increases the likelihood of a false negative by inhibiting the development of the chromogen ***(80)***.
4. Most TBA tests using HPLC neutralize the sample prior to the loading step; however, higher pH causes the adduct to dissociate ***(80)***.
5. Since this method prevents pigments and other substances that react with TBA from affecting the assay, it is reasonable that its values are lower compared with those obtained using other colorimetric methods.
6. **Caution:** Do not use azide as a preservative for buffers with the immunoperoxidase system as it is an inhibitor of horseradish peroxidase.
7. **Caution:** The light emission is very intense, and any movement between the film and the membrane will cause artifacts on the film.
8. Weak or no signal:
    a. Insufficient amount of protein: Increase protein quantity.
    b. Poor transfer: Check orientation of the membrane and gel with respect to the electrodes. Increase transfer time and stain the gel after transfer with Gel Code, Blue Stain Reagent (Pierce, cat. no. 24590) to determine the optimal time required to transfer most of the proteins from the gel to the membrane. In parallel, stain the blotting membrane. Use prestained markers to check efficiency of transfer.
    c. Transfer efficiency could also be improved by omitting methanol from the transfer buffer.
    d. Insufficient quantities of antibodies: Increase antibody concentration or incubation times.

   e. Short exposure time to the chemiluminescent reagents: Increase exposure time.
9. Spots within the protein bands:
   a. Poor protein transfer (*see* **Note 8**).
   b. Unevenly hydrated membrane: After transfer, keep the membranes hydrated during the whole assay.
   c. Bubbles between the film and the membrane.
10. High background:
   a. Inadequate washing: Wash sufficiently, especially after the peroxidase conjugate step.
   b. Inadequate blocking: Increase blocking time; try other blocking solutions.
   c. Too high concentration of antigen or antibodies: Optimize conditions.
11. It is advised to sacrifice the animals and homogenize the tissues on the same day of the detection.
12. Owing to the instability of GSH and its tendency to be oxidized to GSSG when exposed to air, it is advisable to measure GSH levels as close as possible to the homogenization step.
13. For narrow peaks, 0.1–0.2% trifluoroacetic acid can be added. Water (50–100 mL/1 L buffer) may be added for better separation.
14. The efficiency of the colorimetric detector allows almost 100% of the analyte to be electrolyzed and detected by the electrode. In contrast, when using an amperometric mode, only 5% is electrolyzed, and a significant amount of the sample is lost. A major advantage of the colorimetric cell is the fact that it generates less background current by removing impurities from the mobile phase.
15. When assaying numerous samples, replace the buffer after about 30 detections.

Acknowledgment

We wish to thank the National Parkinson Foundation (Miami) for their support of this work.

References

1. Youdim, M. B. H., Ben-Shachar, D., and Riederer, P. (1993) The possible role of iron in the etiopathology of Parkinson's disease. *Mov. Disord.* **8,** 1–12.
2. Gotz, M. E., Kunig, G., Riederer, P. and Youdim, M. B. H. (1994) Oxidative stress: free radical production in neural degeneration. *Pharmacol. Therap.* **63,** 37–122.
3. Jenner, P. and Olanow, C. W. (1996) Oxidative stress and the pathogenesis of Parkinson's disease. *Neurol. Suppl.* **47,** 161–170.
4. Youdim, M. B. H. and Riederer, P. (1997) Understanding Parkinson's Disease. *Sci. Am.* **276,** 52–59.
5. Jenner, P. (1998) Oxidative mechanisms in nigral cell death in Parkinson's disease. *Mov. Disord. Suppl.* **13,** 24–34.

6. Riederer, P., Sofic, E., Rausch, W. D., Schmidt, B., Reynolds, G. P., Jellinger, K., and Youdim, M. B. H. (1989) Transition metals, ferritin, glutathione, and ascorbic acid in parkinsonian brains. *J. Neurochem.* **52,** 515–520.
7. Youdim, M. B. H., Ben-Shachar, D., Eshel, G., Finberg, J. P., and Riederer, P. (1993) The neurotoxicity of iron and nitric oxide. Relevance to the etiology of Parkinson's disease. *Adv. Neurol.* **60,** 259–266.
8. Gerlach, M., Ben-Shachar, D., Riederer, P., and Youdim, M. B. H. (1994) Altered brain iron as a cause of neurodegeneration? *J. Neurochem.* **63,** 793–807.
9. Olanow, C. W. and Youdim, M. B. H. (1996) Iron and neurodegeneration: prospects for neuroprotection, in *Neurodegeneration and Neuroprotection in Parkinson's Disease* (Olanow, C. W., Jenner, P., and Youdim, M. B. H., eds.), Academic Press, London, pp. 55–67.
10. Gassen, M. and Youdim, M. B. H. (1997) The potential role of iron chelators in the treatment of Parkinson's disease and related neurological disorders. *Pharmacol. Toxicol.* **80,** 159–166.
11. Jellinger, K. A. (1999) The role of iron in neurodegeneration: prospects for pharmacotherapy of Parkinson's disease. *Drug Aging* **14,** 115–140.
12. Gutteridge, J. M. and Halliwell B. (1990) The measurement and mechanism of lipid peroxidation in biological systems. *Trend. Biochem. Sci.* **15,** 129–135.
13. Ben-Shachar, D. and Youdim, M. B. H. (1991) Intranigral iron injection induces behavioral and biochemical "parkinsonism" in rats. *J. Neurochem.* **57,** 2133–2135.
14. Sengstock, G. J., Zawia, N. H., Olanow, C. W., Dunn, A. J., and Arendash, G. W. (1997) Intranigral iron infusion in the rat. Acute elevations in nigral lipid peroxidation and striatal dopaminergic markers with ensuing nigral degeneration. *Bio. Trace Elem. Res.* **58,** 177–195.
15. Ben-Shachar, D., Eshel, G., Riederer, P., and Youdim, M. B. H. (1992) Role of iron and iron chelation in dopaminergic-induced neurodegenaration: implication for Parkinson's disease. *Ann. Neurol. Suppl.* **32,** S105–S110.
16. Cadet, J. l., Katz, M., Jackson-Lewis, V. and Fahn. S. (1989) Vitamin E attenuates the toxic effects of intrastriatal injection of 6-hydroxydopamine (6-OHDA) in rats; Behavioral and biochemical evidence. *Brain Res.* **476,** 5–10
17. Ben-Shachar, D., Eshel, G., Finberg, J. P., and Youdim, M. B. H. (1991) The iron chelator desferrioxamine (Desferal) retards 6-hydroxydopamine induced generation of nigrostriatal dopamine. *J. Neurochem.* **56,** 1441–1444.
18. Biewenga, G. P., Haenen, R. G., and Bast, A. (1997) The pharmacology of the antioxidant lipoic acid. *Gen. Pharmacol.* **29,** 315–31.
19. Rosler, M., Retz, W., Thome, J., and Riederer, P. (1998) Free radicals in Alzheimer's dementia: currently available therapeutic strategies. *J. Neural. Transm. Suppl.* **54,** 211–219.
20. Sappey, C., Boelaert, J. R., Legrand-Poels, S., Forceille, C., Favier, A., and Piette, J. (1995) Iron chelation decreases NF-kB and HIV type 1 activation due to oxidative stress. *AIDS Res. Hum. Retroviruses* **11,** 1049–1061.
21. Lin, M., Rippe R. A., Niemela, O., Brittenham, G., and Tsukamoto, H. (1997) Role of iron in NF-kB activation and cytokine gene expression by rat hepatic macrophages. *Am. J. Physiol.* **272,** G1355–G1364.

22. Youdim, M. B. H., Grunblatt, E., and Mandel, S. (1999) The pivotal role of iron in NFkB activation, inflammatory processes and dopaminergic neurodegeneration: prospect for neuroprotection. *Ann. NY Acad. Sci.,* **890,** 7–25.
23. Youdim, M. B. H., Ben-Shachar, D., Yehuda, S., and Riederer, P. (1990) The role of iron in the basal ganglia. *Adv. Neurol.* **54,** 155–162.
24. Cohen, G. and Heikkila, R. E. (1974) The generation of hydrogen peroxide, superoxide radical and hydroxyl radical by 6-hydroxydopamine, dialuric acid, and related cytotoxic agents. *J. Biol. Chem.* **249,** 2447–2452.
25. Glinka, Y. Y. and Youdim, M. B. H. (1995) Inhibition of mitochondrial complexes I and IV by 6-hydroxydopamine. *Eur. J. Pharmacol.* **292,** 329–332.
26. Glinka, Y., Tipton, K. F., and Youdim, M. B. H. (1996) Nature of inhibition of mitochondrial respiratory complex I by 6-hydroxydopamine. *J. Neurochem.* **66,** 2004–2010.
27. Glinka, Y., Gassen, M., and Youdim, M. B. H. (1997) Mechanism of 6-hydroxydopamine neurotoxicity. *J. Neural Transm. Suppl.* **50,** 55–66.
28. Kostrzewa, R. M. and Jacobowitz, D. M. (1974) Pharmacological action of 6-hydroxydopamine. *Pharmacol. Rev.* **26,** 199–288.
29. Linert, W., Herlinger, E., Jameson, R. F., Kienzl, E., Jellinger, K., and Youdim, M. B. H. (1996) Dopamine, 6-hydroxydopamine, iron, and dioxygen-their mutual interactions and possible implication in the development of Parkinson's disease. *Biochem. Biophys. Acta.* **1316,** 160–168.
30. Napolitano, A., Pezzella, A., and Prota, G. (1999) New reaction pathways of dopamine under oxidative stress conditions: nonenzymatic iron-assisted conversion to norepinephrine and the neurotoxins 6-hydroxydopamine and 6,7-dihyhydroxytetrahydroisoquinoline. *Chem. Res. Toxicol.* **12,** 1090–1097.
31. Burns, R. S., Chiue, C. C., Markey, S. P., Ebert, M. H., Jacobowitz, D. M., and Kopin, I. J. (1983) A primate model for parkinsonism: selective destruction of dopaminergic neurons in the pars compacta of the substantia nigra by N-methyl-4-phenyl-1,2,3,6-tetrahydropyridine. *Proc. Natl. Acad. Sci. USA* **80,** 4546–4550.
32. Langston, J. W., Langston, E. B., and Irwin, I. (1984) MPTP-induced parkinsonism in human and non-human primates-clinical and experimental aspects. *Acta Neurolog. Scand. Suppl.* **100,** 49–54.
33. Heikkila, R. E., Manzino, L., Cabbat, F. S., and Duvoisin, R. C. (1984) Protection against the dopaminergic neurotoxicity of 1-methyl-4-phenyl-1,2,5,6-tetrahydropyridine by monoamine oxidase inhibitors. *Nature* **311,** 467–469.
34. Gupta, M. and Wiener, H. L. (1995) Effects of deprenyl on monoamine oxidase and neurotransmitters in the brains of MPTP-treated aging mice. *Neurochem. Res.* **20,** 385–389.
35. Seaton, T. A., Cooper, J. M., and Schapira, A. H. V. (1997) Free radical scavengers protect dopaminergic cell lines from apoptosis induced by complex I inhibitors. *Brain Res.* **777,** 110–118.
36. Chiueh, C. C., Krishna, G., Tulsi, P., Obata, T., Lang, K., Huang, S. J., and Murphy, D. L. (1992) Intracranial microdialysis of salicylic acid to detect hydroxyl radical generation through dopamine autooxidation in the caudate nucleus: Effects of MPP+. *Free Radic. Biol. Med.* **13,** 581–583.

37. Chiueh, C. C., Huang, S. J., and Murphy, D. L. (1992) Enhanced hydroxyl radical generation by 2'-methyl analog of MPTP: reversal by clorgyline and deprenyl. *Synapse* **11,** 346–348.
38. Smith, T. S. and Bennett, J. P., Jr. (1997) Mitochondrial toxins in models of neurodegenerative diseases. I: In vivo brain hydroxyl radicals production during systemic MPTP treatment or following microdialysis infusion of methylpyridinium or azide ions. *Brain Res.* **765,** 183–188.
39. Singer, T. P., Castagnoli, N. Jr., Ramsay, R. R., and Treor, A. J. (1987) Biochemical events in the development of parkinsonism induced by 1-methyl-4-phenyl-1,2,3,6-tetrahydropyridine. *J. Neurochem.* **49,** 1–8.
40. McGeer, E. G. and McGeer, P. L. (1994) Neurodegeneration and the immune system, in *Neurodegenerative Diseases* (Calne, D. B., ed.), Saunders, Phiadelphia, pp. 277–299.
41. Jellinger, K., Paulus, W., Grundke-Iqbal, I., Riederer, P., and Youdim, M. B. H. (1990) Brain iron and ferritin in Parkinson's and Alzheimer's diseases. *J. Neural Transm. Park. Dis. Dement. Sect.* **2,** 327–340.
42. Jellinger, K., Kienzel, E., Rumpelmair, G., Riederer, P., Stachelberger, H., Ben-Shachar, D., and Youdim M. B. H. (1992) Iron-melanin complex in substantia nigra of parkinsonian brains: an e-ray microanalysis. *J. Neurochem.* **59,** 1168–1171.
43. Riederer, P., Janetzky, B., Gerlach, M., Reichmann, H., Mandel, S. and Youdim, M. B. H. (1999) Parkinson's disease, iron, mitochondria, inflammatory responses, and oxidative stress: prospects for neuroprotection. *Neurosci. News* **2,** 83–87.
44. Mogi, M., Harada, M., Riederer, P., Narabayashi, H., Fujita, K., and Nagatsu, T. (1994) Tumor necrosis factor-α (TNF-α) increases both in the brain and in the cerebrospinal fluid from parkinsonian patients. *Neurosci. Lett.* **165,** 208–210.
45. Mogi, M., Harada, M., Narabayashi, H., Inagaki, H., Minami, M., and Nagatsu, T. (1996) Interleukin (IL)-1β, IL-2, IL-4, IL-6 and transforming growth factor-α levels in ventricular cerebrospinal fluid in juvenile parkinsonian and Parkinson's disease. *Neurosci. Lett.* **211,** 13–16.
46. Blum-Degen, D., Muller, T., Kuhn, W., Gerlach, M., Przuntek, H., and Riederer, P. (1995) Interleukin-1β and interleukin-6 are elevated in the cerebrospinal fluid of Alzheimer's and de novo Parkinson's disease patients. *Neurosci. Lett.* **202,** 17–20.
47. Hirsch, E. C. Hunot, S., Damier, P., and Faucheux, B. (1998) Glial cells and inflammation in Parkinson's disease: a role in neurodegeneration? *Ann. Neurol.* **44 (suppl 1),** S115–S120.
48. Lode, H. N., Bruchelt, G., Rieth, A. G., and Niethammer, D. (1990) Release of iron from ferritin by 6-hydroxydopamine under anaerobic conditions. *Free Rad. Res. Commun.* **11,** 153–158.
49. Oestreicher, E., Sengstock, G. J., Riederer, P., Olanow, C. W., Dunn, A. J., and Arendash, G. W. (1994) Degeneration of nigrostriatal dopaminergic neurons increases iron within the substantia nigra: a histochemical and neurochemical study. *Brain Res.* **660,** 8–18.
50. Mochizuki, H., Imai, H., Endo, K., Yokomizo, K., Murata, Y., Hattori, N., and Mizuno, Y. (1994) Iron accumulation in the substantia nigra of 1-methyl-4-phenyl-1,2,3,6-tetrahydropyridine (MPTP) induced hemiparkinsonism in monkeys. *Neurosci. Lett.* **168,** 251–253.

51. Temlett, J. A., Landsberg, J. P., Watt, F., and Grime, G. W. (1994) Increased iron in the substantia nigra compacta of the MPTP-lesioned hemiparkinsonian african green monkey: evidence from proton microprobe element microanalysis. *J. Neurochem.* **62,** 134–146.
52. Han, J., Cheng, F. C., Yang, Z., and Dryhurst, G. (1999) Inhibitors of mitochondrial respiration, iron (II), and hydroxyl radical evoke release and extracellular hydrolysis of glutathione in rat striatum and substantia nigra: potential implications to Parkinson's disease. *J. Neurochem.* **73,** 1683–1685.
53. Reed, D. J., Babson, J. R., Beatty, P. W., Brodie, A. E., Ellis, W. W., and Potter, D. W. (1980) High-performance liquid chromatography analysis of nanomoles levels of glutathione, glutathione disulfide, and related thiols and disulfides. *Anal. Biochem.* **106,** 55–62.
54. Dexter, D. T., Carter, C. J., Wells, F. R., Javoy-Agid, F., Agid, Y., Lees, A., Jenner, P., and Marsden, C. D. (1989) Basal lipid peroxidation in substantia nigra is increased in Parkinson's disease. *J. Neurochem.* **52,** 381–389.
55. Kohn, H. I. and Liversedge, M. (1944) *J. Pharmacol. Exp. Ther.* **83,** 292.
56. Kosugi, H., Kato, T., and Kikugawa, K. (1987) Formation of yellow, orange and red in the reaction of alk-2-enals with 2-thiobarbituric acid. *Anal. Biochem.* **165,** 456–464.
57. Gutteridge, J. M. C. (1986) Aspects to consider when detecting and measuring lipid peroxidation. *Free Rad. Res. Commun.* **1,** 173–184.
58. Bird, R. P., Hung, S. S. O., Hadley, M., and Draper, H. H. (1983) Determination of malonaldehyde in biological materials by high-pressure liquid chromatography. *Anal. Biochem.* **128,** 240–244.
59. Draper, H. H. and Hadley, M. (1990) Malondialdehyde determination as index of lipid peroxidation. *Methods Enzymol.* **186,** 421–431.
60. Esterbauer, H., Lang, J., Zadranec, S., and Slater, T. F. (1984) Detection of malonaldehyde by high-performance liquid chromatography. *Methods Enzymol.* **105,** 319–328.
61. Largilliere, C. and Melancon, S. B. (1988) Free malondialdehyde determination in human plasma by high-performance liquid chromatography. *Anal. Biochem.* **170,** 123–126.
62. Chirico, S. (1994) High-performance liquid chromatography-based thiobarbituric acid tests. *Methods Enzymol.* **233,** 314–318.
63. Floor, E. and Wetzel, M. G. (1998) Increased protein oxidation in human substantia nigra pars compacta in comparison with basal ganglia and prefrontal cortex measured with an improved dinitrophenylhydrazine assay. *J. Neurochem.* **70,** 268–275.
64. Davies, K. J. A., Delsignore, M. E., and Lin, S. W. (1987) Protein damage and degradation of oxygen radicals II: modification of amino acids. *J. Biol. Chem.* **262,** 9902–9907.
65. Levine, R. L. (1983) Oxidative modification of glutamine synthetase I. Interaction is due to loss of one histidine residue. *J. Biol. Chem.* **258,** 11.823–11.827.
66. Stadtman, E. R. (1993) Oxidation of free amino acids and amino acid residues in proteins by radiolysis and by metal-catalyzed reactions. *Ann. Rev. Biochem.* **62,** 797–821.
67. Levine, R. L., Garland, D., Oliver, C. N., Amici, A., Climent, I., Lenz, A. G., Ahn, B. W., Shaltiel, S., and Stadtman, E. R. (1990) Determination of carbonyl content in oxidatively modified proteins. *Methods Enzymol.* **186,** 464–478.

68. Reznick, A. Z. and Packer, L. (1994) Oxidative damage to proteins: spectrophotometric method for carbonyl assay. *Methods Enzymol.* **233,** 357–363.
69. Lyras, L., Evans, P. J., Shaw, P. J., Ince, P. G., and Halliwell, B. (1996) Oxidative damage and motor neuron disease difficulties in the measurement of protein carbonyls in human brain tissue. *Free Rad. Res.* **24,** 397–406.
70. Nakamura, A. and Goto, S. (1996) Analysis of proteins carbonyls with 2,4-dinitrophenylhydrazine and its antibodies by immunoblot in two-dimentional gel electrophoresis. *J. Biochem.* **119,** 768–774.
71. Tamarit, J., Cabiscol, E., and Ros, J. (1998) Identification of the major oxidatively damaged proteins in Escherichia Coli cells exposed to oxidative stress. *J. Biol. Chem.* **273,** 3027–3032.
72. Fahey, R. C. and Newton, G. L. (1987) Determination of low-molecular-weight using monobromobimane fluorescent labeling and high-performance liquid chromatography. *Methods Enzymol.* **143,** 85–96.
73. Rabenstein, D. L. and Saetre, R. (1977) Mercury-based electrochemical detector of liquid chromatography for the detection of glutathione and other sulfur-containing compounds. *Anal. Chem.* **49,** 1036–1039.
74. Mefford, I. and Adams, R. N. (1978) Determination of reduced glutathione in guinea pig and rat tissue by HPLC with electrochemical detection. *Life Sci.* **23,** 1167–1173.
75. Blum-Degen, D., Haas, M., Pohli, S., Harth, R., Romer, W., Oettel, M., Riederer, P., and Gotz, M. E. (1998) Scavengers protect IMR 32 cells from oxidative stress-induced cell death. *Toxicol. Appl. Pharm.* **152,** 49–55.
76. Krien, P. M., Margou, V., and Kermici, M. (1992) Electrochemical determination of femtomole amounts of free reduced and oxidized glutathione. *J. Chromatog.* **576,** 255–261.
77. Pikul, J., Leszczynski, D. E. and Kummerow, F. A. (1983) *J. Agric. Food Chem.* **31,** 1338.
78. Towbin, H., Staehelin, T., and Gordon, J. (1979) Electrophoretic transfer of proteins from polyacrylamide gels to nitrocellulose sheets: Procedure and some applications. *Proc. Natl. Acad. Sci. USA* **76,** 4350–4354.
79. Sinnhuber, R. O., Yu, I. C., and Yu, T. C. (1958) *Food Res.* **23,** 620.
80. Rice-Evans, C. A., Diplock, A. T., and Symons, M. C. R. (1991) *Techniques in Free Radical Research*, Elsevier, Amsterdam.

III

Molecular Aspects of Basal Ganglia Function

11

Quantification of Tyrosine Hydroxylase mRNA

Hiroshi Ichinose, Tamae Ohye, Takahiro Suzuki, Hidehito Inagaki, and Toshiharu Nagatsu

1. Introduction

The main biochemical characteristic of Parkinson's disease (PD) is reduction of the neurotransmitter dopamine and the dopamine-synthesizing enzyme system, including tyrosine hydroxylase (TH, tyrosine 3-monooxygenase, EC 1.14.16.2) and tetrahydrobiopterin (BH_4) co-factor, in nigrostriatal neurons *(1)*. The deficiency in dopamine-synthesizing enzymes is accompanied by cell loss, which is thought to be caused by unknown exogenous environmental factors as well as endogenous genetic factors.

1.1. Tyrosine Hydroxylase

In PD, the decrease in mRNA, protein, and activity of tyrosine hydroxylase (TH) are found specifically in the nigrostriatal dopaminergic regions. TH catalyzes the first step in the biosynthesis of catecholamine neurotransmitters, namely, the formation of L-3,4-dihydroxyphenylalanine (DOPA) from tyrosine *(2,3)*. TH is an iron-containing, tetrahydropterin-requiring monooxygenase. (6*R*)-L-*erythro*-5,6,7,8-tetrahydrobiopterin (BH_4) is the natural cofactor of tetrahydropterin-requiring monooxygenases *(4,5)*. TH is a homotetrameric protein of approximately 240 kDa, consisting of 60-kDa subunits. The catalytic domain is localized in its C-terminal region, and the regulatory domain is localized in the N-terminal region. Phosphorylation of serine residues at the regulatory domain activates TH *(2)*.

1.2. Human TH mRNAs

Four isoforms of TH mRNA are found in humans: type 1 (hTH1), type 2 (hTH2), type 3 (hTH3), and type 4 (hTH4) *(6–11)* (**Fig. 1**, **Table 1**). These

From: *Methods in Molecular Medicine, vol. 62: Parkinson's Disease: Methods and Protocols*
Edited by: M. M. Mouradian © Humana Press Inc., Totowa, NJ

```
                                                                                                   -1
                                                                                             ACTGAGCC
                                      60                                                          120
ATGCCCACCCCCGACGCCACCACGCCACAGGCCAAGGGCTTCCGCAGGGCCGTGTCTGAGCTGGACGCCAAGCAGGCAGAGGCCATCATGGTAAGAGGGCAGGGCGCCCCGGGGCCCAGC
 M  P  T  P  D  A  T  T  P  Q  A  K  G  F  R  R  A  V  S  E  L  D  A  K  Q  A  E  A  I  M  V  R  G  Q  G  A  P  G  P  S
                                     180                                                          240
CTCACAGGCTCTCCGTGGCCTGGAACTGCAGCCCCAGCTGCATCCTACACCCCCACCCCAAGGTCCCCGCGGTTCATTGGGCGCAGGCAGAGCCTCATCGAGGACGCCCGCAAGGAGCGG
 L  T  G  S  P  W  P  G  T  A  A  P  A  A  S  Y  T  P  T  P  R  S  P  R  F  I  G  R  R  Q  S  L  I  E  D  A  R  K  E  R
                                     300                                                          360
GAGGCGGCGGTGGCAGCAGCGGCCGCTGCAGTCCCCTCGGAGCCCGGGGACCCCCTGGAGGCTGTGGCCTTTGAGGAGAAGGAGGGGAAGGCCGTGCTAAACCTGCTCTTCTCCCCGAGG
 E  A  A  V  A  A  A  A  A  A  V  P  S  E  P  G  D  P  L  E  A  V  A  F  E  E  K  E  G  K  A  V  L  N  L  L  F  S  P  R
                                     420                                                          480
GCCACCAAGCCCTCGGCGCTGTCCCGAGCTGTGAAGGTGTTTGAGACGTTTGAAGCCAAAATCCACCATCTAGAGACCCGGCCCGCCCAGAGGCCGCGAGCTGGGGGCCCCCACCTGGAG
 A  T  K  P  S  A  L  S  R  A  V  K  V  F  E  T  F  E  A  K  I  H  H  L  E  T  R  P  A  Q  R  P  R  A  G  G  P  H  L  E
                                     540                                                          600
TACTTCGTGCGCCTCGAGGTGCGCCGAGGGGACCTGGCCGCCCTGCTCAGTGGTGTGCGCCAGGTGTCAGAGGACGTGCGCAGCCCCGCGGGGCCCAAGGTCCCCTGGTTCCCAAGAAAA
 Y  F  V  R  L  E  V  R  R  G  D  L  A  A  L  L  S  G  V  R  Q  V  S  E  D  V  R  S  P  A  G  P  K  V  P  W  F  P  R  K
                                     660                                                          720
GTGTCAGAGCTGGACAAGTGTCATCACCTGGTCACCAAGTTCGACCCTGACCTGGACTTGGACCACCCGGGCTTCTCGGACCAGGTGTACCGCCAGCGCAGGAAGCTGATTGCTGAGATC
 V  S  E  L  D  K  C  H  H  L  V  T  K  F  D  P  D  L  D  L  D  H  P  G  F  S  D  Q  V  Y  R  Q  R  R  K  L  I  A  E  I
                                     780                                                          840
GCCTTCCAGTACAGGCACGGCGACCCGATTCCCCGTGTGGAGTACACCGCCGAGGAGATTGCCACCTGGAAGGAGGTCTACACCACGCTGAAGGGCCTCTACGCCACGCACGCCTGCGGG
 A  F  Q  Y  R  H  G  D  P  I  P  R  V  E  Y  T  A  E  E  I  A  T  W  K  E  V  Y  T  T  L  K  G  L  Y  A  T  H  A  C  G
                                     900                                                          960
GAGCACCTGGAGGCCTTTGCTTTGCTGGAGCGCTTCAGCGGCTACCGGGAAGACAATATCCCCCAGCTGGAGGACGTCTCCCGCTTCCTGAAGGAGCGCACGGGCTTCCAGCTGCGGCCT
 E  H  L  E  A  F  A  L  L  E  R  F  S  G  Y  R  E  D  N  I  P  Q  L  E  D  V  S  R  F  L  K  E  R  T  G  F  Q  L  R  P
                                    1020                                                         1080
GTGGCCGGCCTGCTGTCCGCCCGGGACTTCCTGGCCAGCCTGGCCTTCCGCGTGTTCCAGTGCACCCAGTATATCCGCCACGCGTCCTCGCCCATGCACTCCCCTGAGCCGGACTGCTGC
 V  A  G  L  L  S  A  R  D  F  L  A  S  L  A  F  R  V  F  Q  C  T  Q  Y  I  R  H  A  S  S  P  M  H  S  P  E  P  D  C  C
                                    1140                                                         1200
CACGAGCTGCTGGGGCACGTGCCCATGCTGGCCGACCGCACCTTCGCGCAGTTCTCGCAGGACATTGGCCTGGCGTCCCTGGGGGCCTCGGATGAGGAAATTGAGAAGCTGTCCACGCTG
 H  E  L  L  G  H  V  P  M  L  A  D  R  T  F  A  Q  F  S  Q  D  I  G  L  A  S  L  G  A  S  D  E  E  I  E  K  L  S  T  L
                                    1260                                                         1320
TCATGGTTCACGGTGGAGTTCGGGCTGTGTAAGCAGAACGGGGAGGTGAAGGCCTATGGTGCCGGGCTGCTGTCCTCCTACGGGGAGCTCCTGCACTGCCTGTCTGAGGAGCCTGAGATT
 S  W  F  T  V  E  F  G  L  C  K  Q  N  G  E  V  K  A  Y  G  A  G  L  L  S  S  Y  G  E  L  L  H  C  L  S  E  E  P  E  I
                                    1380                                                         1440
CGGGCCTTCGACCCTGAGGCTGCGGCCGTGCAGCCCTACCAAGACCAGACGTACCAGTCAGTCTACTTCGTGTCTGAGAGCTTCAGTGACGCCAAGGACAAGCTCAGGAGCTATGCCTCA
 R  A  F  D  P  E  A  A  A  V  Q  P  Y  Q  D  Q  T  Y  Q  S  V  Y  F  V  S  E  S  F  S  D  A  K  D  K  L  R  S  Y  A  S
                                    1500                                                         1560
CGCATCCAGCGCCCCTTCTCCGTGAAGTTCGACCCGTACACGCTGGCCATCGACGTGCTGGACAGCCCCCAGGCCGTGCGGCGCTCCCTGGAGGGTGTCCAGGATGAGCTGGACACCCTT
 R  I  Q  R  P  F  S  V  K  F  D  P  Y  T  L  A  I  D  V  L  D  S  P  Q  A  V  R  R  S  L  E  G  V  Q  D  E  L  D  T  L
                                    1620                                                         1680
GCCCATGCGCTGAGTGCCATTGGCTAGGTGCACGGCGTCCCTGAGGGCCCTTCCCAACCTCCCCTGGTCCTGCACTGTCCCGGAGCTCAGGCCCTGGTGAGGGGCTGGGTCCCGGGTGCC
 A  H  A  L  S  A  I  G ***
                                    1740                                                         1800
CCCCATGCCCTCCCTGCTGCCAGGCTCCCACTGCCCCTGCACCTGCTTCTCAGCGCAACAGCTGTGTGTGCCCGTGGTGAGGTTGTGCTGCCTGTGGTGAGGTCCTGTCCTGGCTCCCAG
                                    1860
GGTCCTGGGGGCTGCTGCACTGCCCTCCGCCCTTCCCTGACACTGTCTGCTGCCCCAATCACCGTCACAATAAAAGAAACTGTGGTCTCT(A)n
```

Table 1
Characteristics of the Four Isoforms of Human Tyrosine Hydroxylase

Type	Base pairs of coding region	Amino acids	Molecular mass
1	1491	497	55,533
2	1503	501	55,973
3	1572	524	58,080
4	1584	528	58,521

different mRNAs are produced through alternative mRNA splicing from a single gene per haploid DNA (**Fig. 2**). Compared with type 1 TH mRNA, a 12-bp sequence is inserted in type 2, and an 81-bp sequence is inserted in type 3. Insertion of both the 12- and 81-bp segments, totaling 93 bp, results in type 4 TH mRNA.

Not only human TH but also monkey TH exists in multiple forms ***(12,13)***. Marmosets, macaques (*Macaca irus, Macaca fuscata*), gibbons, orangutans, gorillas and chimpanzees all produce type 1 and type 2 TH isoforms ***(13)***. Comparison among the genomic DNA sequences of various primates reveals that accumulated mutations have created a new exon, resulting in the two new TH isoforms (hTH3 and hTH4) in humans. In contrast to human and monkey TH, various nonprimate mammals such as rats ***(14)*** and mice ***(15)*** only have the type 1 isoform.

The human TH gene is composed of 14 exons interrupted by 13 introns, spanning about 8.5 kb ***(10)*** (**Fig. 2**). Type 4 TH has the entire nucleotide sequence of the coding region. The 12-bp insert in types 2 and 4 is derived from the 3'-terminal portion of exon 1, and the 81-bp insert in types 3 and 4 is encoded by exon 2. The N-terminal region is encoded by the 5'-portion of exon 1, and the remaining region from exon 3 to exon 14, is common to all four mRNA types. In human tissues, types 1 and 2 mRNAs are abundant; types 3 and 4 are expressed at low levels.

1.3. TH in Parkinson's Disease

In PD, reductions in TH mRNA, protein, and enzymatic activity in nigrostriatal regions are considered to be due to cell death of dopaminergic

---

Fig. 1. *(opposite page)* Nucleotide sequence and deduced amino acid sequence of type 4 human TH cDNA. Type 2 human TH cDNA lacks the 81-bp (27-amino acid) insert on the solid line, and type 3 lacks the 12-bp (4-amino acid) insert on the dotted line. Type 1 human TH cDNA lacks the 93-bp (31-amino acids) insert on both the solid and dotted lines. (Data from **refs. *6*** and ***8***.)

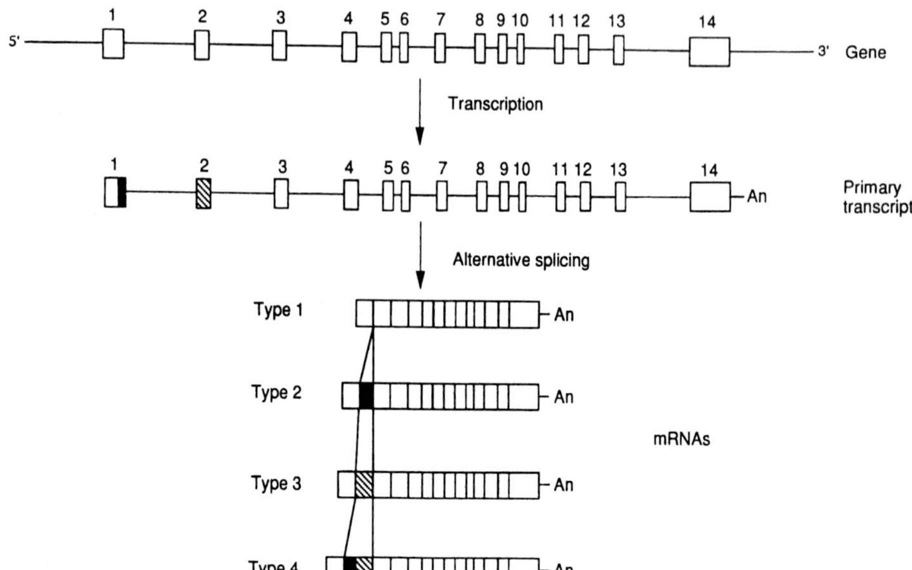

Fig. 2. Schematic diagram demonstrating regulation of the alternative splicing pathway generating four types of human TH mRNA from a single gene. The 3'-terminal portion of exon 1, which corresponds to the 12-bp insertion sequence, is indicated by a solid box. The hatched box shows exon 2, which encodes the 81-bp insertion sequence. (Data from **refs.** ***6*** and ***10***.)

neurons but may occur even before cell death. mRNA, protein, and activity of TH are decreased nearly in parallel. However, some compensatory mechanism to increase TH activity may occur. The level of TH protein is decreased more markedly than TH activity. Thus, the homospecific activity, i.e., activity per protein, is increased in the substantia nigra or striatum in PD ***(16)***. This is contrary to constant homospecific activity of TH in the striatum of parkinsonian mice produced by 1-methyl-4-phenyl-1,2,3,6-tetrahydropyridine (MPTP) ***(17,18)***. We have measured the four isoforms of human TH mRNA by a quantitative method using reverse transcription-polymerase chain reaction (RT-PCR) in the substantia nigra of control subjects and parkinsonian patients ***(19)***. Parkinsonian nigral tissues had very low levels of all four TH isoforms compared with those of control brains. We have also measured the levels of types 1 and 2 TH mRNA in the substantia nigra, locus coeruleus, and adrenal gland of normal (*Macaca fascicularis*) and MPTP-lesioned parkinsonian monkeys ***(20)***. In parkinsonian monkeys, marked decreases in TH mRNA types 1 and 2 were observed specifically in the substantia nigra, whereas modest decreases were found in the locus coeruleus and adrenal gland. Since multiple TH mRNAs are present only in humans and monkeys ***(21)***, MPTP-induced parkinsonism in monkeys is a better model of the human disease for TH studies than MPTP-induced parkinsonism in mice (*see* **Notes 1–5**).

2. Materials

2.1. Preparation of Total Cellular RNA

1. Diethyl pyrocarbonate (DEPC)-treated water: Dissolve 1 mL DEPC in 1 L distilled water. Shake, allow to stand for 2 h at room temperature (RT), and autoclave.
2. Phenol/chloroform (1/1).
3. GTC Solution : 4 *M* guanidium thiocyanate, 0.1 *M* Tris-HCl (pH 7.5), 0.5% sodium-*N*-lauroyl sarcosinate. Just before use, add 1% β-mercaptoethanol and 0.1% Antifoam A (Sigma).
4. CsCl solution: 5.7 *M* CsCl, 0.01 *M* EDTA.
5. 3 *M* sodium acetate solution (pH 5.2).
6. TES buffer: 10 m*M* Tris-HCl, 1 m*M* EDTA, pH 8.0, DEPC-treated water, 5% sodium-*N*-lauroyl sarcosinate. Just before use, add 5% Tris-HCl-saturated phenol.
7. Ethanol.
8. 70% ethanol.

2.2. Reverse Transcription

1. Ribonuclease inhibitor (Takara Shuzo, Japan).
2. 0.1 *M* dithiothreitol (DTT).
3. Moloney murine leukemia virus (MMLV) reverse transcriptase (RT; Bethesda Research Laboratories).
4. Random hexamer.
5. 1.25 m*M* dNTPs.
6. 10X transcription buffer: 0.1 m*M* Tris-HCl, pH 8.3, 15 m*M* $MgCl_2$, 0.1% gelatin.
7. 50 m*M* $MgCl_2$.
8. DEPC-treated water.

2.3. PCR

1. 10X amplification buffer: 0.1 m*M* Tris-HCl, pH 8.3, 15 m*M* $MgCl_2$, 0.1% gelatin.
2. 1.25 m*M* dNTPs.
3. Perfect match polymerase enhancer (Stratagene).
4. Sense and antisense primers (**Table 2**): Sense primer is labeled with a fluorescent marker (5'-carboxyfluorescein; FAM).
5. *Thermus aquaticus* (Taq) DNA polymerase (PE Biosystems). Store at –20°C.
6. Apparatus: GeneAmp PCR system 9600 (PE Biosystems).

2.4. Agarose Gel Electrophoresis

1. Sea Plaque GTG agarose (FMC Products, Rockland, ME).
2. 10X TBE buffer: 0.89 *M* Tris-HCl, 0.89 *M* boric acid, 20 m*M* sodium EDTA.

3. Genescan-1000 (PE Biosystems).
4. Apparatus: Gene Scanner 362 (PE Biosystems).

3. Methods

3.1. Preparation of Total Cellular RNA

1. Introduce the tissue (substantia nigra, locus coeruleus, or adrenal gland) into a sterile homogenizer containing 3.4 mL GTC solution (*see* **Note 6**). After homogenization, transfer the homogenate to a fresh tube, and draw it into a hypodermic syringe fitted with an 18-gage needle. Layer the sample onto 1.6 mL of CsCl solution.
2. Centrifuge at 20°C at 150,000*g* (36,000 rpm) for 12–16 h with an Sw55 Ti rotor (Beckman).
3. Remove the supernatant and add 100 µL 70% ethanol. Invert the tube and drain off the ethanol.
4. Dissolve the RNA in a small volume of TES buffer. Transfer the RNA to a fresh tube.
5. Purify the RNA with phenol-chloroform extraction and ethanol precipitation.
6. Quantify the RNAs by absorbance at 260 nm.

3.2. Synthesis of cRNAs for an Internal Standard

1. Synthetic cRNAs, in which a short synthetic oligonucleotide (5'-GAACTA CCAAAGGCCTTTGGTAGTTCTGCA-3' for types 1 and 2; 5'-CCGGAA TTCCGG-3' for types 3 and 4) is artificially inserted at a restriction site in the amplified region of type 2 or type 4 TH cDNA, are used as internal standards.
2. Four types of TH cRNAs are synthesized from cDNAs and used for calculation of the absolute amounts of mRNAs (*see* **Table 2**).

3.3. Reverse Transcription

1. The reverse-transcription mixture for one preparation contains: 1 µL 100 pmol/µL random primer, 0.1 µL 110 U ribonuclease inhibitor, 1 µL 0.1 *M* DTT, 2 µL 10X transcription buffer, 8 µL 1.25 m*M* dNTPs, 1 µL 50 m*M* $MgCl_2$, 1 µL internal cRNA (for types 1 and 2: 10 or 1 pg/µL; for types 3 and 4: 0.1 or 0.01 pg/µL), 1 µL MMLV-RT (200 U/µL), and 3.1 µL DEPC water.
2. Add 1.8 µL total RNA (1 µg), or 1 µL standard cRNAs and 1 µg of human liver total RNA to reverse transcription mixture, mix gently, and incubate for 1 h at 37°C. After incubation, heat at 95°C for 5 min, and cool rapidly on ice.

3.4. PCR

1. Prepare a PCR mix for assays (sample and standard). The PCR mix *(22)* for one preparation contains 2 µL 10X amplification buffer, 2 µL 1.25 m*M* dNTPs, 1 µL perfect match polymerase enhancer, 1 µL each of 10 pmol/µL sense and antisense primers (**Table 2**), 0.15 µL Taq DNA polymerase (5 U/µL), and 12.85 µL H_2O.
2. Add 5 µL cDNA to 20 µL PCR mix.
3. Start PCR; this is programmed as follows: 94°C for 3 min, and 94°C for 30 s, 60°C for 1 min for 18 cycles (type 1), 23 cycles (types 2 and 3), or 26 cycles (type 4) (*see* **Notes 7** and **8**).

Table 2
Primer Sequences for Human TH mRNA Detection by RT-PCR
(A) Oligonucleotide Primer Sequences For TH mRNA Amplification by RT-PCR

Primer	Sequence(5'–3')	Exon	Position[a]
HS-4 *sense*	5'-dTGTCTGAGCTGGACGCCAAGCAG-3'	1	53–75
HA-3 *antisense*	5'-dCTCCTCAAAGGCCACAGCCTCCA-3'	2	296–318
HA-2 *antisense*	5'-dTGCAGTTCCAGGCCACGGAGAGC-3'	3	128–150

(B) Length of DNA Fragment (bp)

Primer combination	Type 1	Type 2	Internal standard for types 1 and 2	Type 3	Type 4	Internal standard for types 3 and 4
HS-4/HA-3	173	185	207			
HS-4/HA-2				86	98	110

[a]Nucleotides are numbered based on human TH type- 4 cDNA, with the first base of the ATG codon designated as +1.

3.5. Separation and Quantification of mRNA

1. Prepare a 2% Sea Plaque agarose gel with TBE buffer.
2. Mix 4 µL of each PCR product with 3 µL of Genescan-1000 and apply onto 2% Sea Plaque agarose gel.
3. Perform the electrophoresis in TBE buffer.
4. Quantify the fluorescence intensity of each amplified product by Gene Scanner 362 (*see* **Notes 9** and **10**).

4. Notes

1. Using this RT-PCR technique, the total TH mRNA content (all four isoforms) in control human brain (substantia nigra) is about 5.5 ± 1.4 amol of TH mRNA/µg of total RNA. The mean relative ratios of types 1:2:3:4 are about 45:50:2:3, respectively. Parkinsonian brains have very low levels of all four TH mRNAs in the nigra compared with control brains. Brain samples from patients with schizophrenia do not show a significant difference in TH mRNA levels compared with those from controls. The relative ratio of the four TH isoforms is similar among control, parkinsonian and schizophrenic brains. The individual variability in mean TH mRNA content does not correlate with age at death or with postmortem delay ***(19)***.
2. Total TH mRNA (type 1 plus type 2) levels in the adrenal gland, substantia nigra, and locus coeruleus of monkeys (*Macaca fascicularis*) are about 22, 16, and 0.1 amol of TH mRNA/µg of total RNA, respectively. The ratio between TH mRNA type 2/type 1 in both brain regions and in the adrenal gland ranges from 1.1 to 1.6 ***(20)***. In the substantia nigra of control human brains, this ratio is about 1.1 ***(19)***, which is similar to that of monkeys.

3. Marked (98%) decreases in TH mRNA types 1 and 2 without changes in their ratio are observed in the substantia nigra from MPTP-treated monkeys ***(20)***. In contrast, only modest reductions (25%) in TH mRNA types 1 and 2 are observed in the locus coeruleus and adrenal gland. These observations are consistent with our finding of a decrease in human TH mRNA types 1–4 in the substantia nigra of PD patients with no changes in their ratios ***(19)***.
4. Haycock ***(23)*** reported the production of TH isoform-specific antioligopeptide antibodies and demonstrated the presence of all four isoform proteins in human adrenal medulla and brain. He quantified each isoform in the human adrenal medulla with quantitative immunolabeling assays and estimated the ratio of isoforms as 43:40:10:7 for types 1–4, respectively. This estimation is in agreement with our quantification of the four types of TH mRNA ***(19)***, since we observed that the levels of types 3 and 4 in the adrenal gland are higher than those in brain.
5. Dumas et al. ***(24)*** found three new species of human TH mRNA in the adrenal medulla of patients with progressive supranuclear palsy (PSP) in addition to hTH1–hTH4. These isoforms are produced by skipping of exon 3. We have not yet identified these new hTH mRNAs in the substantia nigra from control or PSP patients (H. Ichinose, I. Kanazawa, T. Nagatsu et al., unpublished data).
6. Nothing is amplified using RNA extracted from human frontal cortex as negative control.
7. Amplify samples with 18 cycles for types 1 and 2, or with 23 cycles for types 3 and 4, respectively, and then increase the number of amplification cycles for those samples whose signals are not sufficiently high at the lower cycles.
8. Hot-start PCR is recommended to avoid amplification of misannealed products. The PCR apparatus is preheated to 94°C before putting sample tubes.
9. The linearity between fluorescence intensity of the amplified cDNA and the amount of mRNA introduced into the reaction mixture is studied with cRNA standards of TH mRNAs.
10. A similar quantification can be performed with a Gene-Scan program using models 373, 377, or 310 DNA sequencers.

References

1. Nagatsu, T. (1993) Biochemical aspects of Parkinson's disease. *Adv. Neurol.* **60,** 165–174.
2. Nagatsu, T., Levitt, M., and Udenfriend, S. (1964) Tyrosine hydroxylase. The initial step in norepinephrine biosynthesis. *J. Biol. Chem.* **239,** 2910–2917.
3. Nagatsu, T. (1995) Tyrosine hydroxylase: human isoforms, structure and regulation in physiology and pathology, in *Essays in Biochemistry*, vol. 30 (Apps, D. K. and Tipton, K. F., eds.), Portland Press, London, pp. 15–35.
4. Kaufman, S. and Fisher, D. B. (1974) Pterin-requiring aromatic amino acid hydroxylase, in *Molecular Mechanisms of Oxygen Activation* (Hayaishi, O., ed.), Academic Press, New York, pp. 285–369.
5. Matsuura, S., Sugimoto, T., Masada, S., Murata, Y., and Iwasaki, H. (1985) Streochemistry of biopterin cofactor and facile methods for the determination of

the stereochemistry of a biologically active 5,6,7,8-tetrahydrobiopterin. *J. Biochem.* **98,** 1341–1348.

6. Nagatsu, T. (1991) Genes for human catecholamine-synthesizing enzymes. *Neurosci. Res.* **12,** 315–345.
7. Grima, B., Lamouroux, A., Boni, C., Julien, J.-F., Javoy-Agid, F., and Mallet, J. (1987) A single human gene encoding multiple tyrosine hydroxylases with different predicted functional characteristics. *Nature* **326,** 707–711.
8. Kaneda, N., Kobayashi, K., Ichinose, H., Kishi, F., Nakazawa, A., Kurosawa, Y., et al. (1987) Isolation of a novel cDNA clone for human tyrosine hydroxylase. Alternative RNA splicing produces four kinds of mRNA from a single gene. *Biochem. Biophys. Res. Commun.* **146,** 971–975.
9. Kobayashi, K., Kaneda, N., Ichinose, H., Kishi, F., Nakazawa, A., Kurosawa, Y., et al. (1987) Isolation of a full-length cDNA clone encoding human tyrosine hydroxylase type 3. *Nucleic Acids Res.* **15,** 6733.
10. Kobayashi, K., Kaneda, N., Ichinose, H., Kishi, F., Nakazawa, A., Kurosawa, Y., et al. (1988) Structures of the human tyrosine hydroxylase gene: alternative splicing from a single gene accounts for generation of four mRNA types. *J. Biochem.* **103,** 907–912.
11. O'Mally, K. L., Anhalt, M. J., Martin, B. M., Kalsoe, J. R., Winfield, S. L., and Ginns, E. I. (1997) Isolation and characterization of the human tyrosine hydroxylase gene: identification of 5' alternative splice sites responsible for multiple mRNAs. *Biochemistry* **26,** 6910–6914.
12. Ichikawa, S., Ichinose, H., and Nagatsu, T. (1990) Multiple mRNAs of monkey tyrosine hydroxylase. *Biochem. Biophys. Res. Commun.* **173,** 1331–1336.
13. Ichinose, H., Ohye, T., Fujita, K., Yoshida, M., Ueda, S., and Nagatsu, T. (1993) Increased heterogeneity of tyrosine hydroxylase in humans. *Biochem. Biophys. Res. Commun.* **195,** 158–165.
14. Lamouroux, A., Blanot, F., Biguet, N. F., and Mallet, J. (1985) Complete coding sequence of rat tyrosine hydroxylase mRNA. *Proc. Natl. Acad. Sci. USA* **82,** 617–621.
15. Ichikawa, S., Sasaoka, T., and Nagatsu, T. (1991) Primary structure of mouse tyrosine hydroxylase deduced from its cDNA. *Biochem. Biophys. Res. Commun.* **176,** 1610–1616.
16. Mogi, M., Harada, M., Kiuchi, K., Kojima, K., Kondo, T., Narabayashi, H., et al. (1988) Homospecific activity (activity per enzyme protein) of tyrosine hydroxylase increases in parkinsonian brain. *J. Neural Transm.* **72,** 77–91.
17. Mogi, M., Harada, M., Kojima, K., Kiuchi, K., Nagatsu, I., and Nagatsu, T. (1987) Effects of repeated systemic administration of 1-methyl-4-phenyl-1,2,3,6-tetrahydropyridine (MPTP) on striatal tyrosine hydroxylase activity and tyrosine hydroxylase content. *Neurosci. Lett.* **80,** 213–218.
18. Reinhard, J. F. Jr., and O'Callaghan, J. P. (1991) Measurement of tyrosine hydroxylase apoenzyme protein by enzyme-linked immunosorbent assay (ELISA): effects of 1-methyl-4-phenyl-1,2,3,6-tetrahydropyridine (MPTP) on striatal tyrosine hydroxylase activity and content. *Anal. Biochem.* **196,** 296–301.
19. Ichinose, H., Ohye, T., Fujita, K., Pantucek, F., Lange, K., Riederer, P., and Nagatsu, T. (1994) Quantification of mRNA of tyrosine hydroxylase and aro-

matic L-amino acid decarboxylase in the substantia nigra in Parkinson's disease and schizophrenia. *J. Neural Transm.* [P-D Sect.] **8,** 149–158.

20. Ohye, T., Ichinose, H., Ogawa, M., Yoshida, M., and Nagatsu, T. (1995) Alterations in multiple tyrosine hydroxylase mRNAs in the substantia nigra, locus coeruleus and adrenal gland of MPTP-treated parkinsonian monkeys. *Neurodegeneration* **4,** 81–85.
21. Nagatsu, T. and Ichinose, H. (1991) Comparative studies on the structure of human tyrosine hydroxylase with those of the enzyme of various mammals. *Comp. Biochem. Physiol.* **98C,** 203–210.
22. Wang, M. A., Doyle, M. V., and Mark, D. F. (1989) Quantitation of mRNA by the polymerase chain reaction. *Proc. Natl, Acad. Sci. USA* **86,** 9717–9721.
23. Haycock, J. W. (1993) Multiple forms of tyrosine hydroxylase in human neuroblastoma cells: quantitation with isoform-specific antibodies. *J. Neurochem.* **60,** 493–502.
24. Dumas, S., Le Hir, H., Bodeau-Péan, S., Hirsch, E., Thermes, C., and Mallet, J. (1996) New species of human tyrosine hydroxylase mRNA are produced in variable amounts in adrenal medulla and are overexpressed in progressive supranuclear palsy. *J. Neurochem.* **67,** 19–25.

12

Immunochemical Analysis of Dopamine Transporters in Parkinson's Disease

Gary W. Miller and Allan I. Levey

1. Introduction

The identification of specific and selective markers of the dopamine-producing neurons that are lost in Parkinson's disease has been a major research focus since Hornykiewicz first reported a dopamine deficiency in the disease *(1)*. Antibodies to dopamine or tyrosine hydroxylase, the rate-limiting enzyme in dopamine synthesis, have been used to identify these neurons. Recently, considerable attention has been given to the plasma membrane dopamine transporter (DAT) and the vesicular monoamine transporter (VMAT2), which are responsible for the transport, packaging, and release of dopamine *(2)*. DAT acts to terminate dopamine transmission by rapid reuptake of dopamine from the synapse, and VMAT2 packages cytoplasmic dopamine into vesicles for storage and subsequent release. We have developed specific antibodies to these transporters and used them to characterize the distribution and expression of DAT and VMAT2 in brain from human idiopathic Parkinson's disease and animal models of the disease. The purpose of this chapter is to describe the immunochemical techniques involved in assessing damage to dopamine neurons in Parkinson's disease and experimental models of the disease.

We employ two separate, yet related, techniques for analyzing DAT and VMAT2 expression in human and experimental animal brain. One procedure is Western blotting, which provides an opportunity to identify specific proteins using antibodies. In the first step proteins are denatured in sodium dodecyl sulfate (SDS) or lithium dodecyl sulfate (LDS) and reducing agents and then separated by molecular mass using acrylamide gel electrophoresis. These proteins are then electrophoretically transferred to a membrane, where they can be probed with specific antibodies. This technique can be performed relatively

From: *Methods in Molecular Medicine, vol. 62: Parkinson's Disease: Methods and Protocols*
Edited by: M. M. Mouradian © Humana Press Inc., Totowa, NJ

inexpensively and does not require any special training. The combination of molecular mass and antigenicity provides a high degree of specific molecular recognition. The second technique, immunocytochemistry, takes advantage of the antibody specificity and couples it with microscopy (light, electron, or confocal) for excellent spatial resolution. Some of the techniques involved in immunocytochemistry require some practice, but most laboratories can establish this method without much difficulty. Over the past few decades investigators have used these approaches to localize the distribution of several proteins including tyrosine hydroxylase, dopa decarboxylase, dopamine receptors, and even dopamine itself.

There is evidence that immunochemical assessment of DAT is more accurate than radioligand-based procedures. A comparison of DAT immunoblotting with radioligand binding using DAT ligands revealed that immunoblotting provided the strongest correlate to actual dopamine levels, and neuronal integrity with ligand binding tended to overestimate the remaining terminals *(3)*. Our laboratories have examined the distribution and expression levels of DAT and VMAT2 levels in caudate, putamen, and nucleus accumbens from control and Parkinson's diseased brains (*see* **Figs. 1** and **2**) *(4)*. The putamen, which is known to be most severely affected in Parkinson's disease, displayed the most drastic loss of DAT immunoreactivity, followed by the caudate and accumbens. Although the putamen also showed the greatest losses of VMAT2 *(5)*, the degree of VMAT2 loss in the caudate and accumbens was similar, which may reflect the presence of residual monoaminergic terminals. Furthermore, the loss of DAT correlated to disease duration, further suggesting the utility of DAT immunoreactivity in assessing progression of dopamine terminal loss *(4)*. These techniques have also been used to examine DAT and VMAT2 immunoreactivity in hemiparkinsonian monkey brain (*see* **Fig. 3**) *(5,6)*. Unilateral administration of 1-methyl-4-phenyl-1,2,3,6-tetrahydropyridine (MPTP) selectively destroys dopamine terminals in the caudate and putamen but spares other monoaminergic regions. Thus, immunochemical analysis of dopamine transporters in idiopathic and experimental Parkinson's disease provides an excellent means of assessing neuronal integrity.

2. Materials

2.1. Immunoblotting

1. Homogenization buffer: 320 m*M* sucrose, 5 m*M* HEPES, pH 7.4. Filter and store at 4°C (*see* **Note 1**).
2. Protease inhibitor stock solutions: 2 mg/mL leupeptin in water; 1 mg/mL pepstatin in methanol; 1 mg/mL aprotinin in water (*see* **Note 2**). Store at –20°C.
3. 4X SDS gel loading buffer: Tris-HCl (200 m*M*), dithiothreitol (400 m*M*), SDS (8%), glycerol (40%), bromophenol blue (0.4%); pH of 1X buffer should be 6.8 (*see* **Note 2**). Buffer can be stored at 4°C for up to 6 mo.

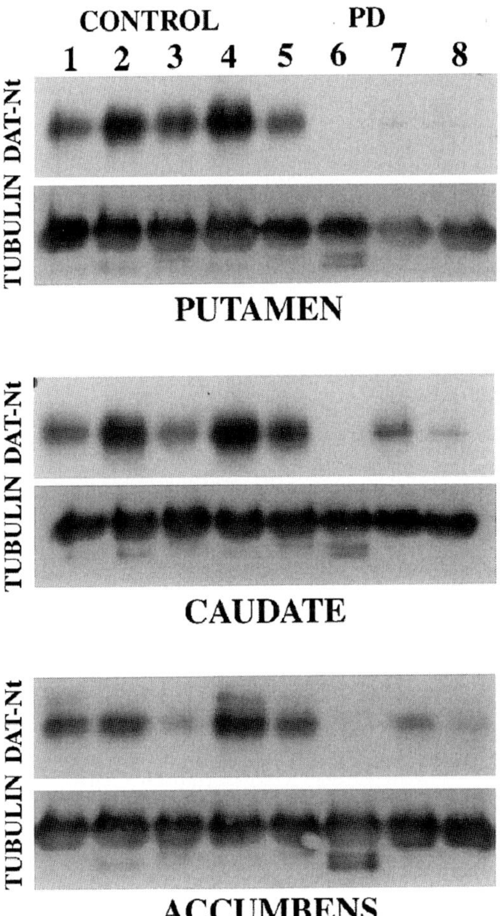

Fig. 1. Western blot analysis of dopamine transporter (DAT) and α-tubulin in the striatum of control (lanes 1–4) and Parkinson's diseased brain (lanes 5–8). Homogenates (20 μg) of microdissected samples from the putamen, caudate, and nucleus accumbens were separated by SDS-PAGE, transferred to PVDF membrane, subjected to immunoblot analysis with DAT Nt or an antibody to α-tubulin, and developed with chemiluminescence. The approximate molecular mass of DAT- and α-tubulin-immunoreactive bands were 85 and 55 kDa, respectively. (Reproduced with permission from **ref.** ***4***.)

4. 20X running buffer: 1 *M* 3-(*N*-morpolino)propane sulfonic acid (MOPS), 1 *M* Tris base, 69.3 m*M* SDS, 20.5 m*M* EDTA, ultrapure water to 500 mL; pH of 1X buffer should be 7.7 (*see* **Note 2**).
5. 20X transfer buffer: 500 m*M* bicine, 500 m*M* Bis-Tris, 20.5 m*M* EDTA, ultrapure water to 125 mL; pH of 1X buffer should be 7.2 (*see* **Note 2**).

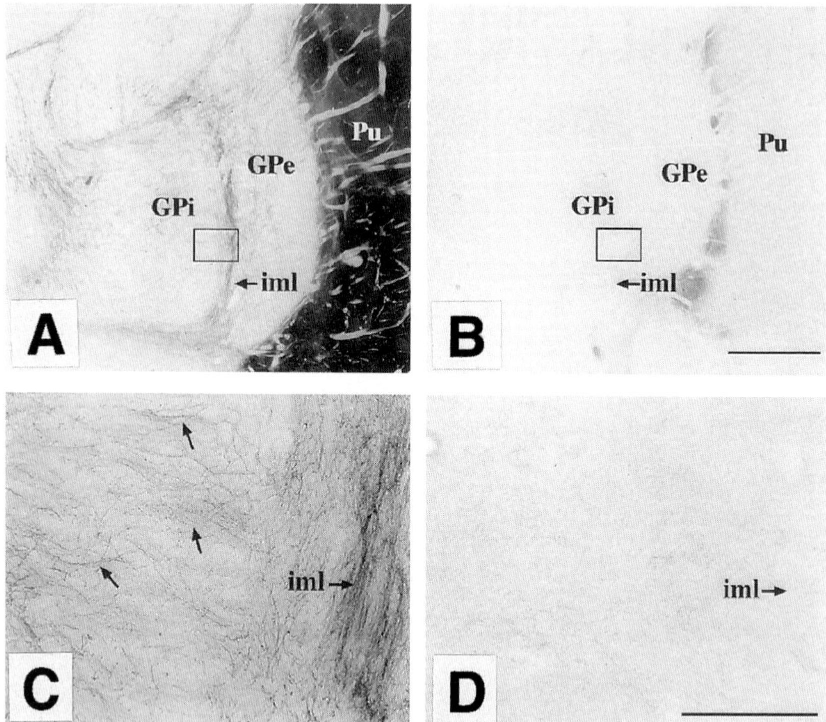

Fig. 2. Loss of dopamine transporter (DAT)-immunoreactive fibers in Parkinson's disease pallidum. **(A)** Control. **(B)** Parkinson's disease. The depletion of DAT-immunoreactive fibers in both the internal (GPi) and external (GPe) globus pallidus corresponds to that seen in the putamen (Pu). Scale bar = 0.5 cm. **(C,D)** High-power photomicrographs of GPi at the border of the internal medullary lamina (iml; from boxed regions in corresponding upper panel). Arrows indicate DAT-immunoreactive fibers. Scale bar = 1 mm. (Reproduced with permission from **ref. *4***.)

6. Molecular weight markers (*see* **Note 2**). Store at –20°C.
7. Tris-bicine gels (*see* **Note 2**).
8. Polyvinylidene difluoride (PVDF) membrane (*see* **Note 2**).
9. Electrophoresis unit for polyacrylamide gel electrophoresis (PAGE) and electrophoretic transfer of proteins (see **Note 2**).
10. Tris-buffered saline containing Tween 20 (TTBS): 135 m*M* NaCl, 2.5 KCl, 25 m*M* Tris-HCl, 0.1% Tween 20, pH 7.4.
11. Blocking solution: 7.5% nonfat dry milk: 7.5 g nonfat dry milk in 100 mL TTBS. Make fresh.
12. Stripping buffer: 8 *M* urea, 100 m*M* 2-mercaptoethanol, 62.5 m*M* Tris-HCl, pH 6.8.
13. Orbital shaker.
14. Rotary mixer (e.g., Nutator; VWR Scientific, West Chester, PA).

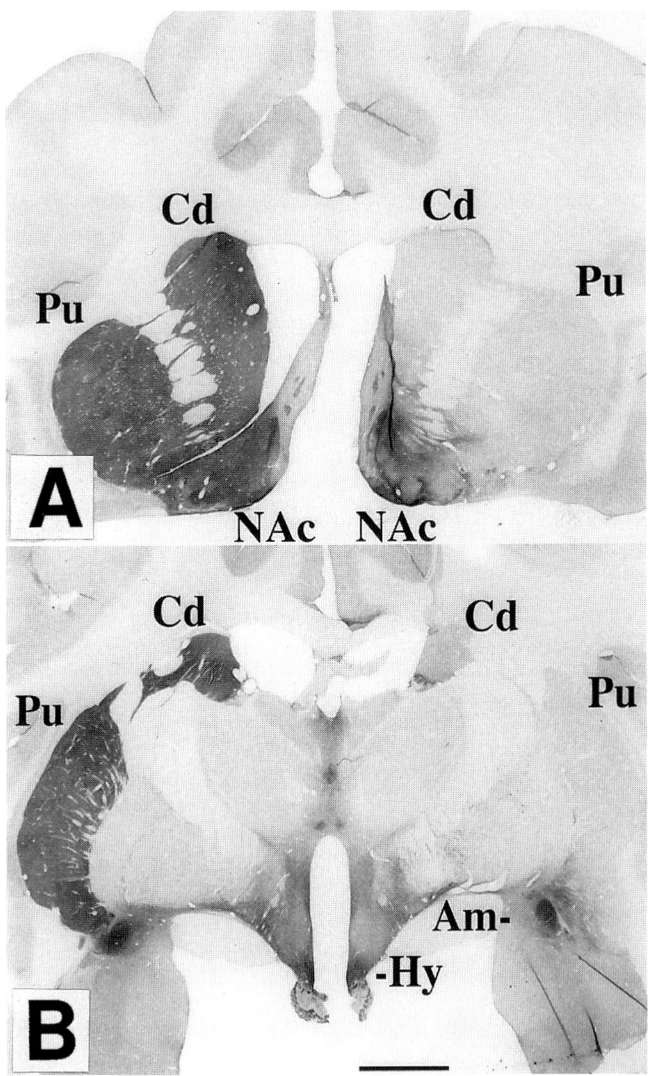

Fig. 3. VMAT2 immunocytochemistry in hemiparkisonian monkey brain. Following a unilateral injection of MPTP and clinical verification of hemiparkisonism, 40-μm brain sections were prepared and incubated in the presence of primary antibody VMAT2-Ct. Immunoreactivity was detected using the avidin-biotin complex method with diaminobenzidine. **(A)** Coronal section at the level of the anterior commissure shows a drastic reduction in VMAT2 immunoreactivity following MPTP. The caudate (Cd) and putamen (Pu) were most severely affected; the nucleus accumbens (NAC) was somewhat preserved. **(B)** Rostral section revealing depletion of VMAT2 immunreactivity in the Cd and Pu, but relative sparing of the amygdala (Am) and hypothalamus (Hy). Scale bar = 0.5 cm. (Reproduced with permission from **ref. 5**.)

2.2. Immunocytochemistry

1. Sliding microtome (*see* **Note 3**).
2. Tris-buffered saline (TBS): 135 m*M* NaCl, 2.5 m*M* KCl, 25 m*M* Tris-HCl, pH 7.4. Store at 4°C.
3. Plastic container with organized dividers to collect brain sections (*see* **Note 3**).
4. Small paint brush (#1, Brain Research Laboratories, Boston, MA).
5. Sodium azide: 1% solution (*see* **Note 4**).
6. 10% Triton X-100 in water. Store at 4°C.
7. 30% hydrogen peroxide. Store at 4°C.
8. Normal goat and human serum. Store at –20°C. Once thawed, store at 4°C (*see* **Note 5**).
9. Avidin/biotin blocking kit (Vector, Burlingame, CA). Store at 4°C.
10. DAT or VMAT2 antibody. Store at –20°C (*see* **Note 6**).
11. Vectastain ABC kit (Vector) containing secondary antibody and biotin-peroxidase complex (*see* **Note 7**)
12. Vector diaminobenzidine kit (*see* **Note 4**).
13. Pyrex pie dish.
14. Ethanol.
15. Hemo-De clearing agent (Fisher Scientific, Pittsburgh, PA).
16. Dishes for incubating tissue and processing slides (Brain Research Laboratories, Boston, MA).
17. Subbed microscope slides and coverslips.
18. Light microscope.
19. Orbital shaker.

3. Methods

3.1. Immunoblotting

1. Isolate tissue from fresh or frozen brain tissue (*see* **Note 3**).
2. Place in ice-cold homogenization buffer containing protease inhibitors (*see* **Note 1**).
3. Homogenize for 10–15 s at maximum speed using a motor-driven tissue homogenizer (e.g., Brinkman Polytron).
4. Centrifuge the sample at 3000*g* for 5 min at 4°C in microcentrifuge.
5. Transfer supernatant to centrifuge tubes and spin at 30,000*g* for 30 min (*see* **Note 8**).
6. Remove supernatant and resuspend the pellet in a small volume of homogenization buffer with protease inhbitors (*see* **Note 8**).
7. Determine protein content using a standard spectrophotometric assay (Lowry, biuret, etc.).
8. Dilute the sample with homogenization buffer and 4X loading dye) for a final concentration of 2 mg/mL (*see* **Note 8**). If quantification of immunoreactive bands will be performed an internal standard curve should be run with each gel using pooled control samples for a curve that spans the predicted range of the samples.
9. Incubate at room temperature for 30 min (*see* **Note 9**).

10. After setting up gel box with 1X running buffer (1 part 20X running buffer, 19 parts ultrapure water) and rinsing the wells, load 10 μL into the wells.
11. Run the gel according to manufacturer's recommendations.
12. Near the end of the run cut a piece of PVDF membrane, and soak it in methanol for 10 s, and then move to transfer buffer for 5 min (*see* **Note 10**).
13. Once the gel is finished running (dye front reaches bottom of gel), remove the gel from the cassette and place it in 1X transfer buffer (1 part 20X transfer buffer, 4 parts methanol, 15 parts ultrapure water) to equilibrate for 5 min. Soak the blotting pads in a separate container containing transfer buffer (we use Pyrex dishes).
14. Prepare the gel-membrane sandwich (*see* **Note 10**).
15. Place the gel-membrane sandwich in the electrophoresis apparatus (*see* **Note 10**).
16. Transfer according to manufacturer's recommendations. (Novex recommends transferring at 30 V for 60 min at room temperature, although additional time may be necessary).
17. Near the end of the transfer, prepare a solution of 7.5% nonfat dry milk in TTBS.
18. Upon completion of transfer, remove the membrane from the sandwich and place in blocking solution for 30–60 min on an orbital shaker.
19. Prepare primary antibody solution (*see* **Note 11**). DAT antibody (Chemicon, Temecula, CA) is used at 1:10,000. Upon receipt we dilute the antibody with an equal volume of glycerol and store at –20°C. This prevents freezing and inhibits bacterial growth. Thus, the glycerol stock is used at 1:5000. VMAT2 (Chemicon) is used at 1:300–1:1000.
20. Place the membrane into a sealable bag, leaving one side open, add primary antibody solution, and seal (*see* **Note 11**).
21. Place on a rotary mixer overnight at 4°C (*see* **Note 11**).
22. Rinse the membrane once in 20 mL TTBS for a few seconds and then rinse 3 × 10 min at room temperature on an orbital shaker.
23. Incubate in secondary antibody solution (*see* **Note 12**) at room temperature on an orbital shaker.
24. Rinse 1 × 10 s and 3 × 10 min at room temperature on an orbital shaker.
25. Develop the blot with a chemiluminescence substrate (*see* **Note 12**).
26. To reprobe the blot with another antibody, strip the blot by incubating for 20 min at 80°C in stripping buffer (*see* **Note 13**).
27. Return to **step 16** and probe with additional antibodies (*see* **Note 13**).

3.2. Immunocytochemistry

Paraformaldehyde-fixed sections should be cut (40–50 μm) on a freezing sliding microtome and collected in cold TBS. Experimental animals should be transcardially perfused for optimal fixation (*see* **Note 14**).

1. Place tissue in divided net well containing TBS (*see* **Note 14**).
2. Block tissue sections in a solution containing 4% normal goat serum (NGS) in 1% Triton X-100, 3% hydrogen peroxide, and avidin (1 drop/10 mL) in TBS for 20 min.
3. Rinse thoroughly in cold TBS (6 × 10 min).

4. Incubate sections in primary antibody solution containing 0.1% Triton X-100, 4% NGS, 4% normal human serum, biotin (1 drop/10 mL), and the affinity-purified antibody (*see* **Note 7**).
5. Rinse sections in TBS for 3 × 10 min
6. Incubate in secondary antibody solution containing 4% NGS, 0.1% Triton X-100, and 1 drop/10 mL Vectastain goat anti-(primary antibody species) antibody for 1 h.
7. Make up tertiary solution containing 4% NGS, biotin-peroxidase complex in TBS and store at 4°C until **step 9**.
8. Rinse 3 × 10 min in cold TBS.
9. Incubate sections in tertiary solution from **step 7** for 1 h at room temperature.
10. Rinse 3 × 10 min in cold TBS.
11. Develop tissue sections in 0.1 *M* Tris-HCl, pH 8.0, with 0.05% diaminobenzidine and 0.01% hydrogen peroxide for 5–6 min (*see* **Note 15**).
12. After 3 × 10 min rinses in TBS, mount the sections on to gelatin-subbed slides. We do this in a shallow glass pie plate with Tris buffer (0.1 *M* Tris-HCl, pH 8.0) with a few drops of 10% Triton X-100 added (**see Note 16**).
13. Air dry.
14. Dehydrate by submersing the slides in increasing concentrations of ethanol, finishing with Hemo-De, and coverslip with Permount (*see* **Note 17**).

4. Notes

1. Buffer should be made fresh weekly due to the possibility of bacterial growth.
2. All the following items are available from Invitrogen (Carlstad, CA): sample buffer (NP0007), running buffer (NP0001), transfer buffer (NP0006), molecular weight markers, gels, and apparatus. Other companies make excellent systems for running and transferring the gels, most notably Bio-Rad (Hercules, CA). Precast gels are also now available from several sources. Purchasing precast gels virtually eliminates the problems of leaky or nonuniform gels that have frustrated many researchers. Many of these gels have a shelf life of up to 1 yr. Tris-glycine gels have been the gels of choice for many years, but newer formats, including the NuPAGE (Tris-bicine) system from Novex have a much longer shelf life and shorter run times. We use conventional loading buffer with the NuPage system, as described under **Subheading 2.**, but Novex also manufactures a loading buffer made specifically for their system.
3. It is highly recommended that a new user of a microtome seek advice from an experienced user or utilize core histology facilities. Several subtleties are beyond the scope of this chapter. Two common problems are not keeping the tissue block frozen throughout the procedure and not maintaining a steady speed of cutting. Dry ice should be added to the stage at frequent intervals, and the blade should move through the tissue in a fluid motion. Using wrist and finger movement to advance the blade through the tissue, rather than moving the shoulder and elbow, will help maintain the fine motor control necessary. Tissue sections should be collected in a divided tray, placing each successive section in the next well and

repeating this throughout the block of tissue. This generates multiple series that can be used to compare different markers in adjacent sections. The more series you have, the farther apart each section within a series is. For monkey and human tissue, though, usually 12 or more series are used. Fresh-frozen tissue sections are typically cut on a cryostat.

4. Sodium azide is very toxic. DAB is a known carcinogen. Wear gloves when working with these reagents.
5. The serum used for the blocking steps should be the same as that of the secondary antibody. Vector Laboratories make secondary antibodies in goat that recognize either rat, rabbit, or mouse; thus we use goat when using these kits. We have found that in human and monkey tissue the addition of 4% human serum helps reduce background.
6. The success of any immunochemical technique is dependent on the quality of the antibodies used. For this reason, it is imperative to use well-characterized antibodies. Before purchasing antibodies check the references provided in the catalogues to see whether the antibodies have been fully characterized. They should have been tested by Western blotting and immuncytochemistry in the species you plan to study. If not, you may want to request a small sample to see whether it works in the species of interest. For more information on characterization of antibodies *see* **ref. *6***. The optimal concentration of each antibody should be determined by titration, but a final concentration of affinity-purified antibody of approx 0.5 μg/mL usually produces excellent results. Exceptional antibodies to both DAT (monoclonal) and VMAT2 (polyclonal) are available from Chemicon.
7. Several companies make detection kits for immunocytochemistry. We have had the most experience with the Vector Vectastain Elite ABC kits. Each kit is designed to recognize a particular species of primary antibody. If one is using a mouse monoclonal primary antibody, one would purchase the mouse kit. The kits contain the particular biotinylated secondary antibody (A) and the components of the avidin-peroxidase complex (B+C). The ABC kits also contain a small amount of blocking serum, which we generally discard.
8. For a small piece of tissue, 500 μL in a microcentrifuge tube works well. The resulting pellet contains membranes and their associated proteins. The supernatant contains cytosolic proteins (e.g., tyrosine hydroxylase). An example of an appropriate amount of buffer would be approx 200–300 μL for a 2–3-mm punch 2–3 mm deep.
9. Do not boil. High temperatures can result in dimerization of transporter proteins.
10. It is very important not to have any bubbles between the gel and PVDF membrane. We have found the following procedure to work well, but other methods also work well. Place a piece of cellophane wrap on the bench (1 × 1 ft). Soak a piece of filter paper in transfer buffer and place on wrap. Then place the PVDF membrane on the filter paper. Pour several milliliters of transfer buffer onto PVDF. The liquid should pool on the membrane. Then, holding the gel from the sides, gently position the middle of the gel in the center of the membrane and let the sides gently down on the membrane, pushing out the buffer. Take another piece

of filter paper and place on top of the gel. Then, using a clean plastic pipet, gently roll across the filter from the center outward. This removes the bubbles from in between the gel and membrane. Remember that the gel is facing up, which means you want the current to run down through the gel into the membrane.

11. We have found that a small amount of nonfat dry milk in the primary antibody solution helps reduce background. We make a 2.5% solution using one-third volume of blocking solution with two-thirds volume TTBS. We recommend an impulse sealer with poylethylene bags. Seal the bag on three sides, add the primary antibody solution (3–5 mL), and seal the open end as you gently push the bubbles out of the bag. We prefer agitating the blot with a rotary shaker.
12. Use an affinity-purifed secondary antibody against the primary antibody coupled to horseradish peroxidase (HRP). Imaging systems can now directly detect chemiluminescence. We have found the Dura Western Substrate from Pierce (Rockford, IL) to work well with these systems. The newer imaging systems can improve quantification since the cameras have a much wider dynamic range than conventional radiographic film.
13. Immunoreactivity will diminish upon stripping. However, we have found it possible to probe the blot a total of three times with good results. We recommend probing the blot for a protein such as tubulin or synaptophysin to confirm equal loading and transfer of proteins.
14. A variety of factors are involved in optimizing the immunocytochemistry procedure, and the reader is referred to more detailed texts *(7–9)*. Paraformaldehyde should be made fresh and used within a day or two. In situ perfusion is recommended for animal tissue. In human tissue the level of fixation will vary widely due to postmortem interval and method of fixation. It is essential that conditions be optimized for each antigen-antibody pair. For example, the antigenicity of some proteins like tyrosine hydroxylase are relatively resistant to variations due to fixation. However, many proteins, including DAT and VMAT2, are quite sensitive to these conditions, and steps such as antigen retrieval may be necessary *(7,**10**)*.

    We like to perform the blocking and rinsing steps in divided containers with mesh bottoms (Brain Research Laboratories). This allows easy changing among solutions without touching tissue. When tissue does need to be transferred from one vessel to the next, we use a Pasteur pipet that has been formed under a flame into a gentle hook.
15. To minimize airborne exposure to diaminobenzidine (DAB), we use the DAB kit from Vector, which already has the DAB in solution and buffer stock and hydrogen peroxide. If color develops within the first minute, it is advisable to reduce the concentrations of primary, secondary, and tertiary complexes.
16. Mounting tissue is labor intensive and tedious. While submersing approximately three-fourths of the subbed slide in the buffer, the tissue sections are moved into position with a paint brush. It is very important to let the tissue float and gently direct it into position. Once the tissue is over the slide correctly, it is gently lifted from the buffer, whereupon it adheres to the slide.

17. Dehydrate in increasing concentrations of ethanol (50, 70, and 95%) and clear in Hemo-De (50% ethanol/50% Hemo-De, 100, 100, and 100%).

References

1. Ehringer, H. H. (1960) Distribution of noradrenaline and dopamine (3-hydroxytyramine) in the human brain and their behavior in diseases of the extrapyramidal system. *Klin. Wochenschr* **38,** 1236–1239.
2. Miller, G. W., Gainetdinov, R. R., Levey, A. I., and Caron, M. G. (1999) Dopamine transporters and neuronal injury. *Trends Pharmacol. Sci.* **20**B 424–429.
3. Wilson, J. M., Levey, A. I., Rajput, A., Ang, L., Guttman, M., Shannak, K., et al. (1996) Differential changes in neurochemical markers of striatal dopamine nerve terminals in idiopathic Parkinson's disease. *Neurology* **47,** 718–726.
4. Miller, G. W., Staley, J. K., Heilman, C. J., Perez, J. T., Mash, D. C., Rye, D. B., et al.(1997) Immunochemical analysis of dopamine transporter protein in Parkinson's disease. *Ann. Neurol.* **41,** 530–539.
5. Miller, G. W., Erickson, J. D., Perez, J. T., Penland, S. N., Mash, D. C., Rye, D. B., et al. (1999) Immunochemical analysis of vesicular monoamine transporter (VMAT2) protein in Parkinson's disease. *Exp. Neurol.* **154,** 138–148.
6. Miller, G. W., Gilmor, M. L., and Levey, A.I. (1998) Generation of transporter specific antibodies. *Meth. Enzymol.* **296,** 407–422.
7. Polak, J. M. (1977) *Introduction to Immunocytochemistry*. Springer, Oxford.
8. Javois, L. C., ed. (1999) *Immunocytochemistry Methods and Protocols,* 2nd ed. Humana, Totowa, NJ.
9. Beesley, J. E., ed. (1993) *Immunocytochemistry: A Practical Approach.* Oxford University Press, Oxford.
10. Ciliax, B. J., Drash, G. W., Staley, J. K., Haber, S., Mobley, C. J., Miller, G. W., et al. (1999) Immunocytochemical localization of the dopamine transporter in human brain. *J. Comp. Neurol.* **409,** 38–56.

13

Dopamine Transporter and Vesicular Monoamine Transporter Knockout Mice

Implications for Parkinson's Disease

Gary W. Miller, Yan-Min Wang, Raul R. Gainetdinov, and Marc G. Caron

1. Introduction

One of the most valuable methods for understanding the function of a particular protein is the generation of animals that have had the gene encoding for the protein of interest disrupted, commonly known as a "knockout" or null mutant. By incorporating a sequence of DNA (typically encoding antibiotic resistance to aid in the selection of the mutant gene) into embryonic stem cells by homologous recombination, the normal transcription of the gene is effectively blocked (**Fig. 1**). Since a particular protein is encoded by two copies of a gene, it is necessary to have the gene on both alleles "knocked out." This is performed by cross-breeding animals with one affected allele (heterozygote) to generate offspring that have inherited two mutant alleles (homozygote). This procedure has been used to generate animals lacking either the plasma membrane dopamine transporter (DAT; **Fig. 2**) or the vesicular monoamine transporter (VMAT2; **Fig. 3**). Both DAT and VMAT2 are essential for dopamine homeostasis and are thought to participate in the pathogenesis of Parkinson's disease *(1–5)*.

DAT acts to terminate dopamine neurotransmission by rapidly removing dopamine from the extrasynaptic spaces. Since altered dopamine neurotransmission is central in the pathophysiology of Parkinson's disease, it is likely that alterations in DAT function may participate in the disease process. Indeed, the ability of DAT to transport potentially toxic molecules that resemble

From: *Methods in Molecular Medicine, vol. 62: Parkinson's Disease: Methods and Protocols*
Edited by: M. M. Mouradian © Humana Press Inc., Totowa, NJ

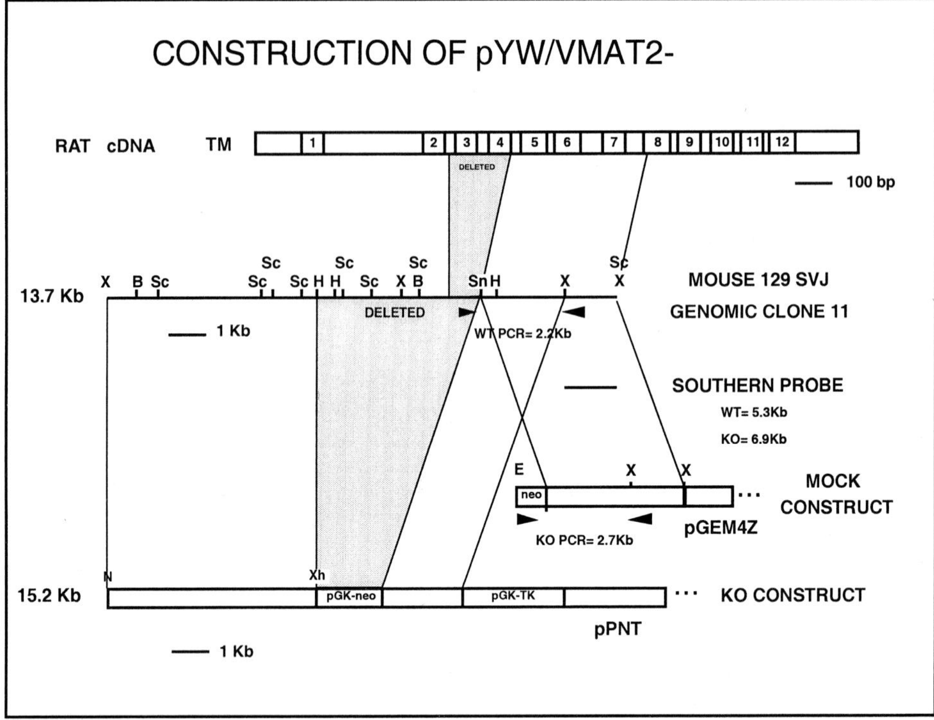

Fig. 1. Maps of the targeting vector and the mock construct. The mouse genomic fragment (clone 11) was isolated from a Stratagene 129 SvJ library by standard colony hybridization using a PCR probe from the 5' end of rat cDNA. The restriction site abbreviations are as follows: H, *Hin*dIII; N, *Not*I; Sc, *Sac*I; Sn, *Sna*I; X, *Xba*I; and Xh, *Xho*I. The region between *Hin*dIII and *Sna*I on clone 11 containing the coding sequence from transmembrane domains 3 and 4 of VMAT2 was deleted and replaced with PGK-neo. The 3' fragment of clone 11 was reserved as an external probe for Southern analysis. To facilitate PCR screening of embryonic stem cell clones, a mock construct containing the *Sna*I/*Xba*I fragment and part of the Neo cassette was generated as a positive control. pPNT and pGEM4Z were used to construct knockout and mock vectors, respectively. (Reproduced with permission from **ref. *1***).

dopamine has implicated DAT expression in dopamine neuron damage. The exclusive expression of DAT on dopamine neurons also makes it an excellent marker of the terminals that degenerate in Parkinson's disease ***(6)***. VMAT2 is expressed in several monoaminergic neuronal cell populations, including dopamine, norepinephrine, and serotonin, and acts to repackage the neurotransmitters into intracellular vesicles. The ability of VMAT2 to sequester putative dopaminergic toxins and the fact that it is a member of the toxin-extruding antiporter gene

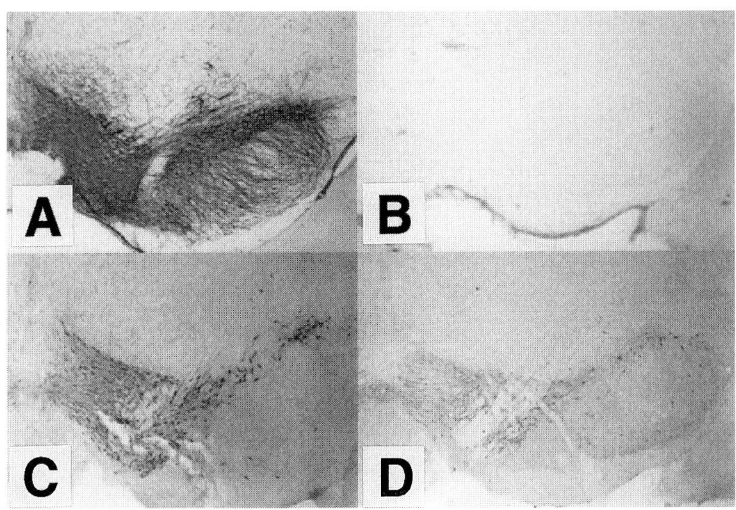

Fig. 2. DAT and VMAT2 expression in wild-type and DAT knockout midbrain. DAT immunoreactivity in wild-type (**A**) and DAT knockout midbrain (**B**). VMAT2 immunoreactivity in wild-type (**C**) and DAT knockout midbrain (**D**). Robust immunoreactivity was observed in the ventral tegmental area and substantia nigra pars compacta and reticulata in the wild-type brain. Note absence of DAT immunoreactivity and modest reduction of VMAT2 immunoreactivity in the DAT knockout.

family *(7)* has given rise to the concept that VMAT2 serves a cytoprotective function *(8)*.

The importance of DAT in neuronal function is highlighted in animals in which DAT has been genetically deleted (DAT KO) *(3)*. In the homozygote DAT KO mice, released dopamine remains in the extracellular space up to 300 times longer than normal. As expected, these animals display behaviors consistent with persistent activation of dopamine receptors, such as hyperlocomotion. Genetic deletion of VMAT2 reveals the essential role of vesicular storage and release of monoamines. Homozygote VMAT2 knockout mice survive for only a few days, whereas heterozygotes appear normal. Studies performed in homozygote pups and heterozygote adults clearly show that the level of VMAT2 expression calibrates the level of vesicular filling *(1,2,4)*. With only 50% of normal VMAT2, heterozygote animals have reduced vesicular filling and release. These alterations in presynaptic monoamine function in the heterozygotes are thought to be responsible for the observed sensitization to the psychostimulants cocaine and amphetamine and to ethanol *(1)*. Knockout animals also appear to parallel the changes that occur in reserpinized animals, suggesting that the adverse actions of this drug are mediated by VMAT2.

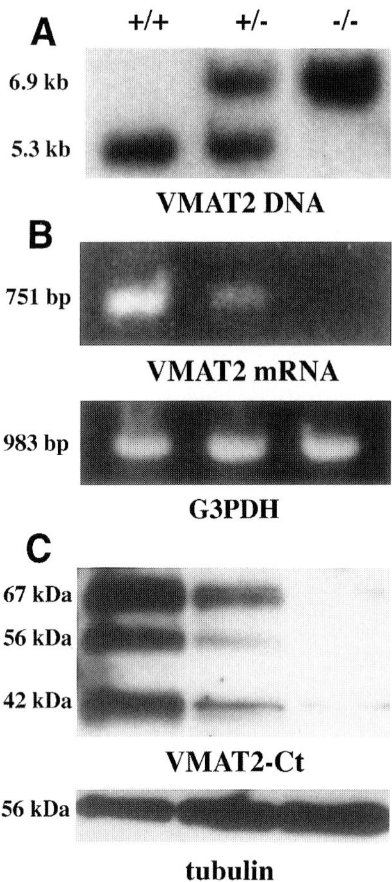

Fig. 3. Characterization of VMAT2 gene disruption. **(A)** Southern blot analysis of mouse genomic DNA. The Southern blot was prepared with 15 μg of genomic DNA per lane and probed with a 1.4-kb 3' external genomic fragment. +/+, wild type littermates; +/–, heterozygote; –/–, homozygote. **(B)** RT-PCR analysis of mouse brain poly(A)$^+$ RNA. For each reverse transcription assay, 0.5 μg of poly(A)$^+$ RNA was used. Equal volumes of cDNA templates were used for each PCR assay. The PCR primers used flank the neomycin cassette for the purpose of detecting potential readthrough of the neomycin DNA. The heterozygote has a reduced amount of transcripts compared with the wild-type littermate; the homozygote is devoid of VMAT2 transcripts. G3PDH was used as internal control. **(C)** Western blot analysis of whole-brain synaptic vesicles. Samples (25 μg) of vesicles were solubilized and separated by SDS-PAGE, transferred to nitrocellulose, subjected to Western blot analysis with anti-VMAT2-Ct (top) or anti-α-tubulin (bottom) antibodies, and developed with chemiluminescence. Molecular mass markers (kDa) are shown to the left. To confirm equal loading and transfer of proteins, the blots were stripped and reprobed with an antibody to α-tubulin. (Reproduced with permission from **ref. *1***).

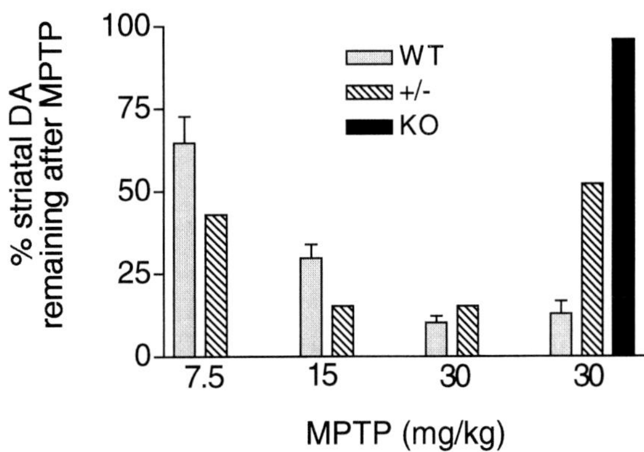

Fig. 4. Effect of MPTP on striatal content of dopamine (DA) in heterozygote VMAT2 knockout (+/-) and DAT knockout mice (KO) mice 2 days after administration. MPTP (7.5, 15, or 30 mg/kg., s.c., b.i.d.) or saline was administered twice a day, 10 h apart. Two days later striatal content of DA was determined by HPLC-EC. At all the doses studied, MPTP produced significant decreases in DA, except in the DAT-/- mice. Data are presented as percent change from animals of the same genotype treated with vehicle. (Data are taken from **refs.** ***12*** and ***13***, with permission).

We have hypothesized that the ratio of DAT to VMAT2 within a particular population of neurons determines vulnerability to several putative neurotoxins, such as 1-methyl-4-phenyl-1,2,3,6-tetrahydropyridine (MPTP) ***(9,10)***. According to this hypothesis, animals with lower than normal DAT expression would be expected to be less susceptible to MPTP, whereas those with lower than normal VMAT2 expression would be expected to be more susceptible to MPTP. Experimental observations demonstrate the predicted results. DAT knockout mice are completely resistant to MPTP-induced nigrostriatal damage (**Fig. 4**) ***(11,12)***. These findings support the concept that DAT is the molecular gateway by which the toxic metabolite of MPTP, 1-methyl-4-phenylpyridirium (MPP^+), enters the nigrostriatal neuron. Heterozygote DAT KO mice, which express approximately 50% of normal DAT, display neurotoxicity that is approximately half of that seen in wild-type mice (**Fig. 4**). Heterozygote VMAT2 knockout mice survive and provide an opportunity to determine whether reduced VMAT2 levels increase susceptibility to neuronal damage. Indeed, VMAT2 heterozygote mice display enhanced vulnerability to MPTP, as evidenced by reductions in nigral dopamine cell counts, striatal dopamine, and dopamine transporter and increase in gliosis ***(2,13)***.

If the expression of DAT and VMAT2 do mediate susceptibility to Parkinson's disease, it is possible that pharmacologic intervention aimed at these transporters may be beneficial. For example, in patients with early stages of the disease, decreasing dopamine uptake may not only increase synaptic and decrease intracellular dopamine concentrations but may also slow the progression of the disease if an endogenous or exogenous toxin is involved. The drug may also be useful in later stages in which side effects, such as dyskinesias, often limit conventional dopaminergic therapies. VMAT2 is another potentially useful target, particularly for neuroprotective agents. For example, potential therapies resulting in increased vesicular uptake by VMAT2 may act to decrease cytosolic dopamine and perhaps prevent oxidation. Data from the knockout animals suggest that pharmacologic strategies aimed at altering the function of DAT and VMAT2 may be beneficial in the treatment of Parkinson's disease. In this chapter, we describe the generation and characterization of null mutant mice for DAT and VMAT2. Furthermore, methods used to analyze susceptibility to the parkinsonism-inducing neurotoxin MPTP are described.

2. Materials

1. 129/SvJ genomic library (Stratagene, La Jolla, CA).
2. Restriction enzymes.
3. A vector containing both PGK-neo and PGK-tk (e.g., pPNT) ***(14)***.
4. 129/SvJ/RW4 ES cells (GenomeSystems).
5. Polymerase chain reaction (PCR) primers for wild-type and mutant alleles, as well as a primer common to genomic sequence located outside the site of disruption (**Fig. 1**).
6. Southern hybridization probes: a probe 3' to the region to be deleted, such that restriction digest will yield a different band size depending on the type of mutation (deletion or insertion).
7. Ganciclovir (Syntex, Boulder, CO) and G418 (Geneticin [G418], Gibco-BRL).
8. High-performance liquid chromatography (HPLC) with electrochemical detector set up (model 5500, Coulochem Electrode Array System [CEAS], ESA, Bedford, MA) for the detection of monoamines.
9. HPLC buffer, pH 3.6: 4 m*M* citrate, 8 m*M* ammonium acetate, 54 μ*M* EDTA, 230 μ*M* 1-octanesulfonic acid (Eastman Kodak, Rochester, NY).
10. Biomax horizontal gel apparatus for running agarose gels (Sigma, St. Louis, MO).
11. Electrophoresis grade agarose (Fisher Scientific, Pittsburg, PA).
12. Qiaex II Gel Extraction kit (Qiagen, Valencia, CA).
13. Qiagen Miniprep kit.
14. Tris-borate EDTA buffer: 45 m*M* Tris-borate, 1 m*M* EDTA.
15. TNES buffer: 50 m*M* Tris, 400 m*M* NaCl, 100 m*M* EDTA, 0.5% sodium dodecyl sulfate (SDS).
16. Proteinase K (20 mg/mL; Roche, Palo Alto, CA).
17. T4 ligase (Promega).
18. Competent *Escherichia coli* cells (Stratagene).
19. Vertical gel apparatus for running Western blot (Novex, San Diego, CA).
20. Electrophoresis power supply (Sigma).

21. Precast 10% polyacrylamide gels (Novex).
22. Running and transfer buffers (Novex).
23. Antibodies to DAT and VMAT2 (Chemicon, Temecula, CA).
24. MPTP (Sigma).
25. Water baths (37°C and 42°C; Fisher Scientific).
26. 37°C shaking incubator (Series 25 Incubator/Shaker; New Brunswick Scientific, Edison, NJ).
27. 37°C incubator for bacterial plates (Fisher Scientific).
28. Poly(A)Pure isolation kit (Ambion, Austin, TX).
29. Retroscript cDNA synthesis kit (Ambion).
30. Thermocycler (MJ Research, Waltham, MA) (*see* **Note 1**).
31. Electroporator (Gene Pulser 165-207; Bio-Rad, Hercules, CA).

3. Methods

3.1. Generation of Mutant Mice

3.1.1. Construction of Vectors

Two regions of homology must be isolated that flank the site targeted for disruption. The neomycin cassette is located between the two regions such that upon homologous recombination, the neomycin cassette will replace the genomic DNA residing between the two regions of homology (deletion-type mutation) (**Fig. 1** and *see* **Note 2**).

1. Isolate fragments from genomic DNA by excising regions of homology using restriction digestion.
2. Run digest on agarose gel, remove band of interest with razor blade, and isolate and purify using Qiaex II gel extraction kit.
3. Ligate first insert DNA fragment into pPNT (linearized with compatible enzymes) with T4 ligase for 12 h at 14°C.
4. Transform ligation reaction into competent cells according to the manufacturer's instructions. Be sure that the water bath for heat shock is precisely 42°C and plate the reaction onto ampicillin treated Luria Bertani culture medium (LB)-agar plates.
5. After incubation at 37°C overnight, pick colonies with toothpicks and incubate in 2 mL ampicillin-treated LB overnight in 37°C shaking incubator.
6. Isolate plasmid DNA using the Qiagen Miniprep kit.
7. Screen for insert DNA by restriction digest or by PCR (*see* **Note 1**).
8. Repeat **steps 3–7** for second insert.
9. We recommend confirming proper insertion of DNA by sequencing.
10. Electroporate purified knockout construct into ES cells (modified for DAT or VMAT2 gene disruption) (*see* **Note 2**).
11. Use positive selection with 400 μg/mL G418 to kill colonies not containing the Neo cassette and negative selection with 5 μg/mL ganciclovir to kill colonies containing the TK insert in DMEM for 10 d (*see* **Note 3**).

12. Edge-scrape surviving clones for three-primer PCR analysis using a Neomycin primer and genomic primers specific to either the DAT or VMAT2 wild-type and mutant alleles (*see* **Note 1**).
13. Expand positive clones and confirm genotypes by Southern blot analysis with high salt purified DNA using a probe external to the 3' end of the KO site.
14. Microinject positive undifferentiated clones individually into C57BL/6 blastocysts and transfer to pseudopregnant females (*see* **Note 2**).
15. Allow chimeric males (identified by agouti coat color) to breed with wild-type C57 mice.
16. Test offsrping for germline transmission by PCR-based genotyping (*see* **Note 1**). Remove a small (0.5-cm) portion of the tail from the mouse. Isolate genomic DNA by incubating the tail sample in 600 μL TNES buffer and 17.5 μL proteinase K solution at 42°C until tissue is completely dissolved.
17. Add 167 μL saturated NaCl, vortex, and centrifuge at 10,000*g* for 10 min.
18. Transfer supernatant to a new tube. Add 800 μL 95% ethanol, invert several times, and centrifuge at 10,000*g* for 15 min at 4°C.
19. Pour off supernatant, being careful not to remove DNA pellet. Rinse with 1 mL 75% ethanol, vortex, and centrifuge at 10,000*g* for 5 min at 4°C.
20. Remove supernatant and allow pellet to dry for 15 min at room temperature. Resuspend the pellet in 200 μL water. Let sit for 30 min at room temperature. One microliter of this sample should serve as a sufficient volume for genotyping.
21. Perform multiplexed PCR using the wild-type and knockout primers. Wild-type animals should display the wild-type band, mutant mice the mutant band, and heterozygotes both bands. Be sure to keep track of lineage for all offspring.
22. Establish a breeding colony consisting of F1 and F2 generation mice. It is recommended that a large number of F1 mice be produced (*see* **Note 4**). Breeding of two F1 heterozygotes yields F2 generation wild-type, heterozygote, and homozygote mice. After the chimeric males are no longer able to generate F1, only F2 mice will be available for breeding. The breeding of two heterozygote F2 mice yields F3 generation animals. Note that the steps in **Subheading 3.2.** should be performed as rapidly as possible to gauge the need for animals. If there is no phenotype, the need for animals is likely to be diminished. The growth of the colony should be coordinated with the phenotypic characterization.

3.2. Phenotypic Characterization of Mice

1. Perform Southern blot analysis on genomic DNA isolated from tail (**Fig. 3**).
2. Confirm deletion of message by reverse transcription (RT)-PCR. Isolate mRNA (Poly[A]Pure kit) from the brain region thought to be enriched in the gene of interest (e.g., midbrain). Generate cDNA using Retroscript or a similar kit. Perform PCR using primers located within the coding region of either DAT or VMAT2 cDNA.
3. To confirm that the protein of interest is reduced (heterozygote) or absent (homozygote knockout) perform Western blotting (*see* Chapter 12).
4. To confirm the functional absence of the protein, pharmacological studies can also be used. We performed binding and uptake assays on striatal tissue from the DAT and VMAT2 knockout mice ***(1,3,13)***.

3.3. Analysis of MPTP Susceptibility

1. MPTP should be dissolved in saline at a final concentration adjusted to inject in a volume of 10 mL/kg.
2. Twice a day (10 h apart), MPTP should be administered (s.c. injections) at 7.5, 15, and 30 mg/kg (total dose 15, 30, or 60 mg/kg, respectively) or vehicle (0.9% NaCl).
3. Two and 7 d following MPTP injection, dissect striata, place one in liquid nitrogen for subsequent processing by HPLC-electrochemical (EC) and the other into homogenization buffer for analysis by Western blotting.
4. For Western blotting, there are many excellent markers of the dopamine system, such as DAT, tyrosine hydroxylase, VMAT2, or dopamine receptors (*see* Chapter 12).
5. Perform HPLC-EC analysis of dopamine, 3,4-dihydroxyphenylacetic acid (DOPAC) and homovanillic acid (HVA) using HPLC with electrochemical detection as previously described ***(12)*** (*see* **Note 5**).
6. On a separate group of animals, analyze glial fibrillary acidic protein (GFAP) expression (a marker of gliosis) by Northern blotting.
7. Isolate mRNA as described above.
8. Perform Northern blotting (50 µg/lane) as previously described ***(15)*** using a pGEM-4 plasmid containing a 216-bp fragment of mouse GFAP.
9. Use a pTRIPLEscript™ vector (Ambion) containing a 115-bp fragment complementary to 28S rRNA as template for in vitro transcription with T7 polymerase.
10. Perform quantitative analysis of Northern blots using phosphorimaging plates and a phosphoimager (Molecular Dynamics Phosphorimager, Sunnyale, CA; and ImageQuant 3.3 software).
11. Confirm equal loading of samples by reprobing the blot for 28S mRNA. Results from GFAP studies can be found in **refs. *12*** and ***13***.

4. Notes

1. For a lab working with only one or two different strains of mice with a moderate amount of cloning, one thermocycler will usually suffice. If more than three lines are being genotyped, additional thermocyclers may be needed. Most manufacturers' units come with a standard 96-well block, which is often more than sufficient for genotyping a few litters. Many companies offer dual blocks (2 × 48) that allow two different programs to be run simultaneously. This is an excellent solution for labs running different PCR reactions. Some newer machines have gone back to the days of capillary tube reactions, but combined with forced air convection these systems can complete 30 cycles of PCR in under 15 min (Rapid Cycler, Idaho Technologies; Light Cycler, Roche). The PCR protocols for these capillary-based machines need to be adapted and optimized for each specific reaction (and setup takes longer), but once they are, the time savings can be significant. Most of the current literature on PCR is based on the heating block and microfuge tube design, which tends to be more reliable. If adaptability is required, look for a thermocycler with interchangeable blocks that permit various types of tubes or slides to be run on the same machine.

2. The design of the knockout construct is perhaps the most challenging part of making a knockout animal and is difficult to explain in a single chapter. Proper design necessitates expertise in molecular biology. However, many of the subsequent steps are relatively straightforward, and we have focused on these. Since the steps from electroporation into ES cells to blastocyst injection are routinely done in a core facility, the methods are intentionally brief. Most universities support such facilities. The amount of effort necessary to perform these procedures by an individual lab is daunting, and such performance is not encouraged ***(16)***. If such facilities are unavailable, it is recommended that one establish a collaboration with an investigator who has access to such a facility. We highly recommend that you submit as pure a sample of DNA as possible to your core facility for electroporation of ES cells. (Cesium chloride gradients generate samples significantly more pure than many kits).

   There are numerous different types of ES cells. The user should be aware of the derivation of the cell lines to be used ***(17)***.
3. Successful integration of the Neomycin resistance gene is determined by the ability of the cells to survive in the antibiotic G418. To confirm targeted homologous recombination, cells are grown in ganciclovir to determine whether the TK gene is absent. The TK gene is located outside the regions of homology. If homologous recombination has occurred, the TK gene will not be inserted. If the TK gene is present, indicating a heterologous recombination event, ganciclovir will kill the cell. This is only one example of the use of positive and negative selection—many other strategies utilize the Neo and TK cassettes for a variety of constructs.
4. The organization of breeding colonies is an often overlooked area in some labs. When working with one transgenic line, it is relatively easy to keep track of the breeding, weaning, and genotyping; however, as additional lines are added, the numbers of mice become cumbersome. A recent review details many of the concerns in establishing transgenic colonies ***(18)***.

   The genetic background on which null mutant and transgenic mice are created is of utmost importance ***(19)***. Most commonly, ES cells from 129/SvJ are injected into C57BL blastocysts to create a chimeric offspring. These chimeras are then bred with pure C57BL blacks. The F1 generation (chimera to pure C57BL) has 50% 129 and 50% C57BL. Crossing of two F1s creates F2 offspring with an unpredictable genetic background. Backcrossing into the pure strain can reduce the representation of a particular genotype, but even after ten backcrossings there remains a small, yet potentially significant amount of DNA from the original breeding. More investigators are examining how to determine whether the resulting behavior and physiologic characteristics are due to the different genetic backgrounds or the specific mutation. For example, some labs are looking into production of knockout mice on pure genetic backgrounds or backcrossing onto a variety of genetic backgrounds. Some of these procedures are costly; however, considering recent concerns about the assessment of mouse behavior, they may be warranted ***(20)***.

5. To perform HPLC, Northern blotting, and Western blotting, we utilize two sets of animals. One group is processed for HPLC and RNA work and the other for HPLC and protein work. Some companies advertise systems that allow simultaneous isolation of RNA and protein, although we have not had success with these procedures.

References

1. Wang, Y. M., Gainetdinov, R. R., Fumagalli, F., Xu, F., Jones, S. R., Bock, C. B., et al. (1997) Knockout of the vesicular monoamine transporter 2 gene results in neonatal death and supersensitivity to cocaine and amphetamine. *Neuron* **19,** 1285–1296.
2. Takahashi, N., Miner, L. L., Sora, I., Ujike, H., Revay, R. S., Kostic, V., et al. (1997) VMAT2 knockout mice: heterozygotes display reduced amphetamine-conditioned reward, enhanced amphetamine locomotion, and enhanced MPTP toxicity. *Proc. Natl. Acad. Sci. USA* **94,** 9938–9943.
3. Giros, B., Jaber, M., Jones, S. R., Wightman, R. M., and Caron, M. G. (1996) Hyperlocomotion and indifference to cocaine and amphetamine in mice lacking the dopamine transporter. *Nature* **379,** 606–612.
4. Fon, E. A., Pothos, E. N., Sun, B. C., Killeen, N., Sulzer, D., and Edwards, R. H. (1997) Vesicular transport regulates monoamine storage and release but is not essential for amphetamine action. *Neuron* **19,** 1271–1283.
5. Sora, I., Wichems, C., Takahashi, N., Li, X. F., Zeng, Z., Revay, R., et al. (1998) Cocaine reward models: conditioned place preference can be established in dopamine- and in serotonin-transporter knockout mice. *Proc. Natl. Acad. Sci. USA* **95,** 7699–7704.
6. Miller, G. W., Staley, J. K., Heilman, C. J., Perez, J. T., Mash, D. C., Rye, D. B., et al. (1997) Immunochemical analysis of dopamine transporter protein in Parkinson's disease. *Ann. Neurol.* **41,** 530–539.
7. Yelin, R. and Schuldiner, S. (1995) The pharmacological profile of the vesicular monoamine transporter resembles that of multidrug transporters. *FEBS Lett.* **377,** 201–207.
8. Liu, Y., Peter, D., Roghani, A., Schuldiner, S., Prive, G. G., Eisenberg, D., et al. (1992) A cDNA that suppresses MPP^+ toxicity encodes a vesicular amine transporter. *Cell* **70,** 539–551.
9. Miller, G. W., Erickson, J. D., Perez, J. T., Penland, S. N., Mash, D. C., Rye, D. B., et al. (1999) Immunochemical analysis of vesicular monoamine transporter (VMAT2) protein in Parkinson's disease. *Exp. Neurol.* **154,** 138–148.
10. Miller, G. W., Gainetdinov, R. R., Levey, A. I., and Caron, M. G. (1999) Dopamine transporters and neuronal injury. *Trends Pharmacol. Sci.* **20,** 424–429.
11. Bezard, E., Gross, C. E., Fournier, M. C., Dovero, S., Bloch, B., and Jaber, M. (1999) Absence of MPTP-induced neuronal death in mice lacking the dopamine transporter. *Exp. Neurol.* **155,** 268–273.
12. Gainetdinov, R. R., Fumagalli, F., Jones, S. R., and Caron, M. G. (1997) Dopamine transporter is required for in vivo MPTP neurotoxicity: evidence from mice lacking the transporter. *J. Neurochem.* **69,** 1322–1325.

13. Gainetdinov, R. R., Fumagalli, F., Wang, Y. M., Jones, S. R., Levey, A. I., Miller, G. W., et al. (1998) Increased MPTP neurotoxicity in vesicular monoamine transporter 2 heterozygote knockout mice. *J. Neurochem.* **70,** 1973–1978.
14. Tybulewicz, V. L., Crawford, C. E., Jackson, P. K., Bronson, R. T., and Mulligan, R. C. (1991) Neonatal lethality and lymphopenia in mice with a homozygous disruption of the c-abl proto-oncogene. *Cell* **65,** 1153–1163.
15. Fumagalli, F., Jones, S. R., Caron, M. G., Seidler, F. J., and Slotkin, T. A. (1996) Expression of mRNA coding for the serotonin transporter in aged vs. young rat brain: differential effects of glucocorticoids. *Brain Res.* **719,** 225–228.
16. Hogan, B., Beddington, R., Costantini, F., and Lacy, E. (1994) *Manipulating the Mouse Embryo: A Laboratory Manual.* Cold Spring Harbor Laboratory Press, Cold Spring Harbor, NY.
17. Simpson, E. M., Linder, C. C., Sargent, E. E., Davisson, M. T., Mobraaten, L. E., and Sharp, J. J. (1997) Genetic variation among 129 substrains and its importance for targeted mutagenesis in mice. *Nat. Genet.* **16,** 19–27.
18. Lake, J. P., Haines, D., Linder, C., and Davisson, M. (1999) Dollars and sense: time and cost factors critical to establishing genetically engineered mouse colonies. *Nature Transgenic Rodents* 8–14.
19. Banbury Conference. (1997) Mutant mice and neuroscience: recommendations concerning genetic background. Banbury Conference on Genetic Background in Mice [see comments]. *Neuron* **19,** 755–759.
20. Crabbe, J. C., Wahlsten, D., and Dudek, B. C. (1999) Genetics of mouse behavior: interactions with laboratory environment. *Science* **284,** 1670–1672.

14

Transcription Mechanisms for Dopamine Receptor Genes

Sang-Hyeon Lee and M. Maral Mouradian

1. Introduction

Transcription regulation is a complex but key control mechanism that underlies differential gene expression during development and in the adult organism. Like all protein coding genes, those encoding dopamine receptors are subject to this form of regulation as well. Modifications in dopamine receptors have been implicated in a number of neurobehavioral disorders, including Parkinson's disease and schizophrenia, as well as in the complications of their long-term therapy ***(1–5)***. Based on clinical pharmacologic observations in parkinsonian and schizophrenic patients, the D_2 dopamine receptor has traditionally been thought to be the main mediator of the motor and behavioral effects of dopamine ***(1,6)***. More recent molecular and neurophysiologic advances, in addition to the availability of receptor-selective pharmacologic agents, have clarified the importance of the D_1 class of dopamine receptors as well ***(7,8)***. The D_{1A} dopamine receptor is one of two dopamine receptors abundantly expressed in the striatum ***(9)***, suggesting that it has a critical role in transmitting the nigrostriatal dopaminergic signal resulting in normal motor function. In the prefrontal cortex, the D_{1A} receptor is more abundantly expressed than the D_2 receptor ***(10)*** and has been shown to modulate memory ***(11)***.

Based on these observations, elucidation of the molecular mechanisms controlling the expression of the D_{1A} dopamine receptor gene is important in our understanding of perturbations in dopaminergic transmission and our therapeutic efforts to modulate this system. To study transcription control of the D_{1A} gene, the 5'-flanking region of the gene was cloned and characterized ***(12,13)***. This gene has a short noncoding exon 1 of about 450 bp, a 116-bp

From: *Methods in Molecular Medicine, vol. 62: Parkinson's Disease: Methods and Protocols*
Edited by: M. M. Mouradian © Humana Press Inc., Totowa, NJ

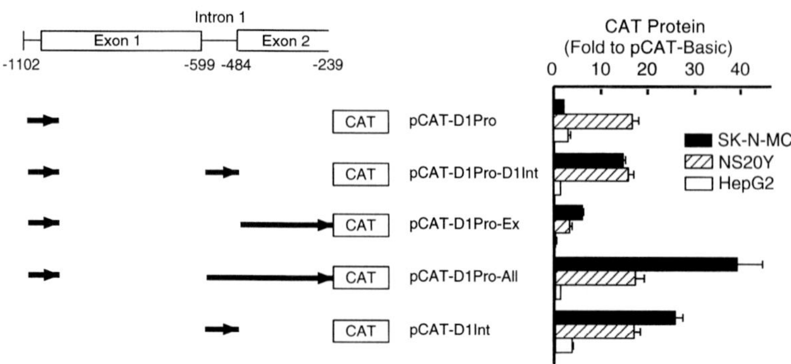

Fig. 1. Transient expression analyses of several CAT constructs of the human D_{1A} dopamine receptor gene. CAT expression plasmids were generated by inserting D1Pro (the upstream promoter region), D1Int (the intron promoter region), Ex (the 5'-end of exon 2), and/or All (the intron combined with the 5'-end of exon 2) into the promoterless plasmid pCAT-Basic.

intron, and a long coding exon 2 (**Fig. 1**). Thus, the 5'-noncoding region of the D_{1A} gene is about 920 bp long. The D_{1A} gene in humans and rats is transcribed from two distinct promoters, one located immediately upstream of exon 1 and another located in the single intron of this gene ***(12–15)***. The upstream promoter is active only in neuronal cells, whereas the intron promoter is active in both neuronal and renal cells. Thus, the kidney expresses only short D_{1A} transcripts lacking exon 1 ***(15)***.

In this chapter, practical methods to study transcription control mechanisms for D_{1A} dopamine receptor gene are discussed as a model for transcription studies for other genes relevant to Parkinson's disease. Promoter activity using the chloramphenicol acetyltransferase (CAT) reporter system as well as confirmation of transcription start sites using the ribonuclease protection assay (RPA) and primer extension are presented.

2. Materials

2.1. Transient Expression Assays

2.1.1. Cells for Study

See **Note 1**. All cell lines are cultured at 37°C in a humidified, 10% CO_2 incubator.

1. Human neuroblastoma cell line SK-N-MC (ATCC no.: HTB-10). Culture medium: 90% minimum essential medium with 2 m*M* *L*-glutamine and Earle's balanced salt solution adjusted to contain 1.5 g/L sodium bicarbonate, 0.1 m*M* nonessential amino acids, and 1.0 m*M* sodium pyruvate, 10% fetal bovine serum.

2. Murine neuroblastoma cell line NS20Y (*see* **Note 2**). Culture medium: 90% Dulbecco's modified Eagle's medium, 10% fetal bovine serum.
3. Human hepatoma cell line HepG2 (ATCC no.: HB-8065). Culture medium: 90% Dulbecco's modified Eagle's medium, 10% fetal bovine serum.

2.1.2. Oligonucleotide Primers

All nucleotide numbers are relative to the first ATG codon (*see* **Fig. 1**) ***(14)***.

2.1.2.1. D_{1A} Upstream Promoter

For the human D_{1A} upstream promoter region (D1Pro, 140 bp long, nucleotides –1102 to –963).

1. Sense: Primer PP-1, 5'-CCCCAAGCTTCCGCGGAACCCCGCCGGCC-3' (inserted *Hin*dIII site underlined).
2. Antisense primer: PP-2, 5'-AACTGCAGCTCGGGCGGCCTTCAGCCCT-3' (inserted *Pst*I site underlined).

2.1.2.2. D_{1A} Intron Promoter

For the human D_{1A} intron promoter region (D1Int, 116 bp long, nucleotides –599 to –484).

1. Sense: PP-3, 5'-AACTGCAGGGATCCGTAGGTGGCTCGGACGGGCT-3' (inserted *Pst*I site underlined).
2. Antisense: PP-4, 5'-GCTCTAGACTTAAAAAGCAAAAGGAAAA-3' (inserted *Xba*I site underlined).

2.1.2.3. Exon 2

For the 5'-end of exon 2 (Ex, 246 bp long, nucleotides –484 to –239).

1. Sense: PP-5, 5'-AACTGCAGGGATCCGCGTTTGGAGAGCTGCTGAG-3' (inserted *Pst*I site underlined)
2. Antisense: PP-6, 5'-GCTCTAGATGCAGGTCACTGTCTTGGGCA-3' (inserted *Xba*I site underlined).

2.1.2.4. Exon 2 and Intron

For the intron combined with the 5'-end of exon 2 (All, 361 bp long, nucleotides –599 to –239).

1. Sense: PP-3.
2. Antisense: PP-6.

2.1.3. PCR Reactions

1. Template DNA (5 ng/μL): pCATD1-1102 (*see* **Note 3**).
2. 10 m*M* dNTP mix: PCR Nucleotide Mix (Boehringer Mannheim).

4. 10X *Taq* reaction buffer: 500 m*M* KCl, 100 m*M* Tris-HCl buffer, pH 8.3, 15 m*M* $MgCl_2$ (Boehringer Mannheim).
5. *Taq* DNA polymerase (5 U/μL; Boehringer Mannheim).
6. Mineral oil.

2.1.4. Analysis of PCR Products

1. Agarose.
2. 10X Tris borate EDTA (TBE) buffer: 108 g Tris base, 55 g boric acid, and 7.5 g EDTA. Make up with ddH_2O to 1 L and autoclave. Store at room temperature.
3. 10X DNA loading dye: 0.5% bromophenol blue, 0.5% xylene cyanol, and 60% glycerol in ddH_2O.
4. Ethidium bromide (10 mg/mL stock).

2.1.5. Phenol/Chloroform/Isoamyl Alcohol Extraction

1. Phenol/chloroform/isoamyl alcohol solution (25:24:1): 25 mL 0.1 *M* Tris-HCl (pH 8.0), buffer-saturated phenol, 24 mL chloroform, 1 mL isoamyl alcohol.
2. Glycogen (DNase-, and RNase-free, Boehringer Mannheim).
3. 5 *M* lithium chloride (LiCl).
4. 95% and 70% ethanol.
5. TE buffer: 10 m*M* Tris-HCl, pH 7.5, 1 m*M* EDTA, pH 8.0. Autoclave and store at room temperature.

2.1.6. Restriction Enzyme Digestions and Dephosphorylation

1. pCAT-Basic plasmid (Promega).
2. *Hin*dIII (10 U/μL), *Pst*I (10 U/μL), and *Xba*I (10 U/μL) (all from Boehringer Mannheim).
3. 10X restriction enzyme B buffer for *Hin*dIII: 100 m*M* Tris-HC, pH 7.5, 50 m*M* $MgCl_2$, 1 *M* NaCl, and 2-mercaptoethanol.
4. 10X restriction enzyme H buffer for *Pst*I, and *Xba*I: 500 m*M* Tris-HCl, pH 7.5, 100 m*M* $MgCl_2$, 1 *M* NaCl, and 10 m*M* dithioerythritol (DTE).
5. Bacterial alkaline phosphatase (BAP) (150 U/μL; Life Technologies).
6. 10X dephosphorylation buffer: 100 m*M* Tris-HCl, pH 8.0.

2.1.7. Ligation

1. T4 DNA ligase (1 U/μL) (Boehringer Mannheim).
2. 10X ligase buffer: 500 m*M* Tris-HCl, pH 7.6, 100 m*M* $MgCl_2$, 10 m*M* DTT, 50% (w/v) polyethylene glycol-8000.
3. 10 m*M* ATP (Boehringer Mannheim).

2.1.8. Transformation

1. *Escherichia coli* strain DH5α.
2. Calcium chloride solution: 50 m*M* $CaCl_2$, 10 m*M* Tris-HCl, pH 8.0. Autoclave and chill on ice.

3. Luria Bertani (LB) medium: 8 g bactotryptone (Difco), 5 g yeast extract (Difco), and 5 g NaCl. Make up with ddH_2O to 1 L and autoclave. Store at room temperature.
4. 1000X ampicillin solution: 50 mg/mL in sterilized ddH_2O. Store at –20°C.
5. LB agar (amp) plate: 8 g bactotryptone (Difco), 5 g yeast extract (Difco), 5 g NaCl, and 1.2 g Bacto agar (Difco). Make up to 1 L and autoclave. Cool to approx 50°C and add 1 mL 1000X ampicillin solution. Pour 25–30 mL of the medium into each Petri dish. After cooling down completely, store at 4°C.

2.1.9. Transfection

1. 1X Phosphate-buffered saline (PBS): 10 m*M* phosphate buffer, pH 7.4, 120 m*M* NaCl, and 2.7 m*M* KCl. Make up with ddH_2O to 1 L and autoclave. Store at 4°C.
2. 2X HEPES-buffered saline (HBS): 11.9 g HEPES acid, 16.4 g NaCl, and 0.21 g Na_2HPO_4. Make up with ddH_2O to 900 mL. Adjust pH to 7.05 with 5 *M* NaOH and then make up to 1 L (*see* **Note 4**). Sterilize by a filter. Make 14-mL aliquots and store at –20°C.
3. 2.5 *M* $CaCl_2$ in ddH_2O; sterilize by a filter.
4. CAT constructs.
5. pCMV-βGal plasmid (Clontech), a β-galactosidase expression plasmid driven by the cytomegalovirus (CMV) promoter.

2.1.10. CAT Assay

1. 1X Tris-EDTA-NaCl (TEN) solution: 40 m*M* Tris-HCl, pH 7.5, 1 m*M* EDTA, and 150 m*M* NaCl in ddH_2O. Store at 4°C.
2. 250 m*M* Tris-HCl, pH 7.8.
3. CAT-ELISA kit (Boehringer Mannheim): CAT proteins produced by the introduced promoter fragments are measured by CAT enzyme-linked immunosorbent assay (ELISA) using a CAT-ELISA kit.
   Kit components:
   a. 1X washing solution (need 3.6 mL/well): dilute 10X washing solution with ddH_2O. Store at 4°C.
   b. Sample buffer: ready-to-use solution. Store aliquots at –20°C.
   c. Anti-CAT-digoxigenin (DIG) stock solution (final concentration: 0.2 mg/mL): Dissolve lyophilized anti-CAT-DIG (100 µg) with 0.5 mL ddH_2O. This can be stored at 4°C for 6 mo.
   d. Anti-CAT-DIG working solution (need 200 µL/well): dilute 100 µL anti-CAT-DIG stock solution with 9.9 mL sample buffer. Make immediately before use.
   e. Anti-DIG-peroxidase (POD) stock solution (final concentration: 20 U/mL): dissolve lyophilized anti-DIG-POD (10 U) with 0.5 mL ddH_2O. This can be stored at 4°C for 6 mo.
   f. Anti-CAT-POD working solution (need 200 µL/well): dilute 75 µL anti-CAT-DIG stock solution with 9.925 mL sample buffer. Make immediately before use.
   g. POD-substrate (need 200 µL/well): ready-to-use solution. Store at 4°C (light-protect).

h. Microtiter plate (MTP)-modules: Anti-CAT-coated; ready-to-use.

2.1.11. β-Galactosidase Activity

1. 100X Mg solution: 0.1 *M* $MgCl_2$ and 4.5 *M* β-mercaptoethanol.
2. 0.1 *M* sodium phosphate, pH 7.5: 41 mL 0.2 *M* $Na_2HPO_4 \cdot 7H_2O$, 9 mL 0.2 *M* $NaH_2PO_4 \cdot H_2O$, and 50 mL ddH_2O.
3. 1X *o*-nitrophenyl-*p*-D-galactopyranoside (ONPG) solution: Dissolve 4 mg of ONPG (Sigma) in 1 mL 0.1 *M* sodium phosphate, pH 7.5, buffer.
4. Stop solution: 1 *M* Na_2CO_3. Store at room temperature.

2.2. Ribonuclease Protection Assay

2.2.1. Preparation of Total RNA From Cells

1. Cultured cells.
2. RNAzol B (Tel Test).
3. Chloroform.
4. Isopropanol.
5. Ice-cold 70% ethanol.
6. Diethylpyrocarbonate (DEPC)-treated water.

2.2.2. Primers for RT-PCR

For a riboprobe that excludes intron 1 (*see* **Fig. 2**) (E1E2, 200 bp long, nucleotides –647 to –599 and –483 to -334).

1. RT: Primer RT1-0, 5'-TCCTGGGCCTCTGCTCTGCT-3'.
2. Sense: RT1-1, 5'-AA<u>CTGCAG</u>GTCCACATTCCAAGCTCCAG-3' (inserted *Pst*I site underlined).
3. Antisense: RT1-2, 5'-GC<u>TCTAGA</u>GGCCTCTGCTCTGCTAGTCA-3' (inserted *Xba*I site underlined).

2.2.3. RT-PCR

1. DEPC-treated water.
2. 5X first strand buffer: 250 m*M* Tris-HCl, pH 8.3, 375 m*M* KCl, and 15 m*M* $MgCl_2$.
3. 0.1 *M* DTT.
4. 10 m*M* dNTP mix: PCR Nucleotide Mix (Boehringer Mannheim).
5. RNase inhibitor (10–50 U/μL; Boehringer Mannheim).
6. SuperScript II RT (200 U/μL; Life Technologies).
7. 10X *Taq* reaction buffer: 500 m*M* KCl, 100 m*M* Tris-HCl, pH 8.3, 15 m*M* $MgCl_2$ (Boehringer Mannheim).
8. *Taq* DNA polymerase (5 U/μL; Boehringer Mannheim).
9. Mineral oil.

2.2.4. Analysis of PCR Products

See **Subheading 2.1.4.**

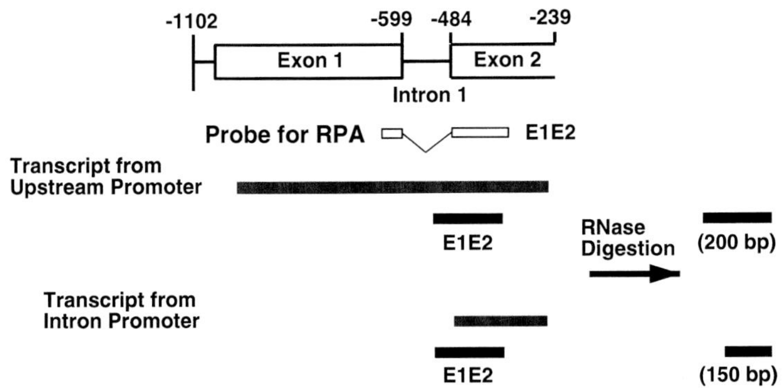

Fig. 2. Design of a riboprobe (E1E2) for RPA. E1E2 was generated using RT-PCR by excluding the intron 1 region of the human D_{1A} dopamine receptor gene. If the probe E1E2 binds to a long transcript driven by the upstream promoter, a 200 bp-long band is protected. On the other hand, if the probe E1E2 binds to a short transcript driven by the intron promoter, a 150 bp-long band is protected.

2.2.5. Phenol/Chloroform/Isoamyl Alcohol Extraction

See **Subheading 2.1.5.**

2.2.6. Restriction Enzyme Digestion and Dephosphorylation

1. pGEM-3Zf(-) (Promega).
2. *Pst*I (10 U/µL) and *Xba*I (10 U/µL) (both from Boehringer Mannheim).
3. 10X restriction enzyme H buffer for *Pst*I, and *Xba*I: 500 m*M* Tris-HCl, pH 7.5, 100 m*M* $MgCl_2$, 1 *M* NaCl, and 10 m*M* DTE.
4. BAP: 150 U/µL (Life Technologies).
5. 10X dephosphorylation buffer: 100 m*M* Tris-HCl, pH 8.0.
6. TE buffer: 10 m*M* Tris-HCl, pH 7.5, 1 m*M* EDTA, pH 8.0. Autoclave and store at room temperature.

2.2.7. Ligation

See **Subheading 2.1.7.**

2.2.8. Transformation

See **Subheading 2.1.8.**

2.2.9. Generating Probe by In Vitro Transcription

2.2.9.1. Linearization of the Probe Construct

1. *Hin*dIII (10 U/µL) (Boehringer Mannheim).
2. 10X restriction enzyme B buffer for *Hin*dIII: 100 m*M* Tris-HCl, pH 7.5, 50 m*M* $MgCl_2$, 1 *M* NaCl, and 2-mercaptoethanol.

3. Phenol/chloroform/isoamyl alcohol solution (25:24:1): 25 mL 0.1 *M* Tris-HCl buffer (pH 8.0)-saturated phenol, 24 mL chloroform, 1 mL isoamyl alcohol.
4. Glycogen (DNase-, RNase-free; Boehringer Mannheim).
5. 5 *M* LiCl.
6. 95% and 70% ethanol.
7. TE buffer: 10 m*M* Tris-HCl, pH 7.5, 1 m*M* EDTA, pH 8.0. Autoclave and store at room temperature.

2.2.9.2. In Vitro Transcription and Purification

1. MAXI script in vitro transcription kit (Ambion) (*see* **Note 5**).
2. [α-^{32}P]CTP (800 Ci/mmol, Amersham).
3. DEPC-treated water.
4. 0.5 *M* EDTA.
5. Nuctrap Push column (Stratagene).
6. Syringe.

2.2.10. Preparation of the Marker DNA

1. ϕX174 *Hin*fI digested DNA (Promega).
2. 10X forward reaction buffer: 700 m*M* Tris-HCl, pH 7.6, 100 m*M* $MgCl_2$, 1 *M* KCl, and 10 m*M* 2-mercaptoethanol.
3. T4 polynucleotide kinase (10 U/µL; Boehringer Mannheim).
4. [γ-^{32}P]ATP (6,000 Ci/mmol; Amersham).
5. 10X DNA loading dye: 0.5% bromophenol blue, 0.5% xylene cyanol, and 60% glycerol in ddH_2O.

2.2.11. Ribonuclease Protection Assay

1. RPA II kit (Ambion) (*see* **Note 5**). Kit components: 5 *M* ammonium acetate, H_2O (DNase and RNase-free), hybridization buffer, yeast RNA (5.0 mg/mL), RNase digestion buffer, RNase A/RNase T1 mix, RNase inactivation/precipitation solution, gel loading buffer.
2. Ice-cold 95% ethanol (*see* **Note 6**).
3. 8% polyacrylamide, urea gel: 20 mL 20% acrylamide urea solution, 30 mL urea mix, 0.4 mL 10% ammonium persulfate, and 50 µL *N,N,N',N'*-tetramethylethylene diamine (TEMED). Mix rapidly and pour into a preformed gel mold.
4. 10X Tris borate buffer (TBE): 108 g Tris base, 55 g boric acid, and 7.5 g EDTA. Make up with ddH_2O to 1 L and autoclave. Store at room temperature.
5. 20% acrylamide urea solution (*see* **Note 7**): 96.5 g acrylamide, 3.35 g *N,N'*-methylene bisacrylamide, 233.5 g ultra-pure urea, 50 mL 10X TBE, ddH_2O to 500 mL.
6. Urea mix: 233.5 g ultra-pure urea, 50 mL 10X TBE, ddH_2O to 500 mL.
7. 10% ammonium persulfate (*see* **Note 8**).
8. TEMED.
9. Gel running buffer: 1X TBE.

2.3. Primer Extension

2.3.1. Primer Labeling

1. Primer PE-1: An oligonucleotide complementary to nucleotides –413 to –384 in exon 2 (5'-TCTGGTGGTGACAGGAGATTCTCCCCTTCT-3') (*see* **Note 9**).
2. 10X forward reaction buffer: 700 m*M* Tris-HCl, pH 7.6, 100 m*M* $MgCl_2$, 1 *M* KCl, and 10 m*M* 2-mercaptoethanol.
3. T4 polynucleotide kinase (10 U/μL; Boehringer Mannheim).
4. [γ-^{32}P]ATP (6000 Ci/mmol; Amersham).
5. Nuclease-free water.
6. Formamide loading dye: 80% formamide, 10 m*M* EDTA, 0.1% xylene cyanol, and 0.1% bromophenol blue.

2.3.2. Preparation of Sequencing Ladder as a Position Marker

1. Template DNA (1–2 μg): pCATD1-1102 (*see* **Note 3**).
2. Primer PE-1 (0.5 pmol/μL).
3. 10 *M* ammonium acetate.
4. Ice-cold 95% and 70% ethanol.
5. [α-^{35}S]dATP (1000 Ci/mmol; Amersham).
6. T7 sequenase 7-deaza-dGTP DNA sequencing kit (USB). Kit components: Sequenase buffer, 0.1 *M* DTT, dNTP mix (0.5 m*M* dATP, 0.5 m*M* dCTP, 0.5 m*M* 7-deaza dGTP, and 0.5 m*M* dTTP [*see* **Note 10**]), dideoxy termination mixtures, stop solution.
7. Sequenase ver 2.0 (1.5 U/μL; USB).

2.3.3. Primer Extension Reaction

1. Total RNA from cells.
2. Labeled primer PE-1.
3. 2X Primer extension buffer: 100 m*M* Tris-HCl, pH 8.3, at 42°C, 100 m*M* KCl, 20 m*M* $MgCl_2$, 20 m*M* DTT, 2 m*M* dNTP mix, and 1 m*M* spermidine.
4. Nuclease-free water.
5. PreMix solution: 5 μL 2X primer extension buffer, 1.4 μL 40 m*M* sodium pyrophosphate, 1 μL avian myeloblastoma virus (AMV) reverse transcriptase (1 U/μL), 1.6 μL nuclease-free water.
6. Formamide loading dye: 80% formamide, 10 m*M* EDTA, 0.1% xylene cyanol, and 0.1% bromophenol blue.

2.3.4. Sequencing Gel Separation

1. 8% Polyacrylamide, urea gel: 20 mL 20% acrylamide urea solution, 30 mL urea mix, 0.4 mL 10% ammonium persulfate, and 50 μL TEMED. Mix rapidly and pour into a preformed sequencing gel mold.
2. 10X Tris borate buffer (TBE): 108 g Tris base, 55 g boric acid, and 7.5 g EDTA. Make up with ddH_2O to 1 L and autoclave. Store at room temperature.

3. 20% Acrylamide urea solution (*see* **Note 7**): 96.5 g acrylamide, 3.35 g *N,N'*-methylene bisacrylamide, 233.5 g ultra-pure urea, 50 mL 10X TBE, ddH_2O to 500 mL.
4. Urea mix: 233.5 g ultra-pure urea, 50 mL 10X TBE, ddH_2O to 500 mL.
5. 10% ammonium persulfate (*see* **Note 8**).
6. TEMED.
7. Gel running buffer: 1X TBE.

3. Methods

3.1. Transient Expression Assays

3.1.1. Preparation of Insert DNA

To elucidate transcription control mechanisms for D_{1A} dopamine receptor gene, human D_{1A} dopamine receptor promoters are cloned by PCR using corresponding primers (*see* **Subheading 2.1.2.2.**) and inserted into CAT reporter plasmids to yield D_{1A} promoter/CAT reporter constructs.

3.1.1.1. PCR Reactions

1. Reaction mixture:

Template DNA (5 ng/µL)	10 µL
10 m*M* dNTP mix	1 µL
Each oligonucleotide primer (10 pmol/µL)	1 µL
10X *Taq* reaction buffer	5 µL
ddH_2O to final volume of 50 µL	
Taq DNA polymerase (5 U/µL)	0.5 µL

   Add 50 µL of mineral oil, if required.
2. Conditions:

Denaturation	95°C	1 min
Annealing	37°C	1 min
Extension	72°C	1 min
[Denaturation	95°C	1 min
Annealing	55°C	1 min
Extension	72°C	1 min] 30 cycles
Extension	72°C	10 min

3.1.1.2. Agarose Gel (2%) Electrophoresis

1. Add 2 g agarose to 10 mL 1X TBE.
2. Boil and cool down to approximately 50°C.
3. Pour the agarose into an appropriate casting tray.
4. After the agarose is solidified, add 1X TBE to the gel tank.
5. Take 5 µL PCR reaction and add 0.5 µL 10X DNA loading dye.
6. Run on the gel and stain in the ethidium bromide solution (0.01% in ddH_2O).
7. Visualize under an ultaviolet (UV) lamp.

3.1.1.3. Phenol/Chloroform/Isoamyl Alcohol Extraction of PCR Products

1. Transfer PCR reaction mixture to a 1.5-mL tube and fill up to 200 μL using TE buffer.
2. Add 200 μL phenol/chloroform/isoamyl alcohol.
3. Vortex vigorously and centrifuge at 10,000*g* for 5 min at 4°C.
4. Transfer upper phase to a new 1.5-mL tube.
5. Add 1 μL glycogen, 20 μL 5 *M* $LiCl_2$ and 500 μL ice-cold 95% ethanol.
6. Place on dry ice for 30 min and then centrifuge at 10,000*g* for 5 min at 4°C.
7. Remove the supernatant and rinse using 1 mL ice-cold 70% ethanol.
8. Dry for 5–10 min under the vacuum and dissolve in 50 μL TE buffer.

3.1.1.4. Restriction Enzyme Digestion of PCR Products

1. Reaction mixture 1:

Treated PCR product	8 μL
10X restriction enzyme buffer	1 μL
Restriction enzyme for one side	1 μL

2. Incubate at 37°C for 1 h and then fill up to 200 μL using TE buffer.
3. Add 200 μL phenol/chloroform/isoamyl alcohol.
4. Vortex vigorously and centrifuge at 10,000*g* for 5 min at 4°C.
5. Transfer upper phase to a new 1.5-mL tube.
6. Add 1 μL glycogen, 20 μL 5 *M* $LiCl_2$, and 500 μL ice-cold 95% ethanol.
7. Place on dry ice for 30 min and then centrifuge at 10,000*g* for 5 min at 4°C.
8. Remove the supernatant and rinse using 1 mL ice-cold 70% ethanol.
9. Dry for 5–10 min under the vacuum and dissolve in 8 μL TE buffer.
10. Reaction mixture 2:

One side digested PCR product	8 μL
10X restriction enzyme buffer	1 μL
Restriction enzyme for the other side	1 μL

11. Incubate at 37°C for 1 h and then fill up to 200 μL using TE buffer.
12. Add 200 μL phenol/chloroform/isoamyl alcohol.
13. Vortex vigorously and centrifuge at 10,000*g* for 5 min at 4°C.
14. Transfer upper phase to a new 1.5-mL tube.
15. Add 1 μL glycogen, 20 μL 5 *M* $LiCl_2$, and 500 μL ice-cold 95% ethanol.
16. Place on dry ice for 30 min and then centrifuge at 10,000*g* for 5 min at 4°C.
17. Remove the supernatant and rinse using 1 mL ice-cold 70% ethanol.
18. Dry for 5–10 min under the vacuum and dissolve in 10 μL TE buffer.

3.1.2 Preparation of Vector DNA

3.1.2.1. Restriction Digestion of Vector DNA

1. Reaction mixture 1:

Vector DNA (pCAT-Basic, 0.2 μg/μL)	7 μL
10X restriction enzyme buffer	1 μL
Restriction enzyme for one side	1 μL

2. Incubate at 37°C for 1 h and then fill up to 200 μL using TE buffer.
3. Add 200 μL phenol/chloroform/isoamyl alcohol.
4. Vortex vigorously and centrifuge at 10,000*g* for 5 min at 4°C.
5. Transfer upper phase to a new 1.5-mL tube.
6. Add 1 μL glycogen, 20 μL 5 *M* $LiCl_2$, and 500 μL ice-cold 95% ethanol.
7. Place on dry ice for 30 min and then centrifuge at 10,000*g* for 5 min at 4°C.
8. Remove the supernatant and rinse using 1 mL ice-cold 70% ethanol.
9. Dry for 5–10 min under the vacuum and dissolve in 8 μL TE buffer.
10. Reaction mixture 2:

One side digested vector DNA	8 μL
10X restriction enzyme buffer	1 μL
Restriction enzyme for another side	1 μL

11. Incubate at 37°C for 1 h.

3.1.2.2. Dephosphorylation of Digested Vector DNA

1. Reaction mixture:

Digested DNA mixture	10 μL
10X dephosphorylation buffer	10 μL
BAP (150 U/μL)	1 μL
ddH_2O to final volume of 100 μL	

2. Incubate at 60°C for 1 h and then fill out to 200 μL using TE buffer.
3. Add 200 μL phenol/chloroform/isoamyl alcohol.
4. Vortex vigorously and centrifuge at 10,000*g* for 5 min at 4°C.
5. Transfer upper phase to a new 1.5-mL tube.
6. Repeat **steps 3–5**.
7. Add 1 μL glycogen, 20 μL 5 *M* $LiCl_2$, and 500 μL ice-cold 95% ethanol.
8. Place on dry ice for 30 min and then centrifuge at 10,000*g* for 5 min at 4°C.
9. Remove the supernatant and rinse using 1 mL of ice-cold 70% ethanol.
10. Dry for 5–10 min under the vacuum and dissolve in 10 μL TE buffer.

3.1.3. Ligation of DNA

1. Reaction mixture:

Insert DNA	5 μL
Vector DNA	2 μL
10X ligase buffer	1 μL

2. Incubate at 55°C for 5 min.
3. Add 1 μL 10 m*M* ATP and 1 μL T4 DNA ligase (1 U/μL).
4. Incubate at 16°C for 1 h to overnight.

3.1.4. Preparation of Competent Bacterial Cells

1. Inoculate 1 mL of an overnight culture of DH5α cells to 100 mL LB medium.
2. Incubate at 37°C for 2–4 h with shaking.
3. When an optimal density of cells at 660 nm is reached to 0.5–0.6, chill the culture on ice for 5–10 min.
4. Centrifuge the cells at 4000*g* for 5 min at 4°C.

5. Discard the supernatant and resuspend the cells in 50 mL ice-cold calcium chloride solution.
6. Place the cell suspension on ice for 15 min and then centrifuge at 4000*g* for 5 min at 4°C.
7. Discard the supernatant and resuspend the cells in 3 mL ice-cold calcium chloride solution.
8. Store the cells on ice.

3.1.5. Transformation of Ligated DNA

1. Add 5 µL ligated DNA to 50 µL competent cells.
2. Place on ice for 30 min.
3. Give heat shock at 42°C for 30 s.
4. Place immediately back on ice to chill the cells.
5. Add 1 mL LB medium and incubate at 37°C for 1 h with shaking.
6. Centrifuge at 10,000*g* for 5 s and remove 4/5 volume of the supernatant.
7. Resuspend the pellet and spread on an LB agar (amp) plate.
8. Incubate at 37°C overnight.

All CAT constructs should be checked by restriction enzyme digestion and partial sequencing.

3.1.6. Transient Transfections of Cells

See **ref. *16*.**

3.1.6.1. Preparation of Cells

1. Split cells in a 100-mm culture dish with the appropriate media.
2. Incubate the cells in a 10% CO_2 incubator at 37°C for 1–3 d.
3. When the cells are 80% confluent, remove media and wash the cells twice with 5 mL each of 1X PBS.
4. Add 9 mL of the appropriate fresh medium and incubate in a 4% CO_2 incubator at 37°C for 2 h (*see* **Note 11**).

3.1.6.2. Preparation of DNA Precipitates

Several methods to introduce DNA into mammalian cells were tried, but the conventional calcium phosphate transfection method was found to be optimal for these experiments. All plasmids used in transfections were purified by the Plasmid Maxi Kit (Qiagen) according to the supplier's manual. The following instructions are for three dishes.

1. Solution A: 1.5 mL 2X HBS, prepared in a 15-mL conical tube.
2. Solution B:

CAT construct (1 µg/µL)	15 µL
pCMV-βGAL (1 µg/µL)	6 µL
ddH_2O	1329 µL
2.5 *M* $CaCl_2$	150 µL

3. Solution A: Make bubbles using an air pipet. Solution B: Drop slowly into solution A.
4. Vortex for 5 s.
5. Place at room temperature for 20 min.
6. Vortex for 20 s.

3.1.6.3. Transfections

1. Add 1 mL of suspension to each dish prepared in **Subheading 3.1.2.1.**
2. Gently agitate the dish to mix precipitate and medium.
3. Incubate the cells at 37°C in a 4% CO_2 incubator for 4 (NS20Y and OK) or 16 (SK-N-MC, HepG2) h.
4. Remove media and wash the cells twice with 5 mL each of 1X PBS.
5. Add 10 mL of appropriate fresh medium.
6. Incubate the cells at 37°C in a 10% CO_2 incubator for 48 h.

3.1.7. CAT Assay

3.1.7.1. Preparation of Cell Extracts

1. Discard medium and wash the cells twice with 5 mL each of 1X PBS.
2. Add 1.5 mL of 1X PBS to each dish and scrape the cells.
3. Transfer the cells to 2-mL tubes and centrifuge at 3000*g* for 2 min at 4°C.
4. Discard the supernatant and add 1 mL 1X TEN solution.
5. Resuspend the cells and centrifuge at 3000*g* for 2 min at 4°C.
6. Repeat **steps 4** and **5**.
7. Discard the supernatant and add 0.4 mL 1X TEN solution.
8. Resuspend the cells and centrifuge them at 3000*g* for 2 min at 4°C.
9. Suck out the supernatant completely.
10. Add 0.23 mL 250 m*M* Tris-HCl buffer, pH 7.8, and resuspend the cells.
11. Freeze tubes on dry ice for 5 min and thaw at 37°C for 5 min.
12. Repeat **step 11** for three more times.
13. Centrifuge the tubes at 10,000*g* for 5 min at 4°C and transfer the supernatants to the new tubes.

3.1.7.2. CAT-ELISA

1. Take 0.2 mL of each cell lysate and put in each well of MTP-modules.
2. Cover the MTP-modules and incubate the plates at 37°C for 1–2 h.
3. Discard the solution and tap MTP-modules.
4. Wash each well five times with 0.25 mL 1X washing solution (*see* **Note 12**).
5. Discard the solution and tap MTP-modules.
6. Add 0.2 mL anti-CAT-DIG working solution to each well.
7. Cover MTP-modules and incubate them at 37°C for 1 h.
8. Discard the solution and tap MTP-modules.
9. Wash each well five times with 0.25 mL 1X washing solution (*see* **Note 12**).
10. Discard the solution and tap MTP-modules.
11. Add 0.2 mL anti-DIG-POD working solution to each well.

12. Cover MTP-modules and incubate them at 37°C for 1 h.
13. Discard the solution and tap MTP-modules.
14. Wash each well five times with 0.25 mL 1X washing solution (*see* **Note 12**).
15. Discard the solution and tap MTP-modules.
16. Add 0.2 mL POD-substrate solution to each well.
17. Cover MTP-modules and incubate them at room temperate until positive samples show a green color.
18. Measure the intensity of colors using a microplate reader at 405 nm.

3.1.7.3. Measurement of β-Galactosidase Activity

All CAT data are normalized by β-galactosidase activity ***(17)***. Dilute cell extracts with 0.1 *M* sodium phosphate buffer, pH 7.5, (0.25 g total protein/µL).

1. Reaction mixture:

100X Mg solution	3 µL
1X ONPG solution	66 µL
0.1 *M* sodium phosphate buffer, pH 7.5	201 µL
Cell extract	30 µL

2. Incubate the mixture at 37°C for up to 100 min.
3. Add 0.5 mL 1 *M* Na_2CO_3 to stop the reaction.
4. Measure color intensity using a spectrophotometer at 420 nm.

3.2. Ribonuclease Protection Assay

3.2.1. Preparation of Total RNA from Cultured Cells

1. Harvest cells from 100-mm culture dishes to 2-mL tubes.
2. Add 1.8 mL RNAzol B and suspend the cells by vortexing (*see* **Note 13**).
3. Add 0.18 mL chloroform per 1.8 mL homogenate.
4. Shake vigorously for 15 s and place on ice for 5 min.
5. Centrifuge at 10,000*g* for 15 min at 4°C.
6. Transfer the upper layer (0.8 mL) to a fresh tube.
7. Add equal volume (0.8 mL) of isopropanol and place on ice for 15 min.
8. Centrifuge at 10,000*g* for 15 min at 4°C.
9. Remove the supernatant and add 1.6 mL 70% ice-cold ethanol.
10. Vortex for 30 s.
11. Centrifuge at 10,000*g* for 8 min at 4°C.
12. Discard the supernatant and dry for 10 min under the vacuum.
13. Dissolve in 10 µL DEPC-treated water.

3.2.2. Preparation of the Probe Insert by RT-PCR

3.2.2.1. RNA Denaturing

1. Reaction mixture:

Total RNA	1 µg
RT primer (10 pmol/mL)	1 µL

DEPC-treated water to a final volume of 10 mL

2. Incubate at 70°C for 10 min and then place on ice for 5 min.

3.2.2.2. RT Reaction

1. Reaction mixture:

Denatured RNA mix	10 µL
5X first strand buffer	4 µL
0.1 *M* DTT	2 µL
10 m*M* dNTP	1 µL
RNase inhibitor	0.2 µL
SuperScript II RT (200 U/µL)	0.5 µL
DEPC-treated water	2.3 µL

2. Incubate at 42°C for 1 h.
3. Incubate at 95°C for 10 min to denature RT.

3.2.2.3. PCR Reaction

1. Reaction mixture:

RT reaction solution	20 µL
10X *Taq* DNA polymerase buffer	5 µL
10 m*M* dNTP	1 µL
PCR primers (10 pmol/mL)	1 µL each
Taq DNA polymerase (5 U/µL)	0.5 µL
ddH_2O	21.5 µL

   Add 50 µL of mineral oil, if required.
2. Conditions: *see* **Subheading 3.1.1.1.** *(2)*.

All PCR products are electrophoresed on 2% agarose gel and visualized by ethidium bromide staining and UV light (*see* **Subheading 3.1.1.2.**).

3.2.2.4. Phenol/Chloroform/Isoamyl Alcohol Extraction of PCR Products

See **Subheading 3.1.1.3.**

3.2.2.5. Restriction Enzyme Digestion of PCR Products

1. Reaction mixture:

Extracted PCR product	7 µL
10X restriction enzyme H buffer	1 µL
*Pst*I	1 µL
*Xba*I	1 µL

2. Incubate at 37°C for 1 h and then fill up to 200 µL using TE buffer.
3. Add 200 µL phenol/chloroform/isoamyl alcohol.
4. Vortex vigorously and centrifuge at 10,000*g* for 5 min at 4°C.
5. Transfer upper phase to a new 1.5-mL tube.
6. Add 1 µL glycogen, 20 µL 5 *M* $LiCl_2$, and 500 µL ice-cold 95% ethanol.
7. Place on dry ice for 30 min and then centrifuge at 10,000*g* for 5 min at 4°C.
8. Remove the supernatant and rinse using 1 mL ice-cold 70% ethanol.
9. Dry for 5–10 min under the vacuum and dissolve in 10 µL TE buffer.

3.2.3. Preparation of Vector DNA

3.2.3.1. Restriction Digestion of Vector DNA

1. Reaction mixture:

Vector DNA (pGEM-3Zf(–), 0.2 μg/μL)	7 μL
10X restriction enzyme H buffer	1 μL
*Pst*I	1 μL
*Xba*I	1 μL

2. Incubate at 37°C for 1 h.

3.2.3.2. Dephosphorylation of Restriction Enzyme Digested Vector DNA

1. Reaction mixture:

Digested DNA mixture	10 μL
10X dephosphorylation buffer	10 μL
BAP (150 U/μL)	1 μL
ddH_2O to final volume of 100 μL	

2. Incubate at 60°C for 1 h and then fill out to 200 μL using TE buffer.
3. Add 200 μL phenol/chloroform/isoamyl alcohol.
4. Vortex vigorously and centrifuge at 10,000*g* for 5 min at 4°C.
5. Transfer upper phase to a new 1.5-mL tube.
6. Repeat **steps 3–5**.
7. Add 1 μL glycogen, 20 μL 5 *M* $LiCl_2$, and 500 μL ice-cold 95% ethanol.
8. Place on dry ice for 30 min and then centrifuge at 10,000*g* for 5 min at 4°C.
9. Remove the supernatant and rinse using 1 mL ice-cold 70% ethanol.
10. Dry for 5–10 min under the vacuum and dissolve in 10 μL TE buffer.

3.2.4. Ligation of DNA

1. Reaction mixture:

Insert DNA (*Pst*I-*Xba*I digested)	5 μL
Vector DNA (*Pst*I-*Xba*I digested)	2 μL
10X ligase buffer	1 μL

2. Incubate at 55°C for 5 min.
3. Add 1 μL 10 m*M* ATP and 1 μL T4 DNA ligase (1 U/μL).
4. Incubate at 16°C for 1 h to overnight.

3.2.5. Transformation of Ligated DNA

1. Add 5 μL ligated DNA to 50 μL competent cells.
2. Place on ice for 30 min.
3. Give heat shock at 42°C for 30 s.
4. Place immediately back on ice to chill.
5. Add 1 mL LB medium and incubate at 37°C for 1 h with shaking.
6. Centrifuge at 10,000*g* for 5 s at 4°C and remove 4/5 volume of the supernatant.
7. Resuspend the pellet and spread on an LB agar (amp) plate.
8. Incubate at 37°C overnight.

The construct should be checked by restriction enzyme digestion and partial sequencing.

3.2.6. Probe Generation by In Vitro Transcription

3.2.6.1. Linearization of the Probe Construct

1. Reaction mixture:

Probe construct (pGEM-E1E2, 0.5 µg/µL)	20 µL
10X restriction enzyme H buffer	5 µL
ddH_2O	20 µL
*Hin*dIII (10 U/µL)	5 µL

2. Incubate at 37°C for 5 h.
3. Add 170 µL TE buffer.
4. Add 200 µL phenol/chloroform/isoamyl alcohol.
5. Vortex vigorously and centrifuge at 10,000*g* for 5 min at 4°C.
6. Transfer upper phase to a new 1.5-mL tube.
7. Add 20 µL 3 *M* sodium acetate and 600 µL ice-cold 95% ethanol.
8. Place on dry ice for 30 min and then centrifuge at 10,000*g* for 5 min at 4°C.
9. Remove the supernatant and rinse using 1 mL ice-cold 70% ethanol.
10. Dry for 5–10 min under the vacuum and dissolve in 10 µL TE buffer.

3.2.6.2. In Vitro Transcription

1. Reaction mixture:

Linearized DNA template (0.5 µg/µL)	2 µL
10X RNA polymerase buffer	2 µL
10 m*M* ATP	1 µL
10 m*M* GTP	1 µL
10 m*M* UTP	1 µL
[α-^{32}P]CTP (800 Ci/mmol)	5 µL
T7 RNA polymerase (5 U/µL) + RNase inhibitor (5 U/µL)	2 µL
RNase-free water	6 µL

   Prepare at room temperature.
2. Incubate at 37°C for 30 min.
3. Add 1 µL DNase I (2 U/µL).
4. Incubate 37°C for 15 min to digest template DNA.
5. Add 1 µL 0.5 *M* EDTA and 50 µL DEPC-treated water.

3.2.6.3. Purification of Riboprobe

1. Add 70 µL DEPC-treated water to a Nuctrap Push Column (Stratagene).
2. Push the syringe to pass water through the column.
3. Load the sample (70 µL) onto the column.
4. Push the syringe to pass the sample through the column and collect the flowthrough.
5. Add 70 µL DEPC-treated water.

6. Push the syringe to pass water through the column and collect the flowthrough.
7. Take 1 μL of the flowthrough and mix with 5 mL cocktail.
8. Measure specific activity of the probe and dilute to 2–8 × 10^4 cpm.

3.2.7. Preparation of Marker DNA

1. Reaction mixture:

φX174 *Hin*fI digested DNA	1 μL
10X forward reaction buffer	1 μL
[γ-^{32}P]ATP (6000 Ci/mmol)	1 μL
T4 oligonucleotide kinase (10 U/μL)	1 μL

2. Incubate at 37°C for 30 min and then at 90°C for 2 min.
3. Add 30 μL of gel loading buffer (use 5 μL for each loading).

3.2.8. Ribonuclease Protection Assay

3.2.8.1. Hybridization of the Probe and Sample RNA

1. Reaction mixture:

Labeled probe (2–8 × 10^4 cpm)	1 μL
Total RNA (5–8 μg/μL)	10 μL
or yeast RNA (for control, 5 mg/mL)	10 μL

2. Add 1 μL 5 *M* ammonium acetate and 25 μL ice-cold ethanol.
3. Place on dry ice for 20 min and centrifuge at 10,000*g* for 20 min at 4°C.
4. Remove the supernatant and add 20 μL of solution A.
5. Vortex and flush.
6. Incubate at 90°C for 4 min.
7. Vortex and flush.
8. Incubate at 45°C overnight.

3.2.8.2. RNase Digestion of the Probe/Sample RNA Hybrid

1. Dilute RNase A/RNase T1 mix to 1 in 200–400 with RNase digestion solution.
2. Add 200 μL diluted RNase A/RNase T1 mix to the hybridized sample prepared as in **Subheading 3.2.8.1.**
3. Incubate at 37°C for 30 min.
4. Add 300 μL RNase inactivation/precipitation solution and 100 μL ice-cold 95% ethanol.
5. Place on dry ice for 15 min.

3.2.8.3. Separation and Detection of Protected Fragments

1. Centrifuge the sample at 10,000*g* for 15 min at 4°C.
2. Remove the supernatant carefully and completely using automatic pipet.
3. Add 8 μL of gel loading buffer and vortex for 1 min.
4. Flush and incubate at 90°C for 4 min.
5. Vortex and flush again.
6. Load samples and marker DNA on 6% polyacrylamide/urea gel and run at 250 V for 1 h (**Fig. 3**).

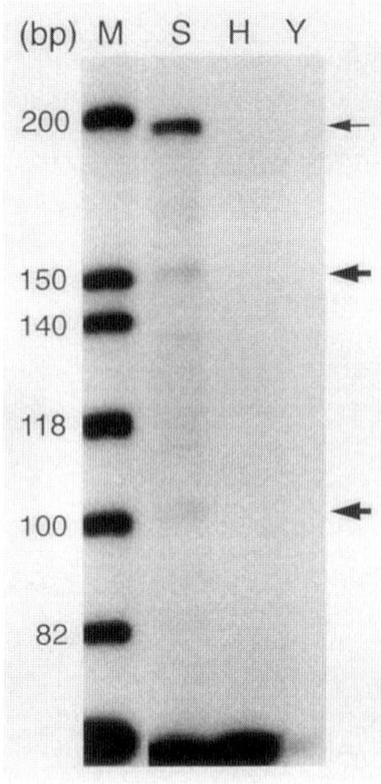

Fig. 3. Detection of transcription start sites driven by the intron promoter using RPA. A labeled antisense RNA probe transcribed from a D_{1A} cDNA that excludes the intron (pGEM-E1E2) was hybridized with RNA from SK-N-MC (S, positive control cell line), HepG2 (H, negative control cell line), and yeast (Y, negative control) cells. The sizes of the protected bands were compared with concurrently electrophoresed labeled ϕX174 *Hin*fI DNA marker (M). Two bands protected by RNA transcribed by the intron promoter are indicated by thick arrows. The strong band protected by RNA transcribed by the D_{1A} upstream promoter in SK-N-MC cells is indicated by a thin arrow.

7. Wash the gel in the ddH_2O for 30 min to remove urea.
8. Place a filter paper on the gel and dry for 30 min under the vacuum.
9. Expose in the cassette with an X-ray film at –80°C.

3.3. Primer Extension

3.3.1. Total RNA Preparation

For preparation of total RNA From Cultured cells, *see* **Subheading 3.2.1.**

3.3.2. Primer Labeling

1. Reaction mixture:

Primer PE-1 (10 pmol/mL)	2 µL
10X forward reaction buffer	1 µL
Nuclease-free water	3 µL

[γ-^{32}P] ATP (6000 Ci/mmol)	3 µL
T4 oligonucleotide kinase (10 U/µL)	1 µL

2. Incubate at 37°C for 10 min and then at 90°C for 2 min.
3. Add 90 µL nuclease-free water.

3.3.3. Preparation of Sequencing Ladder **(18)** *as a Position Marker*

3.3.3.1. Alkaline Denaturation of Sequencing Template

1. Add 2 µL 2 *N* NaOH to 1–2 µg of template DNA and make up with ddH_2O to 20 µL.
2. Incubate at room temperature for 5 min.
3. Add 8 µL 10 *M* ammonium acetate and 100 µL ice-cold 95% ethanol.
4. Place on dry ice for 10 min.
5. Centrifuge at 10,000*g* for 10 min at 4°C and discard the supernatant.
6. Add 200 µL ice-cold 70% ethanol.
7. Place on dry ice for 5 min.
8. Centrifuge at 10,000*g* for 10 min at 4°C and discard the supernatant.
9. Dry for 5–10 min under the vacuum.

3.3.3.2. Annealing

1. Add 1 µL primer PE-1 (0.5 pmol/µL; *see* **Subheading 2.3.1.**) to denatured DNA template.
2. Add 2 µL sequenase buffer and 6 µL ddH_2O.
3. Vortex to dissolve DNA.
4. Incubate at 65°C for 2 min and cool down slowly to room temperature for 30 min.
5. Chill on ice.

3.3.3.3. Labeling Reaction

1. Reaction mixture:

Annealed DNA	9 µL
0.1 M DTT	1 µL
dNTP mix	2 µL
[α-^{35}S]dATP	0.5 µL (5 µCi)
Sequenase (1.5 U/µL)	2 µL

2. Incubate at 15°C for 2–5 min.

3.3.3.4. Termination Reactions

1. Label four tubes as A, C, G, and T and add 2.5 µL of corresponding dideoxy termination mixture.
2. Prewarm these tubes to 42°C.
3. Add 3.5 µL each of labeling reaction mixture.
4. Incubate at 42°C for 2–5 min.
5. Add 4 µL of stop solution.
6. Mix well and place on ice.
7. Incubate at 80°C for 5 min and chill on ice before loading.
8. Use 3 µL for each load.

3.3.4. Primer Extension

1. Reaction mixture:

Total RNA	30 μg
Labeled primer	1 μL
2X primer extension buffer	5 μL
Nuclease-free water to 10 μL	

2. Incubate at 70°C for 20 min.
3. Place at room temperature for 10 min.
4. Place on ice for 1 min.
5. Add 9 μL of PreMix solution.
6. Incubate at 42°C for 30 min.
7. Add 20 μL of gel loading dye.
8. Incubate at 90°C for 10 min.
9. Chill on ice.

3.3.5. Sequencing Gel Separation (**Fig. 4**)

1. Load 20 μL of the sample on an 8% sequencing gel.
2. Electrophorese at 250 V for 2 h.
3. Wash the gel in the ddH_2O for 30 min to remove urea.
4. Place a filter paper on the gel and dry for 30 min under the vacuum.
5. Expose in the cassette with an X-ray film at –80°C.

4. Notes

1. SK-N-MC and NS20Y cells are known to express the D_{1A} dopamine receptor endogenously ***(14)***. The HepG2 cell line is used for negative control.
2. The NS20Y cell line is not commercially available. This is a kind gift from Dr. Marshall Nirenberg (NHLBI, NIH, Bethesda, MD).
3. This CAT construct has a part of the 5'-noncoding region of the human D_{1A} dopamine receptor gene, which spans nucleotides from –1102 to –239 ***(13)***.
4. For efficient transfection, pH should be 7.05. Transfection efficiency of each new batch should be checked by mixing 0.5 mL 2X HBS with 0.5 mL 250 m*M* $CaCl_2$ and vortexing. A fine precipitate should develop.
5. RNA is very sensitive to even a little amount of RNase contamination. Thus, we strongly recommend the use of RNase free reagents from a certified source.
6. Open a new bottle of 95% ethanol and label it "RNA use only." This should be handled with gloves to keep it RNase free.
7. Acrylamide is highly toxic. Use gloves and a mask.
8. Freshly dissolved in ddH_2O.
9. The oligonucleotide primer should be 30 to 40 mer and should be expected to produce approximately a 100-bp-long product.
10. Band compressions of dGTP could be prevented by using 7-deaza dGTP ***(19)***.
11. While the transfection is in progress, the pH of the medium may turn acidic. Lower CO_2 concentration (4%) in the incubator makes the medium pH 7.2–7.4, which is helpful for efficient transfection.

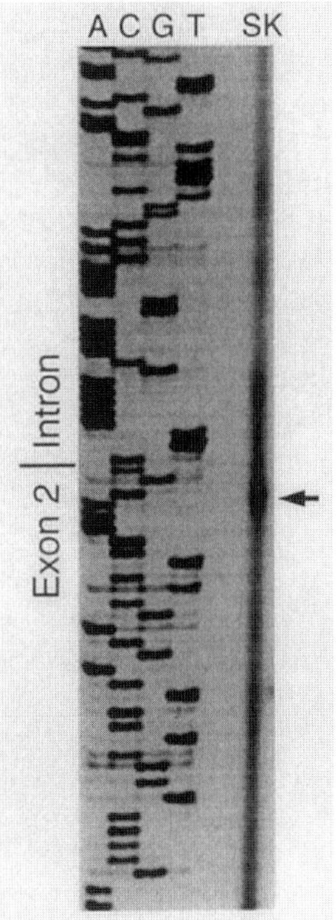

Fig. 4. Identification of transcription start sites driven by the intron promoter using primer extension analysis. The primer (bases -384 to -413 in exon 2) was labeled at the 5'-end, hybridized with RNA from SK-N-MC (SK) cells and extended by AMV reverse transcriptase. The sizes of the extended products were determined by comparing them with the DNA sequencing products of a genomic fragment sequenced using the same primer. Primer extension analysis shows multiple transcription initiation sites. The start site at the junction of intron and exon 2 is indicated by an arrow.

12. The 1X washing solution should be left in the wells for at least 30 s/wash in each wash step.
13. Make sure the cells are completely homogenized.

References

1. Lee, T, Seeman, P., Rajput, A., Farley, I. J., and Hornykiewicz, O. (1978) Receptor basis for dopaminergic supersensitivity in Parkinson's disease. *Nature (London)* **273,** 59–61.
2. Lee, T, Seeman, P., Tourtellotte, W. W., Farley, I. J., and Hornykiewicz, O. (1978) Binding of ^{3}H-neuroleptics and 3H-apomorphine in schizophrenic brains. *Nature (London)* **274,** 897–900.

3. Muller, P. and Seeman, P. (1978) Dopaminergic supersensitivity after neuroleptics: time-course and specificity. *Psychopharmacology* **60,** 1–11.
4. Mouradian, M. M., Juncos, J. L., Fabbrini, G., Schlegel, J., Bartko, J. J., and Chase, T. N. (1988) Motor fluctuations in Parkinson's disease: central pathophysiological mechanisms, Part II. *Ann. Neurol.* **24,** 372–378.
5. Mouradian, M. M., Heuser, I. J. E., Baronti, F., and Chase, T. N. (1990) Modification of central dopaminergic mechanisms by continuous levodopa therapy for advanced Parkinson's disease. *Ann. Neurol.* **27,** 18–23.
6. Seeman, P., Ulpian, C., Bergeron, C., Riederer, P., Jellinger, K., Gabriel, E., et al. (1984) Bimodal distribution of dopamine receptor densities in brains of schizophrenics. *Science* **225,** 728–731.
7. Chipkin, R. E., Iorio, L. C., Coffin, V. L., MaQuade, R. D., Berger, J. G., and Barnett, A. (1988) Pharmacological profile of SCH39166: a dopamine D_1 selective benzonaphthazepine with potential antipsychotic activity. *J. Pharmac. Exp. Ther.* **247,** 1093–1102.
8. Taylor, L. A., Tedford, C. E., and McQuade, R. D. (1991) The binding of SCH 39166 and SCH 23390 to 5-HT_{1C} receptors in porcine choroid plexus. *Life Sci.* **49,** 1505–1511.
9. Boyson, S. J., McGonigle, P., and Molinoff, P. B. (1986) Quantitative autoradiographic localization of the D1 and D2 subtypes of dopamine receptors in rat brain. *J. Neurosci.* **6,** 3177–3188.
10. Lidow, M. S., Goldman-Rakic, P. S., Gallager, D. W., and Rakic, P. (1991) Distribution of dopaminergic receptors in the primate cerebral cortex: quantitative autoradiographic analysis using [^{3}H]raclopride, [^{3}H]spiperone and [^{3}H]SCH23390. *Neuroscience* **40,** 657–671.
11. Williams, G. V. and Goldman-Rakic, P. S. (1995) Modulation of memory fields by dopamine D_1 receptors in prefrontal cortex. *Nature* **376,** 572–575.
12. Minowa, M. T., Minowa, T., Monsma, F. J., Jr., Sibley, D. R., and Mouradian, M. M. (1992). Characterization of the 5' flanking region of the human D_{1A} dopamine receptor gene. *Proc. Natl. Acad. Sci. USA* **89**, 3045–3049.
13. Minowa, M. T., Minowa, T., and Mouradian, M. M. (1993). Activator region analysis of the human D_{1A} dopamine receptor gene. *J. Biol. Chem.* **268**, 23,544–23,551.
14. Lee, S.-H., Minowa, M. T., and Mouradian, M. M. (1996) Two distinct promoters drive transcription of the human D_{1A} dopamine receptor gene. *J. Biol. Chem.* **271**, 25,292–25,299.
15. Lee, S.-H., Wang, W., Yajima, S., Jose, P. A., and Mouradian, M. M. (1997) Tissue-specific promoter usage in human D_{1A} dopamine receptor gene in brain and kidney. *DNA Cell Biol.* **16**, 1267–1275.
16. Graham, F. L. and Van Der Eb, A. J. (1973). A new technique for the assay of infectivity of human adenovirus 5 DNA. *Virology* **52,** 456–467.
17. Sambrook, J., Fritsch, E. F., and Maniatis, T. (1989) *Molecular Cloning: A Laboratory Manual.* Cold Spring Harbor Laboratory Press, Cold Spring Harbor, NY.

18. Sanger, F., Nicklen, S., and Coulson, A.R. (1977) DNA sequencing with chain-terminating inhibitors. *Proc. Natl. Acad. Sci. USA* **74**, 5463–5467.
19. Mizusawa, S., Nishimura, S., and Seela, F. (1986) Improvement of the dideoxy chain termination method of DNA sequencing by use of deoxy-7-deazaguanosine triphosphate in place of dGTP. *Nucleic Acids Res.* **14,** 1319–1324.

15

Detection of DNA/Protein Interactions in Dopamine Receptor Genes

Sang-Hyeon Lee and M. Maral Mouradian

1. Introduction

In the previous chapter, we discussed practical methods to study transcription control mechanisms for the D_{1A} dopamine receptor gene. Since these processes are mediated by a complex set of nuclear regulatory proteins that interact with specific DNA sequences, methods to delineate these interactions are paramount in understanding transcription control. In the case of the D_{1A} gene, we found several consensus binding sites for known transcription factors on the 5'-noncoding region and examined their binding to the nuclear proteins and known transcription factors *(1)*.

In this chapter, we discuss practical methods to detect DNA/protein interactions for the D_{1A} dopamine receptor gene. We localize transcription factor binding sites using gel mobility shift assay and DNase I footprinting.

2. Materials

2.1. Cells for Study (See Note 1.)

All cell lines are cultured at 37°C in a humidified 10% CO_2 incubator.

1. Human neuroblastoma cell line SK-N-MC (ATCC no.: HTB-10). Medium: 90% minimum essential medium with 2 m*M* L-glutamine and Earle's balanced salt solution adjusted to contain 1.5 g/L sodium bicarbonate, 0.1 m*M* nonessential amino acids, and 1.0 m*M* sodium pyruvate, 10% fetal bovine serum.
2. Murine neuroblastoma cell line NS20Y (*see* **Note 2**). Medium: 90% Dulbecco's modified Eagle's medium, 10% fetal bovine serum.

From: *Methods in Molecular Medicine, vol. 62: Parkinson's Disease: Methods and Protocols*
Edited by: M. M. Mouradian © Humana Press Inc., Totowa, NJ

2.2. Preparation of Nuclear Extract

1. Buffer A: 10 m*M* HEPES KOH, pH 7.9, 1.5 m*M* $MgCl_2$, and 9.9 m*M* KCl.
2. Buffer C: 20 m*M* HEPES KOH, pH 7.9, 25% glycerol, 420 m*M* NaCl, 1.5 m*M* $MgCl_2$, and 0.2 m*M* EDTA.
3. Buffer D: 20 m*M* HEPES KOH, pH 7.9, 20% glycerol, 100 m*M* KCl, and 0.2 m*M* EDTA.
4. 1 *M* dithiothreitol (DTT).
5. 0.5 *M* phenylmethylsulfonyl fluoride (PMSF).
6. Cell lysis buffer: 20 m*M* Tris-HCl, pH 7.5, 1 m*M* DTT, 400 m*M* KCl, 10% glycerol, 37.5 μg Leupeptin, and 37.5 μg Aprotinin.

2.3. Gel Mobility Shift Assay

2.3.1. Preparation of Probe

1. DNA fragments for labeling: D1Int, Ex, and All (**Fig. 1**) *(2)*.
2. Random primed DNA Labeling Kit (Boehringer Mannheim).
   a. Reaction mix solution: hexanucleotide mixture in 10X reaction buffer (500 m*M* Tris-HCl buffer, pH 8.0, 100 m*M* $MgCl_2$, and 500 m*M* NaCl).
   b. 0.5 m*M* dATP, 0.5 m*M* dGTP, and 0.5 m*M* dTTP.
   c. Klenow enzyme (5 U/μL).
3. [α-^{32}P]dCTP (3000 Ci/ mmol).
4. Nuctrap Push Column (Stratagene).
5. ddH_2O.

2.3.2. DNA-Protein Binding Reaction and Electrophoresis

1. Nuclear extract (2–3 μg/μL).
2. Labeled probes: 1-5 × 10^4 cpm/μL.
3. Poly dIdC (2 mg/ml, Pharmacia).
4. Competitors: cold probes in 100-fold molar excess relative to the respective probes.
5. Buffer D (*see* **Subheading 2.1.**) *(3)*.
6. 4% Polyacrylamide (29:1) nondenaturing gel: 6.15 mL 30% acrylamide solution, 10 mL 5X Tris glycine buffer, 0.4 mL 10% ammonium persulfate, 33.45 mL ddH_2O, and 50 μL *N,N,N',N'*-tetramethylethylene diamine (TEMED). Mix rapidly and pour into a preformed gel mold.
   a. 5X Tris-glycine buffer: 15.1 g Tris base, and 72.1 g glycine. Make up with ddH_2O to 1 L and autoclave. Store at room temperature.
   b. 30% acrylamide solution (29:1) (*see* **Note 3**): 29 g acrylamide, 1 g *N,N'*-methylene bisacrylamide, ddH_2O to 100 mL.
   c. 10% ammonium persulfate (*see* **Note 4**).
   d. TEMED.
7. Gel running buffer: 1X Tris glycine buffer.

2.4. DNase I Footprinting

2.4.1. Generating Probe by PCR

1. Oligonucleotide primers for the activator region of the human D_{1A} dopamine receptor gene (219 bp long, nucleotides –1220 to –1000) ***(1)***.

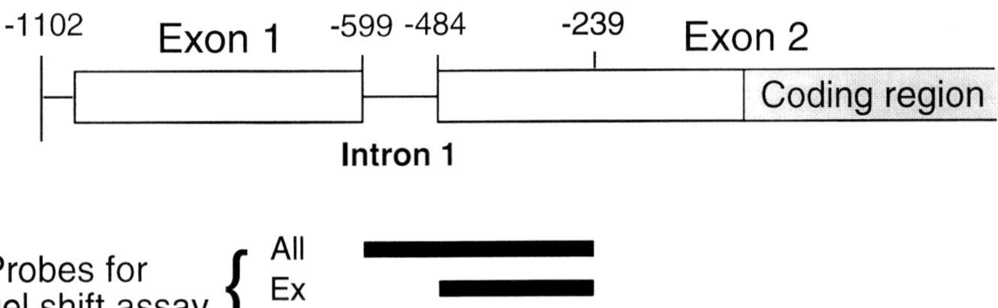

Fig. 1. Schematic structure of the human D_{1A} dopamine receptor gene. The positions of probes used for gel shift assay are indicated below.

   a. Sense primer DF-1: 5'-CTCGCCCGCAGAACCATC-3'.
   b. Antisense primer DF-2: 5'-GCCTCCCCGCAGGCACTG-3'
2. 10X Forward exchange buffer: 700 m*M* Tris-HCl, pH 7.6, 100 m*M* $MgCl_2$, 1 *M* KCl, and 10 m*M* 2-mercaptoethanol.
3. T4 Polynucleotide kinase (10 U/µL; Boehringer Mannheim).
4. [γ-^{32}P]ATP (6000 Ci/mmol, Amersham).
5. Template DNA (5 ng/µL): pCATD1-1220 (*see* **Note 5**).
6. G-25 column: Suspend 1 g Sephadex G-25 resin (Pharmacia) in 5 mL TE buffer. Cut the bottom of a 0.5-mL tube and fill the hole with cotton. Mount the tube into a 1.5-mL tube. Fill the tube with 500 µL suspended G-25 resin. Spin briefly and discard the flowthrough. Centrifuge at 2000*g* for 5 min at room temperature. Mount the tube column into a fresh 1.5-mL tube.
7. 10X *Taq* reaction buffer: 500 m*M* KCL, 100 m*M* Tris-HCl, pH 8.3, 15 m*M* $MgCl_2$ (Boehringer Mannheim).
8. *Taq* DNA polymerase: 5 U/µL (Boehringer Mannheim).
9. 10 m*M* dNTP mix.
10. ddH_2O.
11. Mineral oil.
12. 10X DNA loading dye: 60% glycerol, 0.5% xylene cyanol FF, and 0.5% bromophenol blue in ddH_2O.
13. 5% Polyacrylamide (29:1) nondenaturing gel: 8.3 mL 30% acrylamide solution, 5 mL 10X Tris borate buffer, 0.4 mL 10% ammonium persulfate, 36.3 mL ddH_2O, and 50 µL TEMED. Mix rapidly and pour into a preformed gel mold.
    a. 10X Tris borate buffer (TBE): 108 g Tris base, 55 g boric acid, and 7.5 g EDTA. Make up with ddH_2O to 1 L and autoclave. Store at room temperature.
    b. 30% acrylamide solution (29:1) (*see* **Note 3**): 29 g acrylamide, 1 g *N,N'*-methylene bisacrylamide, ddH_2O to 100 mL.
    c. 10% ammonium persulfate (*see* **Note 4**).
    d. TEMED.
14. Gel running buffer: 1X TBE buffer.
15. TE buffer: 10 m*M* Tris-HCl, pH 7.5, 1 m*M* EDTA, pH 8.0. Autoclave and store at room temperature.

16. 10% sodium dodecyl sulfate (SDS).
17. 3 *M* sodium acetate.
18. Ice-cold 95% and 70% ethanol.

2.4.2. Preparation of Sequencing Ladder

1. Template DNA (1–2 µg): pCATD1-1220 (*see* **Note 5**).
2. 2 *N* NaOH.
3. 10 *M* ammonium acetate.
4. Ice-cold 95% and 70% ethanol.
5. Sequencing primer: Primer DF-2 (0.5 pmol/ml) (*see* **Subheading 2.3.1.**) *(1)*.
6. [α-^{35}S]dATP: 1000 Ci/mmol (Amersham).
7. T7 Sequenase 7-deaza-dGTP DNA sequencing kit (USB). Kit components:
   a. Sequenase buffer.
   b. 0.1 *M* DTT.
   c. dNTP mix: 0.5 m*M* dATP, 0.5 m*M* dCTP, 0.5 m*M* 7-deaza dGTP, and 0.5 m*M* dTTP (*see* **Note 6**).
   d. Dideoxy termination mixtures.
   e. Stop solution.
8. Sequenase version 2.0 (1.5 U/µL; USB).

2.4.3. DNase I Footprinting

1. DNase I: 1 U/µL.
2. 10 m*M* Tris-HCl buffer, pH 8.0.
3. Nuclear extract: 2–3 µg/µL.
4. Buffer D (*see* **Subheading 2.1.**) *(3)*.
5. 1 *M* NaCl.
6. Poly dIdC: 2 mg/mL (Boehringer Mannheim).
7. Labeled probe: 1–5 × 10^4 cpm/µL.
8. ddH_2O.
9. 100 m*M* $MgCl_2$.
10. 10 m*M* $CaCl_2$.
11. Stop mix: 100 m*M* Tris-HCl buffer, pH 8.0, 100 m*M* NaCl, 1% *N*-lauroylsarcosine, sodium salt, 10 m*M* EDTA, pH 8.0, and 25 µg/mL sonicated calf thymus DNA.
12. Phenol/chloroform/isoamyl alcohol solution (25:24:1).
    a. 25 mL 0.1 *M* Tris-HCl (pH 8.0) buffer-saturated phenol.
    b. 24 mL chloroform.
    c. 1 mL isoamyl alcohol.
13. 3 *M* sodium acetate.
14. Ice-cold 95% and 70% ethanol.
15. Formamide loading dye: 80% formamide, 10 m*M* EDTA, 0.1% xyl-ene cyanol, and 0.1% bromophenol blue.
16. Filter papers.
17. Cassette and X-ray film.

18. 8% polyacrylamide sequencing gel: 20 mL 20% acrylamide urea solution, 30 mL urea mix, 0.4 mL 10% ammonium persulfate, and 50 μL TEMED. Mix rapidly and pour into a preformed sequencing gel mold.
    a. 10X Tris borate buffer (TBE): 108 g Tris base, 55 g boric acid, and 7.5 g EDTA. Make up with ddH_2O to 1 L and autoclave. Store at room temperature.
    b. 20% Acrylamide urea solution (*see* **Note 3**): 96.5 g acrylamide, 3.35 g *N,N'*-methylene bisacrylamide, 233.5 g ultra-pure urea, 50 mL 10x TBE, ddH_2O to 500 mL.
    c. Urea mix: 233.5 g ultra-pure urea, 50 mL 10X TBE, ddH_2O to 500 mL.
    d. 10% Ammonium persulfate (*see* **Note 4**).
    e. TEMED.
19. Gel running buffer: 1X TBE.

3. Methods

3.1. Preparation of Nuclear Extract

Chill all buffers on ice before use.

3.1.1. Preparation of Nuclear Extract from Cells

See **ref.** *3*.

1. Collect cell pellet from ten large dishes (150 mm).
2. Add 10 mL buffer A and 5 μL 1 *M* DTT.
3. Place on ice for 10 min.
4. Centrifuge at 2000*g* for 10 min at 4°C and discard the supernatant.
5. Add 4 mL buffer A and 2 μL 1 *M* DTT.
6. Resuspend the cells and transfer to a type B homogenizer (Dounce).
7. Homogenize the cells with 25 strokes.
8. Transfer the cell lysate to a new tube.
9. Wash homogenizer with 2 mL buffer A and 0.5 μL 1 *M* DTT and pool to the cell lysate.
10. Centrifuge at 4000*g* for 10 min and discard the supernatant.
11. Add 4 mL buffer A and 2 μL 1 *M* DTT.
12. Centrifuge at 10,000*g* for 20 min at 4°C and discard the supernatant.
13. Add 1 mL buffer C, 0.5 μL 1 *M* DTT, and 1 μL 0.5 M PMSF.
14. Resuspend the pellet and transfer to a type B homogenizer (Dounce).
15. Homogenize the suspension with 25 strokes
16. Transfer the lysate to a new 1.5-mL tube.
17. Wash homogenizer with 0.3 mL buffer C and pool to the lysate.
18. Stir gently in the cold room for 30 min.
19. Centrifuge at 10,000*g* for 30 min at 4°C.
20. Transfer the supernatant in a dialysis tube.
21. Dialyze against 70 mL Buffer D, 50 μL 1 *M* DTT, and 100 μL 0.5 *M* PMSF in the cold room for 5 h.
22. Centrifuge at 10,000*g* for 20 min at 4°C.
23. Make 50-μL aliquots and store them at –80°C.

3.1.2. Preparation of Nuclear Extract from One-Dish Cells

See **ref. 4**.

1. Collect cell pellet from one dish (100 mm).
2. Add 100 µL cell lysis buffer.
3. Freeze on dry ice for 5 min.
4. Thaw at 37°C for 5 min.
5. Repeat **steps 3** and **4** twice.
6. Centrifuge at 10,000*g* for 5 min at 4°C.
7. Transfer the supernatant to new tubes (use approx 4 µL for each experiment).
8. Store at –80°C.

3.2. Gel Mobility Shift Assay

See **Fig. 2**.

3.2.1. Probe Making

Use the Random Primed DNA Labeling Kit (Boehringer Mannheim).

1. Denature DNA fragment at 100°C for 10 min and chill on ice.
2. Reaction mixture:

Denatured DNA (25 ng/µL)	2 µL
Reaction mix solution	2 µL
dATP	1 µL
dGTP	1 µL
dTTP	1 µL
[α-^{32}P]dCTP (3000 Ci/mmol)	5 µL
ddH$_2$O	7 µL
Klenow enzyme	1 µL

3. Incubate at 37°C for 30 min and then at 90°C for 5 min.
4. Add 50 µL ddH$_2$O.
5. Add 70 µL ddH$_2$O to a Nuctrap Push Column (Stratagene).
6. Push the syringe to pass ddH$_2$O through the column.
7. Load sample (70 µL) onto the column.
8. Push the syringe to pass the sample through the column and collect the flow-through.
9. Add 70 µL ddH$_2$O to the column.
10. Push the syringe to pass the sample through the column and collect the flowthrough.
11. Take 1 µL the flowthrough and mix with 5 mL cocktail.
12. Measure specific activity.

3.2.3. DNA-Protein Binding Reaction and Separation on a Polyacrylamide Nondenaturing Gel

1. Reaction mixture:

Nuclear extract (3–5 µg/µL)	1 µL
Poly dIdC (2 mg/mL)	1 µL
Competitor (X500) or TE	1 µL

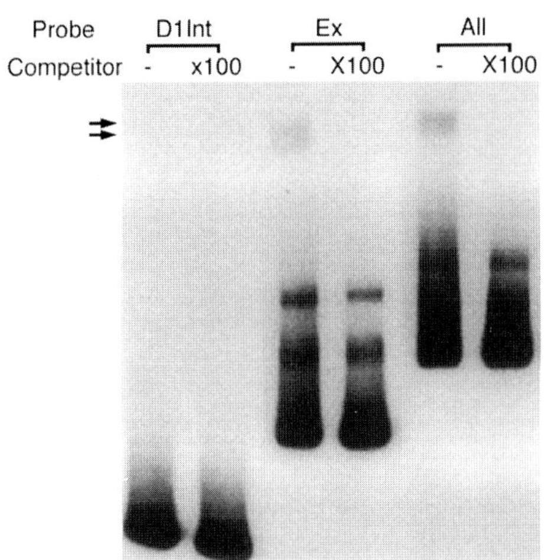

Fig. 2. Gel mobility shift assay with DNA probes, D1Int (the entire intron), Ex (245 bases of exon 2), and All (the entire intron and 245 bases of exon 2) (**Fig. 1**). DNA probes were generated by PCR using ^{32}P-labeled primers for one end and cold primers for the other end with pCAT-D1-1102 as a template. About 5 fmol (>50,000 cpm) of probe and 5 µg of nuclear extract from SK-N-MC cells were used. All probes were purified by PAGE. Competitors indicate the unlabeled fragments corresponding to each probe. Competitors were added in 100-fold molar excess relative to the respective probes. Arrows indicate specific shifted bands seen.

Buffer D	14 µL
ddH_2O	8 µL

2. Place on ice for 20 min.
3. Add 1 µL labeled probe.
4. Place on ice for 20 min.
5. Electrophorese on a 4% polyacrylamide (30:1) nondenaturing gel at 160 V for 1–2 h.
6. Place a filter paper on the gel and dry for 30 min under the vacuum.
7. Expose in the cassette with an X-ray film at –80°C.

3.3. DNase I Footprinting

See **Fig. 3** and **ref. 5**.

3.3.1. Probe Generation by PCR

3.3.1.1. Labeling of Oligonucleotide

1. Reaction mixture:

Primer DF-1 (2 pmol/µL)	1 µL
10X forward exchange buffer	1 µL
[γ-^{32}P]ATP (6000 Ci/mmol)	5 µL
T4 oligonucleotide kinase (10 U/µL)	0.5 µL

2. Incubate at 37°C for 1 h.

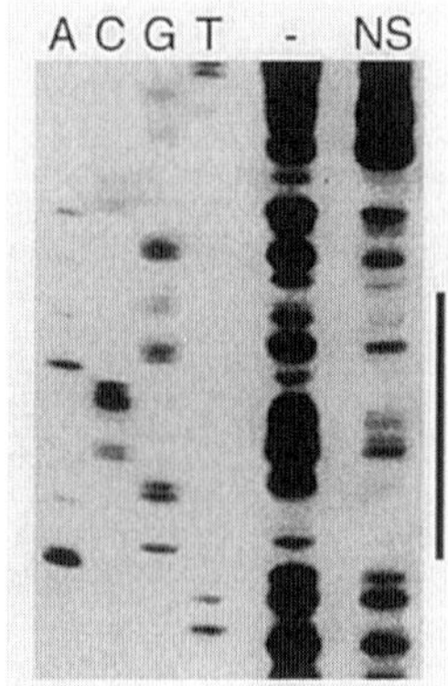

Fig. 3 DNase I footprinting of the human D_{1A} dopamine receptor gene with a nuclear extract from NS20Y cells. Probe was generated by PCR with pCATD1-1220 *(1)* as a template. Forty micrograms of nuclear extract from NS20Y (NS) was used. The sequencing reaction was electrophoresed in parallel. The region of protection is indicated by a solid bar along the right side of the figure.

3. Add 10 µL TE.
4. Load the sample (17.5 µL) onto the G-25 column.
5. Centrifuge at 2000*g* for 5 min at room temperature.
6. Take 1 µL of the flowthrough and mix with 5 mL of cocktail.
7. Measure specific activity.

3.3.1.2. PCR Reaction

1. Reaction mixture:

Labeled primer	15 µL
Cold antisense primer DF-2 (2 pmol/µL)	1 µL
Template (5 ng/µL)	1 µL
10X *Taq* buffer	5 µL
10 m*M* dNTP mix	2 µL
dd H_2O	19.5 µL
Taq DNA polymerase (5 U/µL)	0.5 µL

   Add 50 µL mineral oil, if required.
2. Conditions:

Denaturation	95°C	1 min	
Annealing	37°C	1 min	
Extension	72°C	1 min	
[Denaturation	95°C	1 min	
Annealing	55°C	1 min	
Extension	72°C	1 min]	30 cycles
Extension	72°C	10 min	

3. Add 10 µL 10X DNA loading dye.

4. Electrophorese in a 5% polyacrylamide, nondenaturing gel at 160 V for 1 h.
5. Place a filter paper on the gel.
6. Expose in the cassette with an X-ray film for 30 s.
7. Cut out the labeled part of a gel.
8. Crush a gel piece using a 1-mL syringe and collect gel pieces in a 1.5-mL capped tube.
9. Add 1 mL TE buffer and 10 μL 10% SDS.
10. Incubate at 37°C overnight.
11. Transfer solution to two new tubes (500 μL each).
12. Add 20 μL 3 *M* sodium acetate and 600 μL 95% ice-cold ethanol.
13. Place on dry ice for 30 min.
14. Centrifuge at 10,000*g* for 10 min at 4°C.
15. Discard the supernatant and rinse tubes with 1 mL 70% ice-cold ethanol.
16. Dry up for 5 min and dissolve in 50 μL TE buffer.
17. Take 1 μL of the probe and mix with 5 mL of cocktail.
18. Measure specific activity and dilute the probe to 1–5 × 10^4 cpm/μL.

3.3.2. Preparation of Sequencing Ladder (6) as a Position Marker

3.3.2.1. Alkaline Denaturation of Sequencing Template

1. Add 2 μL 2 *N* NaOH to 1–2 μg template DNA and make up with ddH_2O to 20 μL.
2. Incubate at room temperature for 5 min.
3. Add 8 μL 10 *M* ammonium acetate and 100 μL ice-cold 95% ethanol.
4. Place on dry ice for 10 min.
5. Centrifuge at 10,000*g* for 10 min at 4°C and discard the supernatant.
6. Add 200 μL ice-cold 70% ethanol.
7. Place on dry ice for 5 min.
8. Centrifuge at 10,000*g* for 10 min at 4°C and discard the supernatant.
9. Dry for 5–10 min under the vacuum.

3.3.2.2. Annealing

1. Add 1 μL primer DF-1 (0.5 pmol/μL) to denatured DNA template.
2. Add 2 μL sequenase buffer and 6 μL ddH_2O.
3. Vortex to dissolve DNA.
4. Incubate at 65°C for 2 min and cool down slowly to room temperature for 30 min.
5. Chill on ice.

3.3.2.3. Labeling Reaction

1. Reaction mixture:

Annealed DNA	9 μL
0.1 *M* DTT	1 μL
dNTP mix	2 μL
[α-^{35}S]dATP	0.5 μL
Sequenase (1.5 U/μL)	2 μL

2. Incubate at 15°C for 2–5 min.

3.3.2.4. Termination Reactions

1. Label four tubes as A, C, G, and T, and add 2.5 µL corresponding dideoxy termination mixture.
2. Prewarm these tubes to 42°C.
3. Add 3.5 µL each of labeling reaction mixture.
4. Incubate at 42°C for 2–5 min.
5. Add 4 µL stop solution.
6. Mix well and place on ice.
7. Incubate at 80°C for 5 min and chill on ice before loading.
8. Use 3 µL for each load.

3.3.3. DNase I Footprinting

1. Dilute DNase I to 0.3 U/µL: add 0.7 µL 10 m*M* Tris-HCl buffer, pH 8.0, to 0.3 µL DNase I (1 U/µL) (*see* **Note 7**).
2. Reaction mixture:

Nuclear extract (2–3 µg/µL) or Buffer D	15 µL
Buffer D	25 µL
1 *M* NaCl	5 µL
Poly dIdC (2 mg/mL)	1 µL
Labeled probe (1–5 × 10^4 cpm/µL)	2 µL
ddH_2O	2 µL

3. Place on ice for 15 min.
4. Incubate at 25°C for 2 min.
5. Add 10 µL 100 m*M* $MgCl_2$.
6. Add 40 µL 10 m*M* $CaCl_2$.
7. Add 1 µL diluted DNase I (0.3 U/µL).
8. Place at room temperature for 30 s to 2 min.
9. Add 100 µL stop mix.
10. Add 200 µL phenol/chloroform/isoamyl alcohol solution.
11. Vortex and centrifuge at 10,000*g* for 5 min at 4°C.
12. Take aqueous phase to a new tube.
13. Repeat **steps 10–12**.
14. Add 20 µL 3 *M* sodium acetate and 600 µL 95% ice-cold ethanol.
15. Place on dry ice for 30 min.
16. Centrifuge at 10,000*g* for 5 min at 4°C.
17. Discard the supernatant and rinse a tube with 70% ice-cold ethanol.
18. Dry for 5–10 min and add 8 µL formamide loading dye.
19. Electrophorese in an 8% polyacrylamide sequencing gel at 1200 V for 2 h.
20. Place a filter paper on the gel and dry for 30 min.
21. Expose in a cassette with an X-ray film at –80°C.

4. Notes

1. SK-N-MC and NS20Y cells are known to express D_{1A} dopamine receptor endogenously ***(2)***. The HepG2 cell line is used as negative control.

2. This cell line is not commercially available. It is a kind gift from Dr. Marshall Nirenberg (NHLBI, NIH, Bethesda, MD).
3. Acrylamide is highly toxic. Use gloves and a mask.
4. Freshly dissolved in ddH_2O.
5. This CAT construct has a part of the 5'-noncoding region of the human D_{1A} dopamine receptor gene that spans nucleotides from –1220 to –239 ***(1)***.
6. Band compressions of dGTP could be prevented by using 7-deaza d GTP *(7)*.
7. The optimal amount of DNase I should be checked by pilot experiments.

References

1. Minowa, M. T., Minowa, T., and Mouradian, M. M. (1993) Activator region analysis of the human D_{1A} dopamine receptor gene. *J. Biol. Chem.* **268,** 23,544–23,551.
2. Lee, S.-H., Minowa, M. T., and Mouradian, M. M. (1996) Two distinct promoters drive transcription of the human D_{1A} dopamine receptor gene. *J. Biol. Chem.* **271,** 25,292–25,299.
3. Dignam, J. D., Lebovitz,R. M., and Roeder, R. G. (1983) Accurate transcription initiation by RNA polymerase II in a soluble extract from isolated mammalian nuclei. *Nucleic Acids Res.* **11,** 1475–1489.
4. Ponglikitmongkol, M., White, J. H., and Chambon, P. (1990) Synergistic activation of transcription by the human estrogen receptor bound to tandem responsive elements. *EMBO J.* **9,** 2221–2231.
5. Hennighausen, L. and Lubon, H. (1987) Interaction of protein with DNA *in vitro. Methods Enzymol.* **152,** 721–735.
6. Sanger, F., Nicklen, S., and Coulson, A. R. (1977) DNA sequencing with chain-terminating inhibitors. *Proc. Natl. Acad. Sci. USA* **74**, 5463–5467.
7. Mizusawa, S., Nishimura, S., and Seela, F. (1986) Improvement of the dideoxy chain termination method of DNA sequencing by use of deoxy-7-deazaguanosine triphosphate in place of dGTP. *Nucleic Acids Res.* **14,** 1319–1324.

16

In Situ Hybridization on Brain Tissue

Claas-Hinrich Lammers, Yoshinobu Hara, and M. Maral Mouradian

1. Introduction

In situ hybridization (ISH) is an important method for determining the distribution of mRNA within cells or tissue preparations by hybridization of a nucleic acid probe (either DNA or RNA) with a specific target nucleic acid (usually mRNA) *(1,2)*. Thus, ISH enables the localization of transcripts within cells, tissues, and whole body and allows a neuroanatomic comparison of specific mRNA expression with the respective protein expression. Furthermore, ISH can serve as a tool to detect quantitative changes in gene expression in distinct neuroanatomic areas under various experimental conditions.

In this chapter, we focus on detection of mRNA since currently this is the most widely used ISH approach in experimental neurobiology *(3,4)*. We also discuss the double-labeling approach, which detects two different mRNA species simultaneously in the same cell using a combination of radioactive and nonradioactive probes *(5)*.

The technique of ISH is based on the hybridization of cellular mRNA with a nucleic acid probe (mostly RNA) that has been labeled with a radioisotope or another detectable molecule (e.g., digoxigenin or biotin). The sequence of the antisense riboprobe (RNA probe) is complementary to the target mRNA and will, therefore, anneal specifically to its corresponding sense RNA in a fixed tissue section. Many receptor subtypes for a given neurotransmitter are so highly related both genetically and pharmacologically that ligand binding autoradiography cannot discriminate among the various subtypes. In contrast, an ISH probe could be designed to be highly specific for a particular sequence and does not leave much ambiguity regarding the detected transcript. Therefore, the ISH approach can readily distinguish receptor subtypes as well as their alternate splicing products which is not possible with receptor binding

From: *Methods in Molecular Medicine, vol. 62: Parkinson's Disease: Methods and Protocols*
Edited by: M. M. Mouradian © Humana Press Inc., Totowa, NJ

autoradiography. The signal of radioactive ISH is detected using X-ray film autoradiography, which does not yield adequate resolution at the cellular level, or using liquid nuclear emulsion autoradiography, which does provide cellular resolution. Nonradioactive probes are detected by a specific color reaction at the cellular level.

The advent of molecular biology had a revolutionary impact on our understanding of the function and pathology of neuroanatomic structures important for Parkinson's disease ***(6–8)***. ISH in neurobiology in general and in Parkinson's disease research in particular is used for different purposes: (1) analysis of gene expression of known and newly cloned genes in distinct brain areas at high resolution (**Figs. 1** and **2**); (2) co-localization of either two different mRNA species or of a transcript with its respective protein; (3) study of gene regulation by quantitating changes in mRNA expression with a high degree of anatomic resolution (e.g., differential regulation of dopamine receptor subclasses in animal models of Parkinson's disease ***[9]***). ISH is particularly useful in a tissue such as the brain, which consists of morphologically and biochemically heterogeneous populations of cells.

A number of new ISH techniques have enhanced its sensitivity considerably. These include *in situ* polymerase chain reaction (PCR) ***(10)***, tyramide signal amplification reaction ***(10)***, and fluorescence ISH ***(11)***, which are not covered in this chapter. Several comprehensive reviews on the ISH technique have been published in recent years ***(12–14)***.

2. Materials

2.1. Preparation of Probes

2.1.1. Radioactive and Nonradioactive Labeling of Riboprobes

1. Template (cDNA in plasmid or as a PCR fragment).
2. Transcription kits for either radioactive labeling or digoxigenin labeling:
   a. 10X transcription buffer: 400 m*M* Tris-HCl, 60 m*M* $MgCl_2$, 50 m*M* dithioerythritol, 40 m*M* spermidine, pH 7.2.
   b. 10m*M* adenosine triphosphate (ATP).
   c. 10m*M* cytosine triphosphate (CTP).
   d. 10m*M* guanosine triphosphate (GTP).
   e. 2.5 m*M* digoxigenin-uridine triphosphate (DIG-UTP).
   f. RNase-Inhibitor (20 U/μL).
   g. DNase (10 U/μL; RNase free).
   h. SP6, T3, or T7 RNA polymerase (20 U/μL).
3. [^{35}S]-α-UTP (>1000 Ci/mmol; aqueous, e.g., NEN, NEG-039H).
4. Ethanol, 100 and 70%.
5. 5 *M* dithiothreitol (DTT).
6. 10% sodium dodecyl sulfate (SDS).

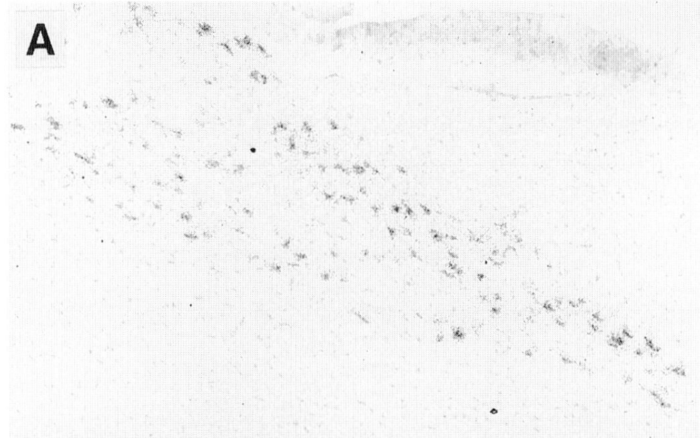

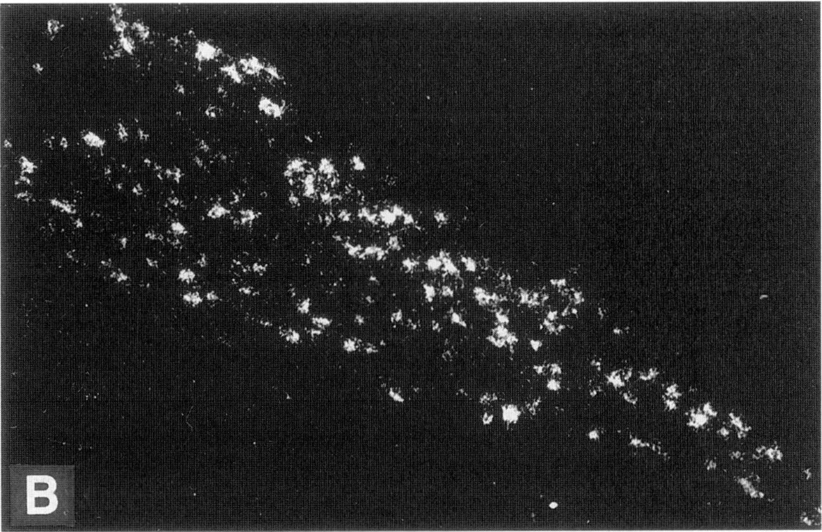

Fig. 1. *In situ* hybridization for tyrosine hydroxylase in substantia nigra. The radiolabeled riboprobe is complementary to nucleotides 1240–1520 in the rat tyrosine hydroxylase cDNA *(24)*, which was a kind gift from Dr. Elaine Lewis of the Oregon Health Sciences University. Both lightfield **(A)** and darkfield **(B)** micrographs of the same section are shown.

7. Phenol/chloroform.
8. Chloroform.
9. 3 *M* sodium acetate, pH 5.2.
10. Dry ice.
11. NucTrap Purification Columns (Stratagene) or Sephadex G50 columns.
12. DIG Nucleic Acid Detection Kit (Boehringer Mannheim).

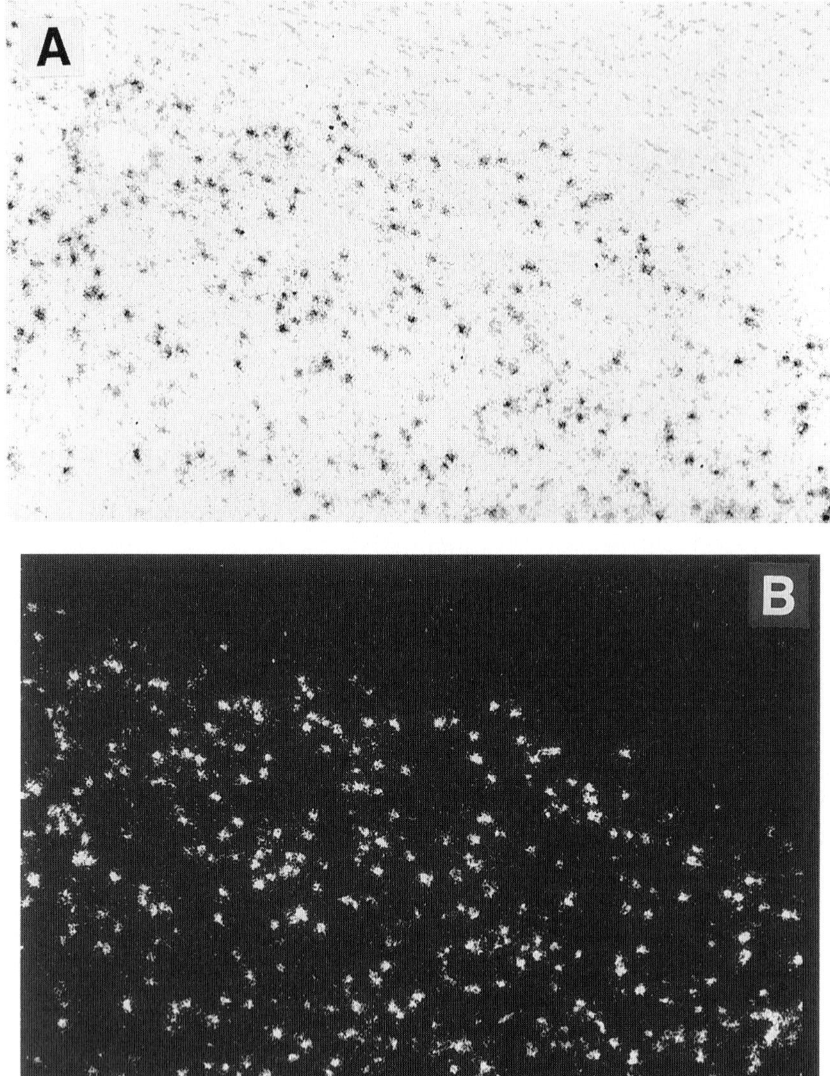

Fig. 2. In situ hybridization for the D_1 dopamine receptor in the striatum. The radiolabeled probe is complementary to nucleotides –602 to –288 of the rat D_1 cDNA *(25)* relative to the initiator ATG and excluding the intron. Both lightfield **(A)** and darkfield **(B)** micrographs of the same section are shown.

2.1.2. Radioactive Labeling of Oligodeoxynucleotide Probes

1. Oligodeoxynucleotide.
2. Terminal deoxynucleotidyl transferase (TdT).

3. 5X tailing buffer.
4. [^{35}S]-α-dATP (>1000 Ci/mmol).
5. Digoxigenine-11-dUTP.
6. NucTrap Purification Columns (Stratagene) or Sephadex G25 columns.

2.2. Preparation of Tissues

1. Dry ice.
2. Silanized slides.
3. Gelatin-coated slides.

2.3. Tissue Fixation and Preparation

1. Paraformaldehyde (4%) (PFA): Add 8 g PFA to 180 mL sterile water and dissolve at 65°C on the day of use. Add 5 drops 1 *M* NaOH, cool to room temperature, and then add 20 mL 10X phosphate-buffered saline (PBS) (*see* **Note 1**).
2. 10X PBS, pH 7.4: 90 g NaCl, 1.22 g KH_2PO_4, 8.15 g Na_2HPO_4, DEPC water to 1 L.
3. 100, 95, 80, and 70% ethanol.
4. Triethanolamine.
5. 0.25% acetic anhydride: 0.25% v/v acetic anhydride, pH 8.0. Per 100 mL, mix 1.49 mL triethanolamine and 420 μL concentrated HCl. Then add and mix 0.25 mL acetic anhydride (*see* **Note 1**).

2.4. Hybridization

1. Hybridization mix (*see* **Note 2**).

	Stock	mL/40 mL	Final conc.
Tris-HCl, pH 7.4	1 *M*	0.95	20 m*M*
EDTA, pH 8.0	250 m*M*	0.19	1 m*M*
NaCl	4 *M*	3.57	300 m*M*
Formamide	100%	23.8	50%
Dextran sulfate (Oncor S4031)	50%	9.52	10%
Denhardt's solution (Sigma D9905)	50X	0.95	1X
DEPC water		1.02	

2. DEPC water: 500 mL sterile distilled water treated with 0.5 mL DEPC. Shake well or stir. Leave overnight at room temperature. Autoclave the next day for 90 min.
3. 10% sodium thiosulfate (should be filtered through Millipore Millex-GV 0.22-μm).
4. 10% SDS.
5. 5 *M* DTT.
6. 20X standard saline citrate (SSC): Dissolve 175.2 g NaCl, 27.6 g $NaH_2PO_4 \cdot H_2O$, and 7.4 g Na_2EDTA in 800 mL DEPC-water. Adjust pH to 7.4 with NaOH and then adjust volume to 1 L with DEPC water.
7. Whatman 3MM chromatography paper.
8. Nunc Sterile Bio-assay dishes (245 × 245 × 30 mm).
9. Formamide.
10. Glass coverslips (no pretreatment needed).

2.5. Detection of Radioactive Probes

1. X-ray film (Kodak Bio-Max MR).
2. Ilford K5.D or Kodak NTB-3 nuclear emulsion. (For double labeling using digoxigenin, Ilford nuclear emulsion should be used.)
3. Coplin jar.
4. Black slide boxes.
5. Desiccant capsules.
6. Kodak D-19 photographic developer (cat no. 1464593).
7. Kodak Fixer (cat no. 1971746).
8. Cytoseal 60 (Stephens Scientific).

2.6. Detection of Digoxigenin-Labeled Probes

1. 20X SSC: Dissolve 175.2 g NaCl, 27.6 g $NaH_2PO_4 \cdot H_2O$, and 7.4 g Na_2EDTA in 800 mL DEPC water. Adjust pH to 7.4 with NaOH and then adjust volume to 1 L with DEPC water.
2. Buffer 1: 100 m*M* Tris-HCl, 150 m*M* NaCl, pH 7.5, at room temperature.
3. Buffer 2: 100 m*M* Tris-HCl, 100 m*M* NaCl, 50 m*M* $MgCl_2$, pH 9.5, at room temperature.
4. Normal goat serum (NGS; Vector).
5. Triton X-100.
6. Sheep polyclonal anti-digoxigenin-alkaline phosphatase (AP; Boehringer Mannheim).
7. Nitroblue tetrazolium chloride (NBT) 75 mg/mL in 70% dimethylformamide (Gibco-BRL).
8. 50 mg/mL 5-bromo-4-chloro-3-indolyl phosphate p-toluidinium salt (BCIP) in 70% dimethylformamide (Gibco-BRL).
9. Levamisole.
10. Cytoseal 60 (Stephens Scientific).

3. Methods

3.1. Choice of Probe and Preparation

The design of a probe that hybridizes specifically to the target sequence but does not cross-hybridize with any other sequences is the most crucial determinant in ISH. The investigator must search and select the most unique sequence for the probe that does not have any similarity with other related genes and does not have long stretches of mono-, di-, or trinucleotide or other repeats. Practically, if the GenBank database is searched with the probe sequence, the probe should not have any significant homology with other genes. The probe should also detect the single gene in genomic Southern hybridization at an appropriate temperature. To preserve good cellular and tissue morphology, it is difficult although not impossible to control the stringent hybridization and washing conditions precisely. Therefore, it would be desirable if the probe could detect the target sequence specifically at a temperature lower than its melting temperature by 10°C. Melting temperature (T_m) is defined as the temperature at which half the duplex molecules dissociate into their constituent single strands. The empirically derived formula ***(15)*** for calculating T_m is: $T_m = 79.8 + 18.5 \log M + 58.4$ (mole fraction GC) + 11.8 (mole fraction GC)^2 – 820/L – 0.5 (% formamide) – % mismatch. If quantitative comparison of different genes is required, the length and GC content of the probes should be similar.

Radioactive and nonradioactive probes can be synthesized in several ways. Most often, single-stranded RNA probes are generated by in vitro transcription with high efficiency, and thus high specific activity, from either T7, T3, or SP6 RNA polymerase promoters. With the availability of transcription vectors, the desired cDNA sequence corresponding to the mature RNA of a particular gene is subcloned into a suitable vector, such as pGEM, pSP, or Bluescript series. The insert is flanked by two different RNA polymerase promoters thus enabling either sense-strand (control) or antisense-strand (probe) RNA to be synthesized. Single-stranded RNA probes are more sensitive than double-stranded DNA probes for several reasons: (1) an RNA probe is free of complementary sense strand to compete for hybridization with the target mRNA; (2) ribonuclease (RNase) treatment following the hybridization step can be used to reduce nonspecific binding; and (3) annealing with the target mRNA is stronger and more stable for RNA probes than for DNA probes. The length of riboprobes can vary from under 100 bp to up to > 1000 bp. Although some protocols recommend breaking up longer probes (e.g., >500 bp) to smaller fragments by alkaline hydrolysis for better tissue penetration and consequently stronger signal, we have successfully used 800-bp riboprobes without such treatment.

Although riboprobes are more sensitive and more reliable than short single-stranded oligodeoxynucleotide probes (typically 20–40 bp), the latter can be useful in certain circumstances. First, oligodeoxynucleotides are easily synthesized and do not require elaborate microbiologic and molecular biologic procedures that are not always available in many laboratories. Second, oligodeoxynucleotides can be useful for specific purposes since it is possible to design probes that distinguish transcripts with relatively small sequence differences, e.g., to study closely related members of a gene family or alternatively spliced RNAs from the same gene such as, D_2 dopamine receptor splice variants ***(16)***. A disadvantage of oligonucleotide probes is that relatively small numbers of labeled nucleotides can be incorporated per molecule of probe, making them less sensitive than longer riboprobes. This limitation can be overcome by using a mixture of oligodeoxynucleotides that are complementary to different regions of the target molecule ***(17–19)***.

The following control procedures can be used to ensure specificity of *in situ* hybridization: (1) co-localization of hybrids formed by different probes complementary to the same mRNA target; (2) competition of hybridization of the labeled probe by unlabeled probe of the same sequence; (3) different distribution of signal with probes against other unrelated transcripts; (4) cautious use of sense probe since occasionally this can detect mRNA transcribed from the complementary DNA strand in the chromosome; or (5) scrambled DNA sequence when using oligonucleotide probes; (6) Northern blot analysis using the probe under the same stringency conditions showing band(s) of expected size(s); (7) pretreatment of tissues with RNase to destroy the targets before subjecting to *in situ* hybridization, as negative control; and (8) co-localization of hybridization signal with appropriate immunoreactive staining for the encoded protein, with notable exceptions (e.g., *see* **ref. *20***).

Two main radioisotopes are currently used for labeling probes. The most widely used radioactive compound for ISH is [^{35}S], which does not require shielding, has a half-life of 87 d allowing probes to be used over a period of 1–2 mo, and does provide a cellular resolution using nuclear emulsion. When using [^{35}S], inclusion of a reducing agent such as DTT is important to protect the sulphur from oxidation, which could result in high background. [^{33}P] is a newer radioisotope with a resolution roughly comparable to that of [^{35}S] and a half-life of 25 d. Since the β-electrons emitted from [^{33}P] are approx 1.5 times more energetic than those emitted from [^{35}S] but have a shorter path length than those from [^{32}P], exposure time is reduced considerably using [^{33}P], especially when detecting low-abundance mRNAs. Similar to [^{35}S], [^{33}P] does not require shielding.

Typically, a plasmid containing the specific cDNA to be transcribed is linearized with a restriction enzyme. It might be useful to restrict a large amount (about 10 μg) of plasmid if that particular probe is to be made repeatedly. Alternatively, PCR fragments of the desired cDNA can be generated using primers containing different RNA polymerase promoter sequences. In this case, PCR fragments are gel-purified and used instead of linearized plasmid. Kits for in vitro transcription are available from different suppliers (such as Promega, Ambion, and Boehringer Mannheim).

3.1.1. Radioisotope Labeling of Riboprobe

1. For radioisotope labeling, mix the following reagents in an Eppendorf tube:
   a. 250 ng linearized template DNA or 10–100 ng PCR product.
   b. 2 μL 10X transcription buffer: 400 m*M* Tris-HCl, 60 m*M* $MgCl_2$, 50 m*M* dithioerythritol, 40 m*M* spermidine, pH 7.2.
   c. 1 μL 10 m*M* ATP.
   d. 1 μL 10 m*M* CTP.
   e. 1 μL 10 m*M* GTP.
   f. 7 μL [^{35}S]-α-UTP (>1000 Ci/mmol).

   g. 1 µL RNase inhibitor.
   h. Add DEPC water to a final volume of 20 µL.
   i. 1 µL RNA polymerase (T7, T3, or SP6).
2. Mix well but do not vortex and incubate at 37°C for 1 h. Add 1 µL DNase, and incubate for an additional 15 min at 37°C to degrade the DNA template.
3. For extraction of the riboprobe, add 60 µL DEPC water and 80 µL phenol/chloroform. Vortex for 30 s and spin for 3 min at 20,800*g* (14,000 rpm).
4. Take the upper layer (80 µL; the RNA probe is in the top aqueous phase) and purify RNA probe with NucTrap Purification Columns (Stratagene) or Spin Column (Sephadex G-50).
5. To determine specific activity, count 1 µL of radiolabeled probe in a scintillation counter. The counts should be in the range of 0.5×10^6 to 2×10^6. Add 5 µL SDS and 1 µL DTT to 100 µL probe and store at –20°C or below until used.

3.1.2. Nonradioactive Labeling of Riboprobe

1. For digoxigenin labeling, mix the following reagents (Boehringer Mannheim) in an Eppendorf tube:
   a. 1 µg linearized template DNA.
   b. 2 µL NTP mix.
   c. 2 µL 10X transcription buffer: 400 m*M* Tris-HCl, 60 m*M* $MgCl_2$, 50 m*M* dithioerythritol, 40 m*M* spermidine, pH 7.2.
   d. 1 µL RNase inhibitor.
   e. Add DEPC water to a final volume of 18 µL.
   f. 2 µL RNA polymerase (T7, T3, or SP6).
   g. Mix well but do not vortex and incubate at 37°C for 2 h.
2. Add 1 µL of DNase and incubate for an additional 15 min at 37°C to degrade the DNA template.
3. For longer storage, LiCl precipitation is recommended. Add 2.5 µL 4 *M* LiCl and 75 µL ice cold ethanol. Mix well and leave at –70°C for at least 30 min followed by centrifugation at 17,900*g* (13,000 rpm) for 15 min. Wash the pellet with ice-cold 70% ethanol, air-dry for a short time, and dissolve in DEPC water. Labeling efficiency and probe concentration can be determined by blotting different dilutions of the probe on a membrane and using a DIG nucleic acid detection kit (Boehringer).

3.1.3. Radioactive and Nonradioactive Labeling of Oligodeoxynucleotide Probes

1. In a sterile Eppendorf tube, add 5 µL 5X tailing buffer, 1 µL oligodeoxynucleotide (35 pmol), and 9 µL ^{35}S-dATP (1000–1500 Ci/mmol; NEN, NEG-034H), adjust volume to 25 µL with distilled water and add 50 U terminal transferase. Mix gently, and do not vortex.
2. Incubate at 37°C for approx 5 min. The exact labeling time varies depending on the batch of isotope or enzyme used.
3. The reaction can be terminated by incubation at 65°C for 10 min.
4. Purify the oligodeoxynucleotide with a Spin Column (Sephadex G-25) or other purification column.

5. Count 1 µL of radiolabeled probe in a scintillation counter. The counts should be in the range of 0.5×10^6 to 3×10^6 dpm/µL. Store at –20°C until used.
6. For digoxigenin-labeled probes, use 1 µL of a 250 m*M* digoxigenin/1 m*M* mix (Boehringer Mannheim). Incubate for 2 h at 37°C. Add 6 µL 10X TE. Use 3–10 µL of probe per 100 µL of hybridization solution.

3.2. Preparation of Tissues for ISH

ISH is performed on fixed tissues to avoid mRNA loss and to preserve the quality of the histologic preparation. Two different approaches to tissue preparation are commonly used for ISH. Samples can either be sectioned frozen with a cryostat, or fixed with a crosslinking fixative and embedded in paraffin wax prior to sectioning. Although paraffin embedding preserves tissue morphology better and sections can be stored almost indefinitely, its disadvantage lies in the multiple preparation steps before the actual ISH. Cryostat sectioning requires less tissue preparation, may be more sensitive for ISH, and storage of sections at –80°C is safe over extended periods, depending on the abundance and stability of the specific message. Therefore, cryostat sectioning is usually preferred over paraffin embedding (for protocols of paraffin embedding, *see* **ref.** ***21***). However, paraffin embedding is the method of choice if good morphology and high resolution are required. When working with mRNA preparations, a major concern is RNase contamination since these are ubiquitous and remarkably stable enzymes, surviving temperatures up to 100°C. Thus, considerable care is required to ensure that all glassware and solutions are RNase free. Glassware should be treated with DEPC and autoclaved. Fill the glassware with freshly prepared 0.1% DEPC water (see above), shake well several times, and leave overnight at room temperature. Next day, autoclave for 90 min to inactivate DEPC (*see* **Note 3**).

1. Tissues for hybridization must be collected and frozen as soon as possible to preventing RNA degradation. After sacrificing the animal, remove the brain as quickly as possible and either freeze it in a beaker containing isopentane chilled by liquid nitrogen or place the brain on dry ice powder until completely frozen. Similarly, postmortem human brain should be recovered as soon as possible and frozen immediately at –80°C.
2. Sections are cut (10–15 µm thickness) on a cryostat at approx –18°C (may need optimization for different tissue types) and thaw-mounted on silanized or gelatin-coated slides. The slides can be placed on a slide warmer at 42°C for several minutes to dry the sections before they are placed at –80°C until use.
3. On the day of ISH, take the slides out of the freezer and allow them to warm up for 10 min at room temperature.
4. Place slides in a rack and immerse in 4% formaldehyde solution at room temperature for 5 min. Rinse twice with 1X PBS and process immediately for hybridization (*see* **Subheading 3.3.1.**).

3.3. Hybridization

Hybridization is usually set up in the late afternoon, which allows overnight incubation. (Complete hybridization requires between 8–18 h.) Probe concentration is usually 1–2 × 10^6 cpm/50 µL, which will saturate target mRNA. Excess probe is removed by RNase treatment and washing. Before hybridization, the probe is heat denatured to remove possible secondary structures that might inhibit hybridization. The use of DTT with [^{35}S]-labeled probes is required to keep them in a reduced state and minimize background. For practical purposes, if a probe is well designed, adjustment of specific hybridization and washing temperatures may not be required. Throughout the hybridization procedure, the use of DEPC water and gloves is recommended to prevent degradation of the target mRNA by RNases. After hybridization, sections are washed several times in salt solutions with the aim of retaining the maximum amount of specifically bound probe while washing off nonspecifically bound probe. Washing, like hybridization, depends on temperature (the higher, the more stringent) and salt concentration (the lower, the more stringent). RNase treatment following hybridization will further reduce nonspecifically bound probe by degrading nonhybridized RNA and leaving hybridized RNA intact. DTT is added to the washing solution to keep the probe in a reduced state to minimize background.

3.3.1. Hybridization Histochemistry with Riboprobes

1. Place the fixed slides in fresh 0.25% acetic anhydride solution for 10 min with gentle rocking to reduce nonspecific binding. Per 100 mL, mix 1.49 mL triethanolamine and 420 µL concentrated HCl. Then add and mix 0.25 mL acetic anhydride. **Caution**: Acetic anhydride is toxic and skin contact or inhalation should be avoided.
2. Wash slides in 2X SSC at room temperature for 5 min twice.
3. Transfer slides through 70% ethanol for 1 min, 80% ethanol for 1 min, 95% ethanol for 1 min, 100% ethanol for 1 min, chloroform for 5 min, 100% ethanol for 1 min, and 95% ethanol for 1 min. Remove the rack from ethanol and allow to air dry.
4. In an Eppendorf tube, add 2 × 10^6 cpm probe plus DEPC water to 8 µL total and add 4 µL nucleic acid mix:

	Stock (mg/mL)	µL/mL	Final conc. (µg/mL)
Salmon sperm DNA	10	250	100
Yeast total RNA Type XI	20	313	250
Yeast tRNA	25	250	250
DEPC water		187	

Heat at 70°C for 5 min, place on ice for 5 min, and add at room temperature:

a. 84 µL hybridization mix.

b. 2 µL 5 *M* DTT (do not add when using digoxigenin, even if double labeling with a radioisotope probe).

c. 1 µL 10% sodium thiosulfate.
d. 1 µL 10% SDS.

5. Place 50–100 µL hybridization solution containing about 1×10^6 cpm/50 µL [^{35}S]-labeled probe on the section and cover with a glass coverslip. When using a digoxigenin probe, a concentration of 2–6 ng/50 µL of probe is recommended. However, trying different concentrations of a digoxigenin probe is advisable when using a probe for the first time to determine the optimum amount for that particular probe. Fifty microliters of hybridization solution is enough to cover two coronal adult rat brain sections under an 18 × 30-mm coverslip. The amount of hybridization solution should be scaled up proportionately if a larger coverslip is used to cover a larger section or if sections tend to dry out with 50 µL of hybridization solution.
6. Hybridize overnight at 55°C in a bioassay dish together with threefold layers of Whatman 3MM paper or tissue paper soaked with distilled water, and seal the dish with a lid to form a moist chamber.
7. The next day, transfer the slides to a slide rack and wash them in 4X SSC, 1 m*M* DTT (40 µL of 5 *M* DTT for 200 mL of solution) at room temperature until coverslips come off. Avoid manual force when removing the coverslips as this may harm the sections. From this step on, DEPC-treated water is no longer required to prepare washing solutions.
8. Rinse slides with 4X SSC, 1 m*M* DTT four times 5 min. Replace with fresh solution each time while shaking.
9. Incubate at 37°C for 30 min in 20 µg/mL RNase A: Dissolve 1 mL 10 mg/mL Rnase in 500 mL prewarmed (37°C) RNase buffer (62.5 mL 4 *M* NaCl, 2.5 mL 2 *M* Tris-HCl, pH 8.0, and 0.5 mL 0.25 *M* EDTA). Add 434.5 mL of distilled water.
10. Rinse the slides twice in 0.1X SSC, 1 m*M* DTT at room temperature for 5 min. Next, wash the slides twice with 0.1X SSC, 1 m*M* DTT at 65°C for 30 min each followed by two 5 min. washes with 0.1X SSC, 1 m*M* DTT at room temperature.
11. The slides are then dehydrated through a graded series of ethanol (70, 80, 95, and 100%; each 1 min) and air-dried.

3.3.2. Hybridization Histochemistry with Oligodeoxynucleotide Probes

1–5. Follow the protocol for riboprobes in **Subheading 3.3.1.**

6. Hybridize overnight at 37°C in a bioassay dish together with threefold layers of Whatmann 3MM paper or tissue paper soaked with distilled water, and seal the dish with a lid to form a moist chamber.
7. The next day, transfer the slides to a slide rack and wash them in 1X SSC, 1 m*M* DTT (40 µL 5 *M* DTT for 200 mL of solution) at room temperature until coverslips come off. Avoid manual force when removing the coverslips as this may harm the sections.
8. Slides are then washed four times in 1X SSC, 1 m*M* DTT at 55°C for 15 min four times, followed by washes in 1X SSC, 1 m*M* DTT at room temperature for 5 min twice.
9. The slides are then dehydrated through a graded series of ethanol (70, 80, 95, and 100%; each 1 min) and air-dried.

3.4. Detection of Radiolabeled Probes

Detection of radiolabeled probes entails apposition of the slides to X-ray film or coating of the sections with nuclear emulsion if higher cellular resolution is required. Radioactive particles from the isotope convert the silver bromide contained in the detector emulsion to metallic silver, which yields a visible image after the process of development and fixation. Several nuclear emulsions are available. Kodak's NBT-2 gives a fine cellular localization, whereas NBT-3 and Ilford's K5 are more sensitive. If sections are double labeled simultaneously with radioisotope- and digoxigenin-labeled probes, the exposure to nuclear emulsion must be performed after detecting the digoxigenin signal. Exposure time for X-ray film and for nuclear emulsion largely depends on the abundance of the particular mRNA. When using a new probe, slides may be initially exposed to an X-ray film for 1 wk. If the signal is too weak, expose again for 2 weeks and so on. Then, using the same slides, proceed with nuclear emulsion exposure.

1. Under safelight conditions (e.g., Kodak Wratten series II safelight), scoop out 40 mL of emulsion with a plastic spatula into a Coplin jar placed in a 41°C water bath for 20–30 min to allow air bubbles to rise. If emulsion coating appears to be too thick, one can dilute the nuclear emulsion 50:50 with distilled water before use. Nuclear emulsion is extremely sensitive to light. Therefore, safelight conditions are of utmost importance since even minor light sources can ruin the experiment (e.g., phosphorescent watches or sparks from electronic devices).
2. Mix emulsion gently and dip a clean blank slide into the emulsion. If uneven coating is seen, allow more time for the emulsion to heat up. If coating is smooth but bubbles are still present, repeat dipping with new blank slides until bubbles disappear.
3. After ensuring a smooth coating and no bubbles, dip the experimental slides briefly into the emulsion and air-dry them upright for several hours in the dark.
4. The emulsion-coated slides are then placed in black slide boxes containing desiccant capsules. Tape the edges with black photography tape and store the boxes at 4°C in the dark for an appropriate time depending on the radioisotope used and the abundance level of the particular transcript. As a rule of thumb, one can estimate a threefold longer exposure time for emulsion detection compared with X-ray film detection.
5. Under safelight conditions, put the slides in racks and pass them through the following solutions at 17°C with gentle agitation every 30 s: Kodak D-19 for 2 min at 14°C; running tap water for 15 s; and Kodak Fixer for 3 min. The developer should be used at 17°C since the temperature affects the size of the silver grains produced; the warmer the developer, the larger the grains.
6. Rinse in running tap water for 10 min If desired, counterstain with hematoxylin/eosin (not when using digoxogenin probes), or any stain of choice, and rinse briefly with water to remove excess stain.

7. Dip very briefly into distilled water, and then 70% ethanol (could reduce the signal of digoxigenin-labeled probes) and place on a slide warmer to dry thoroughly.
8. Coverslip slides with Cytoseal 60 or a similar organic-based mounting medium.

3.5. Hybridization and Detection of Double ISH Localization Using Digoxigenin-Labeled Probes

After localizing a particular mRNA in the brain, the question often arises of which of the cell types express this mRNA and in which functional circuits the cell type is involved. To address such questions, the co-localization of certain mRNAs in the same cell can be addressed by two different techniques. First, since neurons have an average size of 15 µm, very thin brain slices (<5 µm) can be cut to obtain two consecutive slices of the cell on two different slides. Each slide is then processed for ISH with a different probe and, after cellular localization of the mRNAs using nuclear emulsion exposure, individual cells are traced on both slides and compared for their respective signal.

The more sophisticated direct method consists of combining nonradioactive with radioactive ISH on the same brain section (**Fig. 3**). One of the most widely employed nonradioactive ISH techniques uses DIG-UTP-labeled probes, which are subsequently detected using specific antibodies coupled to the enzyme alkaline phosphatase. The color signal is then developed with the enzyme substrate NBT/BCIP. Hybridization signal appears as a blue precipitate over the cytoplasm of the cell. An interesting alternative to this colorimetric method is the use of a gold system (anti-digoxigenin antibody coupled to a gold particle; Boehringer Mannheim), especially for electron microscopy. A nonradioactive method using biotin labeling is also available *(5)*.

1. Follow the ISH protocols from **Subheading 3.3.1., steps 1–5**. Add both radioactive and nonradioactive probes in the hybridization mix at previously determined concentrations.
2. Follow the washing procedures outlined in **Subheading 3.3.1.** for riboprobes (**steps 7–10**) but do not add DTT to the SSC solutions.
3. After the last wash with 0.1X SSC, transfer the slides to buffer 1 for two 5-min washes. To reduce the amount of antibody needed, the use of autoclaved Teflon Coplin jars or slide mailers is recommended.
4. Transfer slides to buffer 1 with 5% NGS and 0.6% Triton X-100 for 30 min.
5. Transfer slides to buffer 1 with 5% NGS, and 0.6% Triton X-100, and 1:2000 anti-digoxigenin-AP for 5 h with gentle rocking (*see* **Note 4**).
6. Transfer the slides to buffer 1 for two 10-min washes.
7. Transfer the slides to buffer 2 for 5 min.
8. Incubate overnight at room temperature in the dark in buffer 2 with 0.34 mg/mL NBT and 0.18 mg/mL BCIP (*see* **Note 5**).
9. Wash the slides in 1X SSC for 30 min four times. These long washes eliminate residual NBT/BCIP, which interacts nonspecifically with nuclear emulsion.

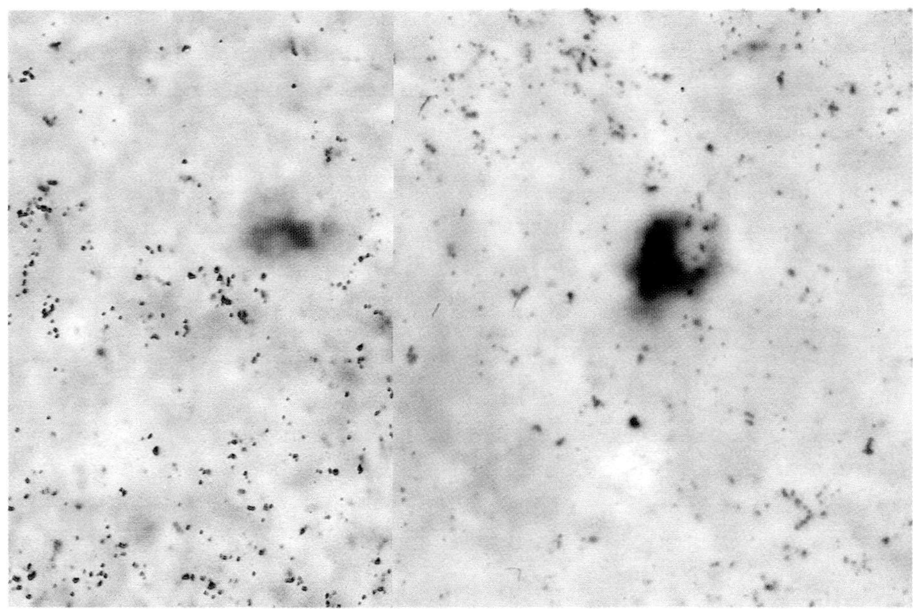

Fig. 3. Co-localization of digoxigenin-labeled D_2 dopamine receptor riboprobe and radiolabeled murine glial derived neurotrophic factor inducible factor (mGIF) riboprobe in the mouse striatum. The D_2 probe was generated by RT/PCR, yielding a 484-bp template including nucleotides 831–1271 ***(26)***. The mGIF riboprobe is complementary to the 578-bp *Hin*dIII-*Pst*I fragment ***(27)***. Left panel shows cells with no co-localization; right panel shows a cell that has both transcripts.

10. Dip briefly in distilled water and air-dry.
11. Proceed the slides to nuclear emulsion exposure (*see* **Note 6**).
12. After development, the slides should be thoroughly dried and coverslipped with Cytoseal 60 or a similar organic-based mounting medium.

3.6. Quantitation of ISH Signals

When comparing mRNA levels in various anatomical locations, different developmental stages, or in response to pharmacologic, physiologic, or surgical manipulations, quantitative ISH allows not only identification of regional changes, but also measurement of the magnitude of these changes. For a reliable quantitative experiment, one should minimize any variation between experimental groups, ideally processing the different tissues in one single ISH. After exposure to X-ray film, optical density, which correlates with the relative amount of target mRNA, is measured with a computer image analysis system. If the sample preparation and all assay conditions are identical between the samples, this approach gives a reliable result of altered gene expression. A quantitative approach, which converts the autoradiographic signal into nanograms per cell, consists of using appropriate standards. Brain homogenates that incorporate known amounts of [^{35}S] *(18)* or commercially available standard strips labeled with [^{14}C] are used for this purpose. The radioactive standard sections are treated in the same way as the tissue sections and exposed to emulsion or film. A less time-consuming, semiquantitative approach in which signal from an affected tissue is compared with signal from an unaffected tissue is widely used. The results are expressed as a ratio of the two signals, control vs experimental, and allow the detection of relative changes in mRNA. Each measurement and signal is corrected for background by subtracting the value of an unlabeled brain region within the same tissue. To exclude potential differences due to experimental procedures, affected and unaffected tissue should be processed in parallel, using the same conditions. It is important to control film exposure times to prevent saturation of film since above a certain time limit (specific for each riboprobe) increases in radioactivity produce little or no further increase in labeling density (for detailed protocols, *see* **refs.** ***12,22,23***).

4. Notes

1. **Caution:** PFA and acetic anhydride are toxic, and skin contact or inhalation should be avoided. Work should be done with mask and gloves, preferably under a hood.
2. All solutions should be prepared with 0.1% DEPC water. Dissolving the mix takes time, and heating is not recommended to facilitate it.
3. RNases are also present on the skin, so gloves should be worn throughout the transcription and hybridization steps. However, wearing masks because of contamination of breath by RNases is usually not necessary, and the likelihood of RNase contamination as the reason for a nonsuccessful experiment is usually overrated.
4. The antibody can be reused several times.
5. Levamisole, up to 1 m*M*, may be added to block most endogenous alkaline phosphatases in brains.
6. When doing double labeling using digoxigenin, one should preferably use Ilford emulsion because Kodak emulsion interfers with the NBT/BCIP reaction.

References

1. Pardue, M. and Gall, J. (1969) Molecular hybridization of radioactive DNA to the DNA of cytological preparations. *Proc. Natl. Acad. Sci. USA* **64,** 600–604.
2. John, H., Birnstiel, M., and Jones, K. (1969) RNA:DNA hybrids at the cytological level. *Nature* **2,** 582–587.
3. Hunot, S., Bernard, V., Faucheux, B., Bossiere, B., Leuguern, E, Brana, C., et al. (1996) Glial cell-line derived neurotrophic factor (GDNF) gene expression in the human brain: a post mortem in situ hybridization study with special reference to Parkinson's disease. *J. Neural. Transm.* **103,** 1043–1052.

4. Joyce, J., Schmutzer, C., Whitty, A., Myers, M., and Bannon, M. (1997) Differential modification of dopamine transporter and tyrosine hydroxyalse mRNAs in midbrain of subjects with Parkinson's, Alzheimer's with parkinsonism, and Alzheimer's disease. *Movement Dis.* **12,** 885–897.
5. Le Moine, C., Normand, E., and Bloch, B. (1995) Use of non-radioactive probes for mRNA detection by in situ hybridization: interests and application in the central nervous system. *Cell Mol. Biol.* **41,** 917–923.
6. Gerfen, C., Engber, T., Mahan, L., Susel, Z., Chase, T., Monsma, F., and Sibley, D. (1990) D1 and D2 dopamine receptor-regulated gene expression of striatonigral and striatopallidal neurons. *Science* **7,** 1429–1432.
7. Schwartz, J.-C., Giros, B., Martres, M.-P., and Sokoloff, P. (1992) The dopamine receptor family: molecular biology and pharmacology. *Sem. Neurosci.* **4,** 99–108.
8. Polymeropoulos, M., Lavedant, C., Leroy, E., Ide, S., Deheija, A., Dutra, A., et al. (1997) Mutation in the α-synuclein gene identified in families with Parkinson's disease. *Science* **276,** 2045–2047.
9. Morissette, M., Goulet, M., Calon, F., Falardeau, P., Blanchet, P., Bedard, P., and Di Paolo, T. (1996) Changes of D1 and D2 dopamine receptor mRNA in the brains of monkeys lesioned with 1-methyl-4-phenyl-1,2,3,6-tetrahydripyridine: correction with chronic administration of L-3,4-Dihydroxyphenylalanine. *Mol. Pharmacol.* **50,** 1073–1079.
10. Komminoth, P. and Werner, M. (1997) Target and signal amplification: approaches to increase the sensitivity of in situ hybridization. *Histochem. Cell. Biol.* **108,** 325–333.
11. Albertson, D., Fishpool, R., and Birchall, P. (1995) Fluorescence in situ hybridization for the detection of DNA and RNA. *Methods Cell Biol.* **48,** 339–364.
12. Eberwine, J., Valentino, K., and Barchas, J. (1994) *In Situ Hybridization in Neurobiology. Advances in Methodology.* Oxford University Press, Oxford.
13. Wisden, W. and Morris, B. (1994) In situ hybridization protocols for the brain, in *Biological Techniques* (Sattelle, D., ed.), Academic Press, London.
14. Wilkinson, D. (1992) *In Situ Hybridization. A Practical Approach. The Practical Approach Series.* (Rickwood, D. and Hames, B., eds.), RL Press, Oxford.
15. Bodkin, D. and Knudson, D. (1985) Assessment of sequence relatedness of double-stranded RNA genes by RNA-RNA blot hybridization. *J. Virol. Methods* **10,** 45–52.
16. Giros, B., Sokoloff, P., Martres, M.-P., Riou, J.-F., Emorine, L., and Schwatz, J.-C. (1989) Alternative splicing directs the expression of two D2 dopamine receptor isoforms. *Nature* **342,** 923–926.
17. Lewis, M., Krause II, R., and Robert-Lewis, J. (1988) Recent developments in the use of synthetic oligonucleotides for in situ hybridization histochemistry. *Synapse* **2,** 308–316.
18. Young III, W. (1992) In situ hybridization with oligodeoxyribonucleotide probes, in *In Situ Hybridzation. A Practical Approach* (Wilkinson, D., ed.), IRL Press, Oxford.
19. Wisden, W. and Morris, B. (eds.) (1994) In situ hybridization with synthetic oligonucleotide probes, in *In Situ Hybridization Protocols for the Brain. (Biological Techniques).* Academic Press, San Diego.

20. Sernia, C. (1995) Location and secretion of brain angiotensin. *Reg. Pept.* **57,** 1–18.
21. Conway, S. J. (1996) In situ hybridization of cells and tissue sections, in *Methods in Molecular Medicine. Molecular Diagnosis of Cancer.* (Cotter, F., ed.), Humana Press, Totowa, NJ, pp. 193–206.
22. Wisden, W. and Morris, B. (eds.) (1994) *In situ Hybridization Protocols for the Brain. (Biological Techniques).* Academic Press, San Diego.
23. Sharif, N. A. (1993) *Molecular Imaging in Neuroscience, A Practical Approach.* IRL, Oxford.
24. Lewis, E. J., Tank, A. W., Weiner, N., and Chikaraishi, D. M. (1983) Regulation of tyrosine hyrdoxylase mRNA by glucocorticoid and cyclic AMP in a rat pheochromocytoma cell line. Isolation of a cDNA clone for tyrosine hyrdoxylase mRNA. *J. Biol. Chem.* **258,** 14,632–14,637
25. Zhou, Q., Li, C., and Civelli, O. (1992) Characterization of gene organization and promoter regions of the rat D1 dopamine receptor gene. *J. Neurochem.* **59,** 1875–1883.
26. Mantmayeur, J., Bausero, P., Amlaiky, N., Maroteaux, ?., Hen, R., and Borelli, E. (1991) Differential expression of the mouse D2 dopamine receptor isoforms. *FEBS Lett.* **278,** 239–243.
27. Yajima, S., Lammers, C.-H., Lee, S.-H., Hara, Y., Mizuno, K., and Mouradian, M. M. (1997) Cloning and characterization of murine glial cell-derived neurotrophic factor inducible transcription factor (MGIF). *J. Neurosci.* **15,** 8657–8666.

17

Regulation of Striatal *N*-Methyl-D-Aspartate Receptor (NMDAR) Function by Phosphorylation of its Subunits in Parkinsonian Rats

Justin D. Oh

1. Introduction

The cardinal signs of Parkinson's disease (PD) reflect striatal dopamine depletion due to the progressive degeneration of neurons arising from the substantia nigra. Initially, treatment with the dopamine precursor levodopa ordinarily confers substantial clinical benefit. Later, however, increasing difficulties arise mainly due to the appearance of motor response fluctuations and dyskinesias complicating the treatment of late-stage PD ***(1–6)***. Available evidence suggests that standard dopaminomimetic treatment regimens promote the intermittent activation of striatal dopaminergic receptors, which under normal conditions operate mainly tonically ***(7)***, and that this nonphysiologic stimulation favors the appearance of the motor fluctuations and dyskinesias ***(8)***.

The cellular mechanisms by which intermittent dopaminergic stimulation leads to motor response complications has only recently become clear. Studies suggest that periodic stimulation of denervated striatal dopaminergic receptors enhances the sensitivity of co-localized glutamatergic receptors of the *N*-methyl-D-aspartate (NMDA) subtype on striatal medium spiny neurons ***(9–11)*** in ways that favor the clinical appearance of parkinsonism motor complications ***(12–14)***. NMDA receptors are heteroligomers of NR1 (a–h) and NR2 (A–D) subunits ***(15,16)***. In rat striatum, medium spiny neurons express NR1 splice variants along with NR2B and to a lesser extent NR2A subunits ***(17)***. It has recently been shown that phosphorylation at tyrosine and serine/threonine residues serves as a major regulatory mechanism for these receptors ***(18,19)*** by modulating channel opening probability and their subcellular distribution and anchoring, respectively ***(7,13,20,21)***.

From: *Methods in Molecular Medicine, vol. 62: Parkinson's Disease: Methods and Protocols*
Edited by: M. M. Mouradian © Humana Press Inc., Totowa, NJ

Since various forms of synaptic plasticity ***(22,23)*** as well as some pathologic states have been linked to a rise in NMDA receptor subunit phosphorylation ***(24)***, it is reasonable to assume that the enhanced NR2A and NR2B tyrosine phosphorylation in the striatum may affect glutamatergic transmission and thus contribute to the motor response alterations associated with chronic levodopa therapy. Current data support the view that the enhancement in tyrosine and serine phosphorylation contributes to the heightened sensitivity of the NMDA receptor complexes and thus to the motor dysfunctions attending dopaminergic denervation and dopaminomimetic therapy ***(25)***. It is conceivable that the pharmaceutical targeting of striatal NMDA receptors that are modified in PD—initially as a consequence of dopaminergic denervation and later due to nonphysiologic dopaminergic stimulation—will ultimately prove to be a safe and effective treatment for all stages of this disorder.

In view of the important functional implications of NMDA phosphorylation in its channel function, continued exploration of the phosphorylation state of NMDAR subunits will be worthwhile. Biochemical methods are presented here for reliable and rapid determination of the presence or absence of phosphorylated residues of the NMDA receptors in striatal tissue. Immunoprecipitation combined with immunoblotting techniques can be useful in assessing the degree of NMDA receptor phosphorylation in the striatum following dopaminergic denervation and subsequent chronic dopaminergic stimulation.

2. Materials

1. Sonication buffer consists of the following: 1.0% ultrapure sodium dodecyl sulfate (SDS), 20 m*M* HEPES, pH, 7.4, 150 m*M* NaCl, 1.0 m*M* EDTA, 1.0 m*M* EGTA, 25 m*M* NaF, 10 m*M* NaPPi, 1.0 m*M* Na_3VO_4, 10 µg/mL leupeptin, aprotinin, pepstatin A, and ddH_2O, containing 10% glycerol, 1.0 m*M* phenylmethylsulfonyl fluoride, 1.5 m*M* $MgCl_2$, and 1 m*M* $ZnCl_2$.
2. Immunoprecipitation buffer consists of the following: 2.7 m*M* KCl, 1.2 m*M* KH_2PO_4, 137 m*M* NaCl, 8.3 m*M* NaH_2PO_4, 5.0 m*M* EDTA and EGTA, 10 m*M* NaPPi, and 50 m*M* NaF.
3. Protein A slurry: Protein A Sepharose (Sigma) and 10% Sephacryl G10 (Pharmacia) in 1% Triton X-100 immunoprecipitation buffer. Sephacryl is added directly to protein A Sepharose and washed several times using 1X cold phosphate-buffered saline (PBS). The mixture is equilibrated and kept in 1% Triton X-100 immunoprecipitation buffer until use.
4. Sample buffer for polyacrylamide gel electrophoresis (PAGE): ddH_2O is added to tissue sample to adjust the concentration of protein; then stock sample buffer and stock reducing agent are added to the final concentration of 1X sample buffer and 1X reducing agent. Composition of the sample buffer: 6.8% Tris base, 6.7% Tri-HCl, 40% sucrose, 8% SDS, 0.06% EDTA, 0.08% Serva blue G250, and 0.03% Phenol Red in sterile ddH_2O.

5. Running buffer for PAGE: 100 mL 10X running buffer is diluted with 900 mL H_2O and 2.5 mL antioxidant (10% ascorbic acid in ddH_20) is added. The running buffer is kept cold until use. The 10X running buffer contains the following: 10.5% 3-(*N*-morpholino) propane sulfonic acid, 6.0% Tris base, 10% SDS, 0.3% EDTA in sterile ddH_2O.
6. Blocking buffer: Add 0.24 g of blocking dry milk powder to 120 mL of 1X PBS (containing 0.06 *M* Na_2HPO_4, 0.017 *M* $NaH_2PO_4H_2O$, and 0.068 *M* NaCl) and microwave to dissolve the powder for about 2 min. Tween 20 (120 µL) is added after cooling the buffer to room temperature.
7. Wash buffer: 10 mL of 10X PBS (containing 0.6 *M* Na_2HPO_4, 0.17 *M* $NaH_2PO_4H_2O$, and 0.68 *M* NaCl) and 0.1 mL Tween 20 is added to dd H_2O to make 100 mL of wash buffer.
8. Transfer buffer: To 850 mL of H_2O, add the following solutions: 50 mL stock transfer buffer, 100 MeOH, and 1 mL antioxidant (10% ascorbic acid).
9. Assay buffer: 20 m*M* Tri-HCl, at pH 9.8, containing 1 m*M* $MgCl_2$.

3. Methods

3.1. Tissue Preparation and Protein Measurement

1. Three weeks after 6-hydroxydopamine (6-OHDA) lesioning or at the end of chronic levodopa treatment, rat brains are removed and striatal tissue from the lesioned (ipsilateral) and intact (contralateral) sides are dissected and frozen rapidly into separate microtubes.
2. Striatal tissues are homogenized by sonication and an aliquot taken for protein determination by the Lowry method (*see* **Note 1**).

3.2. Tissue Homogenization and Sample Preparation

Another aliquot containing approximately 100 µg of striatal tissue is heated for 5 min at 90°C in sonication buffer to solubilize the NMDA receptor proteins completely (*see* **Note 2**).

3.3. Immunoprecipitation

1. Homogenized samples are equilibrated in immunoprecipitation buffer containing 5% Triton X-100 and precleared with 100 µL Protein A slurry, which had been previously washed in the same buffer containing 10 mg/mL bovine serum albumin.
2. Precleared homogenate samples are incubated next for 3 h at 4°C with anti-phosphotyrosine (Boehringer Mannheim; 10 µg), anti-phosphoserine (Sigma; 20 µg), anti-NR2A (CalBiochem; 2 µg), or anti-NR2B (CalBiochem; 2 µg).
3. The immune complexes are then incubated for another 3 h at 4°C with 100 µg of protein A slurry and washed three times with the immunoprecipitation buffer in the following order: (1) with 1.0% Triton X-100; (2) with 1.0% Triton X-100 and 0.5 *M* NaCl; and (3) without Triton X-100. Pellets are finally boiled for 5 min in 100 µL 2X sample buffer.

3.4. Western Blot Analysis and Chemiluminescent Detection

1. Striatal homogenates (14 μg of protein per lane) or immunoprecipitated fractions (20 μg of protein per lane) are subjected to SDS-PAGE on 10% polyacrylamide gels and transferred to a nitrocellulose membrane (Novex, San Diego, CA).
2. Immonoblotting is performed with primary antibodies against phosphotyrosine, phosphoserine, NR2A, or NR2B.
3. Following protein transfer, blots are washed in 1X PBS and then incubated in blocking buffer for 1 h.
4. Blots are incubated with primary antibody for 1 h and then washed with 1X PBS before incubation with secondary antibody-alkaline phosphatase conjugate 1:5,000 in blocking buffer for 30 min.
5. Nitrocellulose membranes are washed three times for 5 min each in wash buffer, two times for 2 min each in assay buffer, and then placed on Saran Wrap on a flat surface (*see* **Note 3**).
6. Nitrocellulose membranes are incubated for 5–10 min in substrate solution containing Nitroblock II (20X chemiluminescent enhancer; TROPIX, Bedford, MA) and CDP Star (0.25 mM CDP-StarTM substrate solution; TROPIX).
7. The membranes are placed in a developing cassette and exposed to X-ray film in a darkroom (*see* **Note 4**).

3.5. Immunoreactive Detection and Quantitative Analysis

1. Immunoreactivity is detected by ECL chemiluminescence (TROPIX). Following immunoreactivity detection, ECL-exposed films are scanned with an image analyzer (NIH Image 1.60 software) and densitometric quantification of immunopositive bands carried out.
2. After background subtraction, values are expressed as the mean percentage of intact striatum (contralateral side) for each immunoblot data. A photograph of ECL-exposed films and a bar graph of densitometric quantification of immunopositive bands are demonstrated in **Fig. 1**.

4. Notes

1. For the spectrophotometric quantification of protein in tissue samples, bicinchoninic acid (BCA) protein assay reagent (Pierce, Rockford, IL) is used. Briefly, working reagent consists of 49 mL buffer solution (containing sodium carbonate, sodium bicarbonate, BCA detection reagent, and sodium tartrate in 0.2 *N* NaOH) and 1 mL of 4% copper sulfate solution. Standard, blank, or striatal tissue samples (10 μL each) and working reagent (200 μL) are loaded into the appropriate microliter plate wells. Samples are mixed well and incubated for 30 min at 37°C. Finally, absorbance is read at 562 nm, and the protein concentration of striatal samples is determined from the standard curve.
2. Prior to the immunoprecipitation procedure, to make sure that NMDA receptor subunits are soluble, striatal homogenate can be extracted with 2% SDS, boiled for 3 min, and left to cool down to room temperature; then 5 vol of cold Triton X-

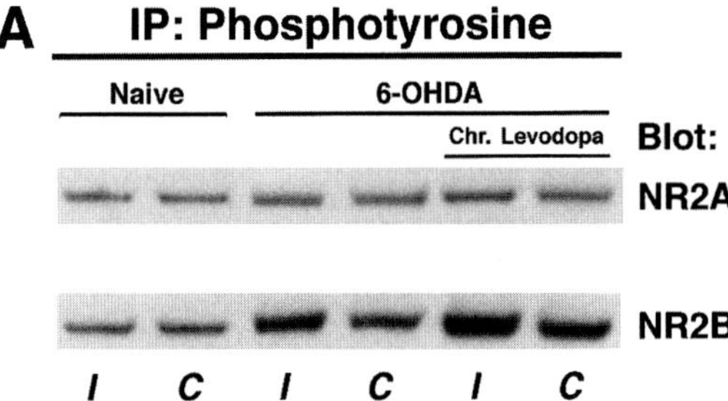

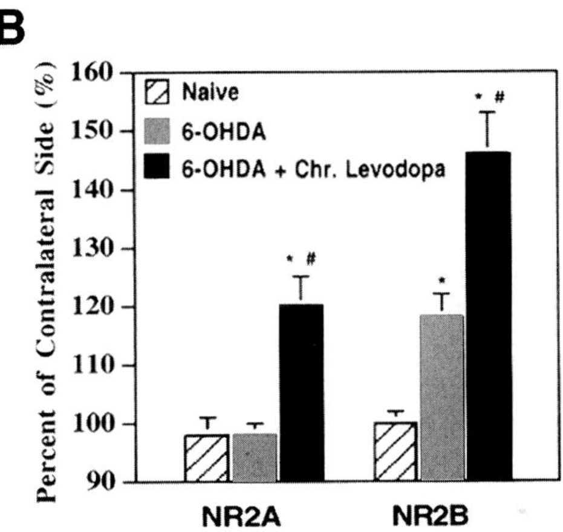

Fig. 1. The effect of 6-OHDA lesioning and subsequent levodopa treatment on tyrosine phosphorylation of NR2 subunits in rat striatum. Modulation of heteromeric NMDAR function following the motor response alterations associated with intermittent levodopa treatment is conferred by modifications in subunit tyrosine phosphorylation. **(A)** Striatal homogenates from naive (lanes 1, 2), 6-OHDA-lesioned (lanes 3, 4), or 6-OHDA lesioned plus levodopa-treated (lanes 5, 6) animals were immunoprecipitated with phosphotyrosine antibodies and the precipitates analyzed by Western blotting with antibodies specific for NR2A or NR2B subunits. **(B)** Bands corresponding to NR2A and NR2B (180 kDa) on immunoblots shown as in A were scanned, their optical density quantified by densitometry, and the value of lesioned side expressed as percent of intact striatum (ipsilateral/contralateral × 100% ± SEM). Data are reported as means ± SEM and analyzed by analysis of variance (ANOVA) followed by Scheffe's posthoc comparison tests. Statistical significance was taken as $p < 0.05$ for all analyses. I, striatum ipsilateral to the lesion; C, striatum contralateral to the lesion.

100 in PBS are added. Add sample buffer and run an aliquot (about 5–10 μg on a minigel) on a Western blot (against NR2A or NR2B antibodies) to make sure your solubilization is working first.

3. Blots can be drained by touching one side of edge on a paper towel without drying the blot too much. Blots should be handled either with forceps or gloves.
4. Blots may be imaged by using standard X-ray film or by phosphorimager. To assess optimum exposure time, initial exposure of 3 min followed by shorter exposure times are recommended.

References

1. Hurtig, H. I. (1997) Problems with current pharmacologic treatment of Parkinson's disease. *Exp. Neurol.* **144,** 10–16.
2. Chase, T. N. (1998) The significance of continuous dopaminergic stimulation in the treatment of Parkinson's disease. *Drugs* **55,** 1–9.
3. Metman, L. V., Locatelli, E. R., Bravi, D., Mouradian, M. M., and Chase, T. N. (1998) Apomorphine responses in Parkinson's disease and the pathogenesis of motor complications. *Neurology* **50,** 574–574.
4. Miyawaki, E. Lyons, K., Pahwa, R., Troster, A. I., Hubble, J., Smith, D., et al. (1997) Motor complications of chronic levodopa therapy in Parkinson's disease. *Clin. Pharmacol.* **20,** 523–530.
5. Chase, T. N. and Oh, J. D. (1999) Striatal mechanisms contributing to the pathogenesis of parkinsonian signs and levodopa-associated motor complications. *Ann. Neurol.* **47(suppl. 1),** S112–S129.
6. Quinn, N. P. (1998) Classification of fluctuations in patients with Parkinson's disease. *Neurology* **51(suppl 2),** S25–S29.
7. Schultz, W. (1994) Behavior-related activity of primate dopamine neurons. *Rev. Neurol. (Paris)* **150,** 634–639.
8. Chase, T. N., Oh, J. D., and Blanchet, P. J. (1998) Neostriatal mechanisms in Parkinson's disease. *Neurology* **51,** S30–S35.
9. Bravi, D., Mouradian, M. M., Roberts, J. W., Davis, T. L., Shon, Y. H., and Chase, T. N. (1994) Wearing-off fluctuations in Parkinson's disease: contribution of postsynaptic mechanisms. *Ann. Neurol.* **36,** 27–31.
10. Kotter, R. (1994) Postsynaptic integration of glutamatergic and dopaminergic signals in the striatum. *Prog. Neurobiol.* **44,** 163–196.
11. Engber, T. M., Papa, S. M., Boldry, R. C., and Chase, T. N. (1994) NMDA receptor blockade reverses motor response alterations induced by levodopa. *NeuroReport* **5,** 2586–2588.
12. Engber, T. M, Papa, S. M., Boldry, R. C., and Chase, T. N. (1994) NMDA receptor blockade reverses motor response alterations induced by levodopa. *NeuroReport* **5,** 2586–2588.
13. Papa, S. M., Boldry, R. C., Engber T. M., Kask, A. M., and Chase, T. N. (1995) Reversal of levodopa-induced motor fluctuations in experimental parkinsonism by NMDA receptor blockade. *Brain Res.* **701,** 13–18.
14. Cepeda, C. and Levine, M. S. (1998) Dopamine and N-methyl-D-aspartate receptor interactions in the neostriatum. *Dev. Neurosci.* **20,** 1–18.
15. Wollmuth, L. P., Kuner, T., Seeburg, P. H., and Sakmann, B. (1996) Differential contribution of the NR1- and NR2A-subunits to the selectivity filter of recombinant NMDA receptor channels. *J. Physilo. (London)* **491,** 779–797.

16. Ozawa, S, Kamiya, H., and Tsuzuki, K. (1998) Glutamate receptors in the mammalian central nervous system. *Prog. Neurobiol.* **54,** 581–618.
17. Chen, Q. and Reiner, A. (1996) Cellular distribution of the NMDA receptor NR2A/2B subunits in the rat striatum. *Brain Res.* **743,** 346–352.
18. Gurd, J. W. (1997) Protein tyrosine phosphorylation: Implications for synaptic function. *Neurochem. Int.* **31,** 635–649.
19. Suen, P. C., Wu, K., Xu, J. L., Lin S. Y., Levine, E. S., and Black, I. B. (1998) NMDA receptor subunits in the postsynaptic density of rat brain: expression and phosphorylation by endogenous protein kinases. *Brain Res.* **59,** 215–228.
20. Rostas, J. A. P., Brent, V. A., Voss, K., Errington, M. L., Bliss, T. V. P, and Gurd, J. W. (1996) Enhanced tyrosine phosphorylation of the 2B subunit of the N-methyl-D-aspartate receptor in long-term potentiation. *Proc. Natl. Acad. Sci. USA* **93,** 10,452–10,456.
21. Sigel, E. (1995) Functional modulation of ligand-gated gaba(a) and NMDA receptor channels by phosphorylation. *J. Recep. Sig. Transduc. Res.* **15,** 325–332.
22. Rosenblum, K., Berman, D. E., Hazvi, S., Lamprecht, R., and Dudai, Y. (1997) NMDA receptor and the tyrosine phosphorylation of its 2B subunit in taste learning in the rat insular cortex. *J. Neurosci.* **17,** 5129–5135.
23. Rosenblum, K., Dudai, Y., and Levin, G. R. (1996) Long-term potentiation increases tyrosine phosphorylation of the N-methyl-D-aspartate receptor subunit 2B in rat dentate gyrus in vivo. *Proc. Natl. Acad. Sci. US.* **93,** 10,457–10,460.
24. Takagi, N., Shinno, K., Teves, L., Bissoon, N., Wallace, M. C., and Gurd, J. W. (1997) Transient ischemia differentially increases tyrosine phosphorylation of NMDA receptor subunits 2A and 2B. *J. Neurochem.* **69,** 1060–1065.
25. Stefani, A., Pisani, A., Bernardi, G., Bonci, A., Mercuri, N. B., Stratta, F., and Calabresi, P. (1995) The modulation of dopamine receptors in rat striatum. *J. Neural. Transm. Supp.* **45,** 61–66.

IV

Molecular Therapies

18

Chronic Intracerebral Delivery of Trophic Factors via a Programmable Pump as a Treatment for Parkinsonism

Richard Grondin, Zhiming Zhang, Dennis D. Elsberry, Greg A. Gerhardt, and Don M. Gash

1. Introduction

The most common treatment for Parkinson's disease (PD) aims at pharmacologically augmenting striatal dopamine (DA) using the DA precursor levodopa. Such treatment provides symptomatic relief, but does not slow or halt continued degeneration of nigral dopaminergic neurons. Considerable effort has been devoted to the search for neurotrophic factors with survival-promoting activities on dopaminergic neurons that could potentially be of therapeutic value in the treatment of PD. One such candidate is glial cell line-derived neurotrophic factor (GDNF).

1.1. The GDNF Story: An overview

1.1.1. Molecular Aspects

GDNF is a glycosylated, disulfide-bonded homodimer distantly related to the transforming growth factor-β (TGF-β) superfamily *(1)*. The purification and cloning of new trophic factors, termed neurturin *(2)*, persephin *(3)*, and artemin *(4)*, all structurally related to GDNF, have established the existence of a new family of neurotrophic factors structurally similar to TGF-β. GDNF is widely expressed throughout the body in many neuronal (e.g., striatum, cerebellum, cortex) *(5–7)* and nonneuronal tissues (e.g., kidney, gut) *(5,8,9)*. GDNF uses a multisubunit receptor system consisting of a glycosyl-phosphatidylinositol (GPI)-anchored membrane protein termed GFRα-1, (α subunit) that can bind GDNF and facilitate its interaction with the tyrosine

From: *Methods in Molecular Medicine, vol. 62: Parkinson's Disease: Methods and Protocols*
Edited by: M. M. Mouradian © Humana Press Inc., Totowa, NJ

kinase Ret receptor (β subunit) ***(10,11)***. Three other GPI-anchored membrane proteins are now known, namely, GFRα-2, -3, and -4 ***(12–16)***.

1.1.2. Trophic Effects in Rodent and Nonhuman Primate Models of PD

In addition to its trophic effects on cultured fetal midbrain DA neurons ***(1,17,18)***, GDNF promotes recovery of the lesioned nigrostriatal DA system and improves motor functions in animal models of PD. Several studies on the restorative effects of GDNF have used rodent models with 6-hydroxydopamine (6-OHDA)- or 1-methyl-4-phenyl-1,2,3,6-tetrahydropyridine (MPTP)-induced lesions of the nigrostriatal DA system. In the 6-OHDA-lesioned rat, GDNF was found to restore a number of functional and morphologic features of the midbrain DA neurons, namely, the number of neurons expressing tyrosine hydroxylase (TH), the number of TH-positive neurites, TH levels, and DA tissue levels ***(19–21)***. In MPTP-treated mice, either striatal or nigral administration of GDNF was shown to improve motor performance and promote recovery of midbrain DA tissue levels ***(22)***. In addition to its neurorestorative effects, GDNF also exhibits neuroprotective properties in rodents as it protects midbrain DA neurons against MPTP toxicity ***(22)***, intranigral and intrastriatal injections of 6-OHDA ***(23)***, neurotoxic doses of methamphetamine ***(24)***, and axotomy-induced degeneration of the medial forebrain bundle ***(25)***.

Based on the rodent data, our group has carried out an extensive series of experiments to study the restorative effects of GDNF in nonhuman primates expressing left hemiparkinsonian features as a result of right intracarotid artery infusions of MPTP ***(26)***. Sterile stereotaxic procedures guided by magnetic resonance imaging (MRI) were used to deliver a single injection of GDNF into the right side of the brain by one of three routes: intranigral (150 μg), intracaudate (450 μg), and intracerebroventricular (450 μg) ***(27)***. Further testing was carried out on the ventricular-treated animals to assess their ability to respond to three repeated doses (100 or 450 μg) 4 wk apart. GDNF recipients showed significant functional improvements from all three routes of administration by 2 wk posttreatment, which continued for the remainder of the 4-wk test period. In this and subsequent experiments, improvements were found in three of the cardinal features of PD: bradykinesia, rigidity, and postural stability. GDNF administered every 4 wk maintained functional recovery. On the lesioned side of GDNF-treated animals, DA levels in the midbrain and globus pallidus were twice as high, and nigral DA neurons were 20% larger on average, with an increase in fiber density. Follow-up experiments have shown dose-dependent improvements in motor functions in MPTP-induced hemiparkinsonian monkeys receiving monthly ventricular injections of 100–1000 μg GDNF ***(28)***. After trophic factor treatment was discontinued, the parkinsonian features in most animals began to return to baseline levels within 60 d.

1.2. Delivery Strategies: The Pump Infusion Approach

Altogether, data collected in cell culture and in animal models of PD provide strong support for a role of GDNF in treating PD. As GDNF does not pass through the blood-brain barrier, it needs to be administered directly into the brain. The first studies conducted by our group evaluated the effects of GDNF on parkinsonian monkeys administered single intracerebral injections spaced 1 mo apart. Efficacious GDNF dose levels using this approach ranged from 100 to 1000 μg/mo. However, monthly injections of high dose GDNF increased the risk of inducing unwanted side effects such as weight loss that limit the clinical applications of this approach ***(27,28)***. Thus, one of the current challenges is to define better delivery systems for GDNF to optimize its actions. These may require continuous or timed infusion of low-dose GDNF into specific brain sites, which may produce the same or enhanced functional improvements as monthly injections with fewer side effects.

Novel methods for chronic delivery or prolonged release of GDNF into the nigrostriatal pathway have already been reported in rodents using biodegradable biomaterial ***(29,30)***, adenovirus vectors ***(31)***, and encapsulated cells genetically engineered to produce GDNF ***(32)***. However, little is known about the effects of chronic delivery of GDNF in nonhuman primates. Such information would help us to design better methods for GDNF treatment and also to lay the foundation for chronic delivery of other molecules into the human brain. Therefore, over the past year, our group has been testing the safety and efficacy of chronically infusing a low dose of GDNF using a SynchroMed implantable pump (model 8616-10; Medtronic, Minneapolis, MN) attached by tubing to a catheter implanted into the right lateral ventricle of monkeys with MPTP-induced left hemiparkinsonian features.

Preliminary results obtained in three animals show that daily infusion of vehicle (citrate/NaCl buffer) for a month has no effect on motor function, whereas 7.5 μg/d of GDNF continuously infused in the lateral ventricle promotes sustained improvement in parkinsonian features over a 12-wk period in these animals ***(33)***. Functional improvement was associated with increased levels of DA in the striatum as well as with increased numbers of DA fibers in the paraventricular region of the caudate nucleus and accumbens. The solution in the pump reservoir can easily be changed by injections through the skin in a fill port, while the rate and the timing (continuous or timed infusion) of delivery are noninvasively reprogrammed through an external computer. Thus he SynchroMed pumps offer a greater range of flexibility and control in delivering trophic factors into specific brain sites compared with other approaches for chronic delivery previously tested in rodents. Here we describe the procedures involved in using the pump infusion approach as a treatment for parkinsonism.

2. Materials

2.1. Animals

Our laboratory uses adult female rhesus monkeys (*Macaca mulatta*) obtained from a commercial supplier (Covance, Alice TX). Throughout the studies, they are housed in individual primate cages and are maintained on a 12-h light/12-h dark cycle. They are fed daily with certified primate biscuits, supplemented with fruits and vegetables, and water is available *ad libitum*. All the procedures performed on nonhuman primates are in strict accordance with the *NIH Guide for the Care and Use of Laboratory Animals* and are approved by institutional animal care and use committees. The surgeries are conducted under sterile field conditions using standard surgical equipment in a sterile surgical suite accredited by the Association for Assessment and Accreditation of Laboratory Animal Care International.

2.2. Recombinant Human GDNF and Vehicle

2.2.1. Storage and Handling

Upon receipt, the vials containing 0.5-mL recombinant human r-metHu GDNF (0.25 mg/mL; Amgen, Thousands Oaks, CA) can be stored frozen at –70°C or thawed by simply placing the vials in a refrigerator (5 ± 3°C) for permanent storage as a refrigerated liquid. Alternatively, if the drug is kept frozen it may be thawed immediately prior to use by transferring to room temperature (20 ± 5°C) for approx 1 hr. Upon receipt, the vials containing 10-mL r-metHu GDNF vehicle (10 m*M* citrate/120 m*M* NaCl buffer, pH 5.5) should be stored and maintained at 2–8°C.

2.2.2. Dilution

The drug must be used immediately following dilution with the vehicle. A concentration of 0.025 mg/mL postdilution is used for chronic delivery of low-dose GDNF. To obtain the proper concentration, use a vial containing 0.5 mL GDNF (0.25 mg/mL) and add 4.5 mL citrate/NaCl buffer. Gently mix the resulting solution. To minimize the risk of contamination, it is recommended that buffer be added to the storage vials using a standard hypodermic needle through the septum rather than opening the vials (*see* **Note 1**). Extended storage and reuse of diluted product is not recommended.

2.3. SynchroMed Pump, Ventricular Catheter, and Accessories

The implantable sterile devices include the pump, pump catheter segment, ventricular catheter, and catheter accessories. The external nonsterile component consists of a computer for programming the pump. The pump can dispense drugs in a variety of ways (e.g., continuous or timed infusion) according to instructions received by radiofrequency from the SynchroMed model 8820 computer using a programming head that is held directly above the implanted pump. The pump is a round titanium disk about 1-in. thick and 3 in. in diameter. The model 8616-10 pump contains a collapsible 10-mL reservoir and a self-sealing silicone septum through which a needle is inserted to refill the pump reservoir. It also contains a bacterial retentive filter (0.22 μm) through which the drug passes as it leaves the reservoir. The pump connects to the ventricular catheter via a pump catheter segment. The pump should not be exposed to temperatures above 43°C or below 5°C.

The ventricular catheter (model no. 8770AS) comes packaged with a metal connector, L-shaped nylon anchor, and nylon screws. A stylet inserted in the catheter lumen provides additional stiffness and control during placement. The ventricular catheter has a hole in the tip with two adjacent side holes for drug delivery. The ventricular catheter as well as the pump catheter segment are made of polyurethane that is elastic and flexible and can be cut to the desired length. The catheter and accessories should not be exposed to temperatures above 57°C or below –34°C.

3. Method

3.1. Preoperative Procedures

3.1.1. MRI Scans

All animals first undergo an MRI scan to provide stereotaxic coordinates for the catheter implantation. The anesthetized animals are placed in an MRI-compatible stereotaxic apparatus and are imaged on a 1.5-T Siemens multinuclear imaging and spectroscopy system using an 8-cm radiofrequency (RF) surface coil placed over the head of the animal. Anteroposterior, lateral, and vertical coordinates for stereotaxic surgery are derived from T1-weighted 2 mm adjacent coronal sections through the brain. The interaural line is identified on the scans by modified ear bars containing vitamin E.

3.1.2. MPTP Lesion

Prior to catheter implantation, the animals are given MPTP to induce stable left hemiparkinsonian features using procedures described in detail elsewhere ***(30)***. Briefly, using standard sterile operating procedures, 0.4 mg/kg MPTP is infused through the right carotid artery via a 27-G butterfly needle at the rate of 2 mL/min.

3.2. Surgery Procedures

After a minimum of 2 mo following MPTP administration, when the parkinsonian features expressed by the animals have stabilized, the catheter is surgi-

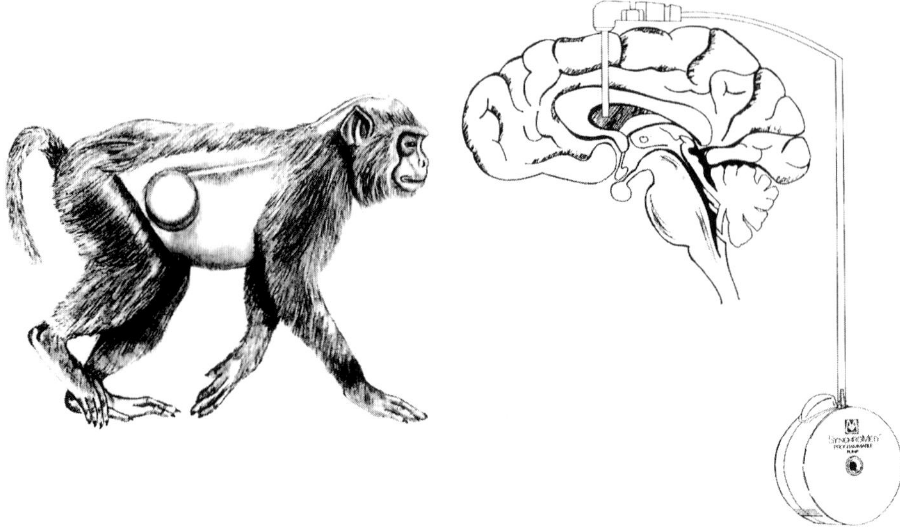

Fig. 1. SynchroMed pump and catheter placement. The titanium-encased, biologically-compatible pump is surgically implanted in the subcutaneous layer of the lateral abdomen and connected to a catheter stereotactically positioned in the lateral ventricle. The pump is refilled by injections through the skin into a portal diaphragm. The rate and timing of delivery are noninvasively programmed from an external computer.

cally positioned and tunneled to the pump that is subcutaneously implanted in the lateral abdominal region (**Fig. 1**). The surgery is performed under sterile field conditions using standard surgical procedures.

3.2.1. Animal Preparation

1. Following induction of anesthesia with intramuscular injection of ketamine HCL (15 mg/kg) and atropine (0.04 mg/kg), anesthetize the animal with isoflurane gas anesthesia (1–3%) using a tracheal tube (4.0 mm I.D.) and position it in the MRI-compatible stereotaxic apparatus.
2. Place the animal in a ventral/lateral position to allow easy access to ventricular and pump incision sites.
3. After the animal is shaved, mark the pump pocket location using a template.
4. Clean the ventricular and pump incision sites with antiseptic (providone-iodine)
5. Cover the animal with sterile drapes.

3.2.2. Catheter Implantation

1. Make an incision through the scalp and the skin, and reflect the muscles overlying the lateral ventricle.

2. Using MRI-guided stereotaxic procedures, drill a hole through the skull directly above the ventricle.
3. Remove the overlying meninges to expose the surface of the brain for penetration of the catheter.
4. Using a stereotaxic holder, implant the indwelling catheter surgically into the right lateral ventricle (*see* **Note 2**).
5. Remove the catheter stylet to verify return of cerebrospinal fluid and placement in the ventricle.
6. Seat the catheter in the groove of the L-shaped nylon device, which is anchored against the skull using two nylon screws.
7. Using the metal tubing connector, connect the ventricular catheter segment to the pump catheter segment and secure it (*see* **Notes 3** and **4**).
8. Suture the scalp incision over the exposed areas per normal procedures.

3.2.3. Pump Preparation and Implantation

1. Palce the pump in a warm bath of sterile saline (35–40°C) for 15 min.
2. Prepare the GDNF/citrate buffer solution as described in **Subheading 2.1.1.**
3. Using a 22-G needle attached to a 10-ml empty syringe, aspirate the contents of the pump reservoir (sterile water) until air bubbles are observed in the syringe.
4. Remove the needle and syringe containing aspirate, while maintaining negative pressure on the syringe.
5. To avoid generation of high fluid pressure, fill the warmed pump by inserting a 22-G needle attached to a 10-mL syringe containing GDNF into the reservoir septum. Inject the solution at an infusion rate not greater than 1 mL/3 s for a maximum of 6 mL at the time of implantation (*see* **Note 5**).
6. Remove the needle and syringe while maintaining a slight positive pressure once the maximum 6 mL of GDNF has been injected.
7. Using a shunt passer, make a tunnel from the abdominal pocket prepared in parallel to the scalp incision.
8. After tunneling subcutaneously, thread the pump catheter segment from the ventricular site to the pump site.
9. Connect the pump catheter segment to a model 8616-10 SynchroMed programmable pump and secure (*see* **Note 3**).
10. Place the warmed and filled pump into the subcutaneous abdominal pocket.
11. Suture the pump subcutaneously into the pocket.
12. Close the abdominal incision per normal procedure and apply dressings (*see* **Notes 6** and **7**).
13. The pump is noninvasively programmed using the SynchroMed model 8820 computer (e.g., rate and timing of delivery, reservoir volume).

3.1. Postoperative Procedures: Pump Refills and Information Update

1. Identify location of the center reservoir fill port.
2. Prepare injection site by cleansing area with an agent such as povidone-iodine.

3. Remove cleansing agent from the skin with alcohol.
4. Attach a three-way stopcock to a 22-G needle and insert through the center fill port.
5. Using a 10-mL empty syringe, withdraw the remaining fluid in the pump reservoir using gentle negative pressure until air bubbles are present in the syringe.
6. Close the three-way stopcock to prevent any air from getting into the pump and remove the syringe containing aspirate.
7. Refill the pump reservoir using a 10-mL syringe containing a fresh solution of GDNF (do not exceed the reservoir capacity at refill, e.g., 10 mL for the Synchro Med model 8616-10; *see* **Note 5**).
8. When filling is complete, maintain a slight positive pressure on the syringe and turn the stopcock to the "syringe off" position.
9. Remove the needle/stopcock/syringe components and discard.
10. Using the external computer, the reservoir volume, and/or other parameters (e.g., rate and timing of delivery) can be noninvasively updated via the programming head held directly above the implanted pump.

4. Notes

1. Vials containing product have a total capacity of nearly 6 mL. The addition of 4.5 mL buffer into an enclosed vial will require purging the excess pressure via a second needle or repeated small volume additions followed by withdrawal of air from the headspace using the same syringe.
2. The putamen is an important processing center in the neural circuitry regulating motor functions. Thus, another possible efficacious site for the chronic delivery of GDNF would be directly into the putamen using intraparenchymal catheters (model no. 87701P3).
3. Do not use chromium or wire sutures, which may damage the catheter, resulting in a disconnection or leakage. Be cautious when using any other type of sutures (e.g., nylon).
4. Leave enough slack in the catheters to allow for head movement.
5. If you encounter unusual resistance before the maximum volume is injected or you are unable to inject fluid, the reservoir valve has been activated.
   a. Discontinue injection and remove syringe and needle from the septum.
   b. Insert a 22-G needle attached to a 10-mL empty syringe through the septum and aspirate until all fluid/air is removed.
   c. Remove needle and syringe with aspirate from the center reservoir and reinsert the needle and syringe containing GDNF.
6. Before suturing, verify that after implantation the pump's center reservoir fill port will be easy to palpate and that the pump catheter segment will not become contorted. Also, verify that the pump catheter segment is secured well away from the center fill port, so that the pump segment will not be punctured by needles used to refill the pump.
7. Consider using peri- and postoperative antibiotics to prevent infection and/or consider using a primate jacket (Lomir Biomedical, Montreal, Canada) to prevent the animal from scratching and infecting the pump incision.

Acknowledgments

The work in the authors' laboratory discussed in this chapter was supported by NIH grant NS35642 and contracts with Amgen Inc. We thank Medtronic Inc. for providing the pumps and associated hardware and software used for chronic infusions. The authors are grateful to Ms. Susan Tucker for the illustration used in this chapter. Richard Grondin holds a postdoctoral fellowship award from the Fond de la Recherche en Santé du Québec (FRSQ).

References

1. Lin, L.-F. H., Doherty, D. H., Lile, J. D., Bektesh, S. and Collins, F. (1993) GDNF: A glial cell line-derived neurotrophic factor for midbrain dopaminergic neurons. *Science* **260,** 1130–1132.
2. Kotzbauer, P. T., Lampe, P. A., Heuckeroth, R. O., Golden, J. P., Creedon, D. J., Johnson, E. M., Jr., et al. (1996) Neurturin, a relative of glial cell line-derived neurotrophic factor. *Nature* **384,** 467–470.
3. Milbrandt, J., de Sauvage, F. J., Fahrner, T. J., Baloh, R. H., Leitner, M. L., Tansey, M. G., et al. (1998) Persephin, a novel neurotrophic factor related to GDNF and neurturin. *Neuron* **20,** 245–253.
4. Baloh, R. H., Tansey, M. G., Lampe, P. A., Fahrner, T. J., Enomoto, H., Simburger, K. S., et al. (1998) Artemin, a novel member of the GDNF ligand family, supports peripheral and central neurons and signals through the GFRα3-Ret receptor complex. *Neuron* **21,** 1291–1302.
5. Choi-Lundberg, D. L. and Bohn, M. C. (1995) Ontogeny and distribution of glial cell line-derived neurotrophic factor (GDNF) mRNA in rat. *Dev. Brain Res.* **85**, 80–88.
6. Springer, J. E., Mu, X., Bergmann, L. W. and Trojanoski, J. Q. (1994) Expression of GDNF mRNA in rat and human nervous tissue. *Exp. Neurol.* **127,** 167–170.
7. Strömberg, I., Bjorklund, L., Johansson, M., Tomac, A., Collins, F., Olson, L., et al. (1993) Glial cell line-derived neurotrophic factor is expressed in the developing but not adult striatum and stimulates developing dopamine neurons in vivo. *Exp. Neurol.* **124,** 401–412.
8. Suter-Crazzolara, C. and Unsicker, K. (1994) GDNF is expressed in two forms in many tissues outside the CNS. *Neuroreport* **5,** 2486–2488.
9. Trupp, M., Rydén, M., Jörnavall, C., Funakoshi, H., Timmusk, T., Arenas, E., et al. (1995) Peripheral expression and biological activities of GDNF, a new neurotrophic factor for avian and mammalian peripheral neurons. *J. Cell. Biol.* **130,** 137–148.
10. Jing, S., Wen, D., Yu, Y., Holst, P. L., Luo, Y., Fang, M., et al. (1996) GDNF-induced activation of the Ret protein tyrosine kinase is mediated by GDNFR-α, a novel receptor for GDNF. *Cell* **85,** 1113–1124.
11. Treanor, J. J. S., Goodman, L., de Sauvage, F., Stone, D. M., Poulsen, K. T., Beck, C. D., et al. (1996) Characterization of a multicomponent receptor for GDNF. *Nature* **382,** 80–83.

12. Baloh, R. H., Tansey, M. G., Golden, J. P., Creedon, D. J., Heuckeroth, R. O., Keck, C. L., Zimonjic, D. B., Popescu, N. C., Johnson, E. M., Jr., and Milbrandt, J. (1997) TrnR2, a novel receptor that mediates neurturin and GDNF signaling through Ret. *Neuron* **18,** 793–802.
13. Buj-Bello, A., Adu, J., Pinon, L. G. P., Horton, A., Thompson, J., Rosenthal, A., et al. (1997) Neurturin responsiveness requires a GPI-linked receptor and the ret receptor tyrosine kinase. *Nature* **387,** 721–724.
14. Naveilhan, P., Baudet, C., Mikaels, A., Shen, L., Westphal H., and Ernfors, P. (1998) Expression and regulation of GFRα-3, a glial cell line-derived neurotrophic factor family receptor. *Proc. Natl. Acad. Sci. USA* **95**, 1295–1300.
15. Worby, C. A., Vega, Q. C., Chao, H. H. J., Seasholtz, A. F., Thompson, R. C., and Dixon, J. E. (1998) Identification and characterization of GFRα-3, a novel co-receptor belonging to the glial cell line-derived neurotrophic receptor family. *J. Biol. Chem.* **273,** 3502–3508.
16. Thompson, J., Doxakis, E., Pinon, L. G. P., Strachan, P., Buj-Bello, A., Wyatt, S., et al. (1998) GFRα-4, a new GDNF family receptor. *Mol. Cell Neurosci.* **11,** 117–126.
17. Lin, L.-F. H., Zhang, T. J., Collins, F., and Armes, L. G. (1994) Purification and initial characterization of rat B49 glial cell line-derived neurotrophic factor. *J. Neurochem.* **63,** 758–768.
18. Hou, J.-G. G., Lin, L.-F. H., and Mytilinenou, C. (1996) Glial cell line-derived neurotrophic factor exerts neurotrophic effects on dopaminergic neurons in vitro and promotes their survival and regrowth after damage by 1-methyl-4-phenylpyridinium. *J. Neurochem.* **66,** 74–82.
19. Hoffer, B. J., Hoffman, A., Bowenkamp, K., Huettl, P., Hudson, J., Martin, D., et al. (1994) Glial cell line-derived neurotrophic factor reverses toxin-induced injury to midbrain dopaminergic neurons in vivo. *Neurosci. Lett.* **182,** 107–111.
20. Bowenkamp, K. E., Hoffman, A. F., Gerhardt, G. A., Henry, M. A., Biddle, P. T., Hoffer B. J., et al. (1995) Glial cell line-derived neurotrophic factor supports survival of injured midbrain dopaminergic neurons. *J. Comp. Neurol.* **355,** 479–489.
21. Lapchak, P. A., Miller, P. J., Collins, F., and Jiao, S. (1997) Glial cell line-derived neurotrophic factor attenuates behavioural deficits and regulates nigrostriatal dopaminergic and peptidergic markers in 6-hydroxydopamine-lesioned adult rats: comparison of intraventricular and intranigral delivery. *Neuroscience* **78,** 61–72.
22. Tomac, A., Lindqvist, E., Lin, L.-F. H., Ogren, S. O., Young, D., Hoffer, B. J., and Olson, L. (1995) Protection and repair of the nigrostriatal dopaminergic system by GDNF in vivo. *Nature* **373,** 335–339.
23. Kearns, C. and Gash, D. M. (1995) GDNF protects nigral dopamine neurons against 6-hydroxydopamine in vivo. *Brain Res.* **672,** 104–111.
24. Cass, W. (1996) GDNF selectively protects dopamine neurons over serotonin neurons against the neurotoxic effects of methamphetamine. *J. Neurosci.* **16,** 8132–8139.
25. Beck, K. D., Valverde, J., Alexi, T., Poulsen, K., Moffat, B., Vandlen, R. A., et al. (1995) Mesencephalic dopaminergic neurons protects by GDNF from axotomy-induced degeneration in the adult brain. *Nature* **373,** 339–341.

26. Ovadia, A., Zhang, Z., and Gash, D. M. (1995) Increased susceptibility to MPTP toxicity in middle-aged rhesus monkeys. *Neurobiol. Aging* **16,** 931–937.
27. Gash, D. M. , Zhang, Z., Ovadia, A., Cass, W. A., Yi, A., Simmerman, L., et al. (1996) Functional recovery in parkinsonian monkeys treated with GDNF. *Nature* **380,** 252-255.
28. Zhang, Z., Miyoshi, Y., Lapchak, P. A., Collins, F., Hilt, D., Lebel, C., et al. (1997) Dose response to intraventricular glial cell line-derived neurotrophic factor administration in parkinsonian monkeys. *J. Pharmacol. Exp. Ther.* **282,** 1396–1401.
29. Cheng, H., Fraidakis, M., Blomback, B., Lapchak, P., Hoffer, B., and Olson, L. (1998) Characterization of a fibrin glue-GDNF slow release preparation. *Cell Transplant.* **7,** 53–61.
30. Cheng, H., Hoffer, B., Strömberg, I., Russell, D. and Olson, L. (1995) The effects of glial cell line-derived neurotrophic factor in fibrin glue on developing dopamine neurons. *Exp. Brain Res.* **104,** 199–206.
31. Choi-Lundberg, D. L., Lin, Q., Chang, Y.-N., Chiang, Y. L., Hay, C. M., Mohajeri, H., et al. (1997) Dopaminergic neurons protected from degeneration by GDNF gene therapy. *Science* **275,** 838–841.
32. Tseng, J. L., Baetge, E. E., Zurn, A. D., and Aebischer, P. (1997) GDNF reduces drug-induced rotational behavior after a medial forebrain bundle transection by a mechanism not involving striatal dopamine. *J. Neurosci.* **17,** 325–333.
33. Grondin, R., Zhang, Z., Beck, K., Hilt, D., Elsberry, D., and Gash, D. M. (1998) Chronic intracerebral infusion of glial cell line-derived neurotrophic factor (GDNF) in parkinsonian rhesus monkeys. *Soc. Neurosci. Abstr.* **24,** 42.

19

Grafting Genetically Engineered Cells into the Striatum of Nonhuman Primates

Krys S. Bankiewicz, Phillip Pivirotto, Rosario Sanchez-Pernaute, and Eugene O. Major

1. Introduction

An emerging new technology based on genetic engineering of viral vectors that can insert genes into the cells of living organisms may play a significant role in treating disorders of the central nervous system (CNS). Most neurodegenerative disorders affect focal regions of the brain. Preventive and/or palliative treatment strategies need to be targeted only to the diseased parts of the brain without affecting other regions. Administration of therapeutic genes specifically to the disease-affected regions of the brain may be more beneficial than current treatment strategies, which are largely based on systemically administering small molecules. The latter can result not only in peripheral side effects but also CNS side effects since the drugs can affect both targeted and nontargeted brain sites. In addition, many therapeutic agents are prevented from entering the brain by the blood-brain barrier (BBB). For these reasons, many otherwise potentially useful proteins, such as trophic factors, cannot be administered systemically *(1)*.

Parkinson's disease is a good example of a focal brain disorder in which slow degeneration of dopamine-producing neurons, mostly in the nigrostriatal pathway, results in neurologic signs. Ex vivo gene transfer techniques can provide an alternative for long-term delivery of therapeutically active proteins to affected regions. One of the advantages of ex vivo gene therapy is the possibility of selecting the cell type that would express the transgene. Prior to grafting into the brain, cells can be tested and optimized in vitro. Furthermore, several genes can be co-expressed, and cell types can be combined in the graft for a

From: *Methods in Molecular Medicine, vol. 62: Parkinson's Disease: Methods and Protocols*
Edited by: M. M. Mouradian

more functional outcome. Major disadvantages are related to graft survival and long-term gene expression and regulation as well as host response to the implant and/or to the transgene product.

In Parkinson's disease, transplantation of genetically modified cells can aim at the following:

1. Dopamine (DA) replacement through grafting of cells engineered to synthesize and release DA in a regulated manner. This requires the introduction, expression, and regulation of multiple genes, i.e., tyrosine hydroxylase (TH), aromatic amino acid decarboxylase (AADC), and guanosine trophosphate (GTP) cyclohydrolase I. The latter is responsible for synthesizing the TH co-factor tetrahydrobiopterin. Ideally, all these genes should be expressed in a cell that has the capacity for DA storage and regulated release/uptake.
2. Protection and/or regeneration of the DA system. This approach aims at protecting intact cells from degeneration or rescuing cells that have already begun to degenerate. Grafted engineered cells might become a continuous source of trophic factors. Several growth factors, such as basic fibroblast growth factor (bFGF), brain-derived neurotrophic factor (BDNF) ***(2,3)*** truncated insulin-like growth factor-1 (tIGF1) ***(3)***, and glial cell line-derived neurotrophic factor (GDNF) ***(4)*** have been shown to exert positive effects on DA neurons. GDNF appears to be most selective ***(5)*** in increasing DA activity and improving clinical signs of parkinsonism in rodent and primate models of PD ***(6,7)***. Neurturin, artemin, and persephin are structurally related to GDNF and also have neurotrophic effects on DA neurons ***(8,9)***.
3. Both approaches could be combined so that a trophic factor-expressing cell population provides support to a DA-producing cell type.

1.1. Selection of Cells

The choice of the cell used as the delivery vehicle must meet several criteria. The cell should not (1) elicit an inflammatory response from the host; (2) migrate in the host brain; and, importantly, (3) form tumors after in vivo placement.

1.1.1. Autologous Cells

Although autologous cells from the patient meet these criteria, it is difficult to prepare such cells with rigorous quality control. For example, evaluation of autologous cells for chromosomal alterations during propagation (for viruses or other microbial contaminants introduced during establishment of the cells and transduction procedures and for phenotypic changes during the multiple mitotic events needed to accomplish stable transgene expression) requires large stocks of cells with homogeneous characteristics. This is not easily accomplished if biopsy tissues from the patient are used. Furthermore, it is unlikely that such candidate cells would be derived from the nervous system, but rather from an anatomically accessible source. Skin fibroblasts have been the primary choice for experimental studies and result in good survival in the striata of 1-methyl-4-phenyl-1,2,3,6-tetrahydropyridine (MPTP)-treated primates. In addition, TH-positive autologous fibroblasts have been detected by immunohistochemistry and *in situ* hybridization several months after implantation ***(10,11)***. However, genetically engineered fibroblasts have not resulted in long-term transgene expression in the rat. One reason that may account for the gradual decline in gene expression has come from cell culture studies suggesting that fibroblast transgene expression is downregulated by the inflammatory cytokines, tumor necrosis factor-α (TNF-α), interleukin-1β (IL-1β), and transforming growth factor-β1 (TGF-β1) ***(12)***. These cytokines are released from macrophages and microglial cells that can invade the fibroblast grafts.

1.1.2. Cell Lines

An alternative to autologous cells would be human-derived cell lines that meet the afore-mentioned criteria. Initially, ex vivo gene transfer to the CNS was based on the use of fibroblastic tumorgenic cell lines or primary fibroblasts. The generation of immortalized lines of CNS-derived neural stem cells has made it possible to obtain clonal, genetically homogeneous neural stem cell lines, which appear more appropriate for ex vivo gene transfer to the CNS. These cells survive and integrate into the surrounding host cytoarchitecture and are neither tumorgenic nor immunogenic. The cell line SVG was immortalized using an SV40 replication origin-defective mutant which synthesizes the viral T protein ***(13,14)***. This protein is responsible for the immortalization of the cells most likely interfering with cell cycle-regulated proteins such as p53 and Rb (retinoblastoma protein). The cells have many phenotypic characteristics of astrocytes, as well as biologic properties of cells typically described as progenitor cells. Clones of SVG cells have been made to express many genes including TH and AADC in an attempt to produce DA. SVG cells can be readily transduced through DNA transfer techniques and can carry multiple copies of a transgene in a viral vector that contains a functional SV40 origin of DNA replication in an episomal state, even with cell division. Viral DNA transfected into these cells can replicate to high copy number and segregate into dividing nuclei as the cell undergoes division. Transgenes can also become integrated into the host cell chromosome if selection is made using a marker such as geneticin (G418). This chapter describes a method for transplanting SVG cells as a model for ex vivo gene transfer into the parkinsonian primate brain.

The use of multiple passes through the cortex has been an established method for the delivery of cell suspensions into target sites. In an effort to increase reproducibility and to minimize surgical procedure time, our method for multiple implants employs a dual-cannula approach guided by an automated, hydraulic-driven micropositioner. Tissue is deposited by an infusion pump while the cannula assembly is slowly withdrawn using a micropositioner. A 2-mm separation between the cannula allows for adequate distribution of cells within the parenchyma, and the custom designed cannulae holder provides independent movement of each cannula for fine dorsoventral adjustments prior to implantation. To provide accurate placement of the implants in the striatum, magnetic resonance imaging (MRI) is used to calculate stereotaxic coordinates *(15,16)* (*see* **Note 1**).

2. Materials

2.1. Cell Culture and Preparation of Cells for Infusion

1. Dulbecco's modified Eagle's medium (DMEM) with 10% fetal bovine serum (FBS).
2. 1% L-glutamine (200 m*M*).
3. 1% gentamycin (50 mg/mL).
4. Phosphate-buffered saline (PBS).

2.2. Preparation of Cannulae and Lines

1. 26-G, 25-mm-long needles (from 24-G venous catheters).
2. Hemostats (two).
3. Temperature-controlled heat gun (Steinel HL 1800 E).
4. Teflon tubing (0.030 × 0.062 in. × 50 ft.).
5. 5-mL syringe (sterile).
6. 0.9% saline.
7. Scalpel blade and holder.
8. Super Glue (Duro quick gel).
9. Tefzel Ferrule 1/16 in. (Upchurch Scientific).
10. Tefzel male Luer-lock (Upchurch Scientific).
11. Tefzel fittings (Upchurch Scientific).
12. Tefzel Union (Upchurch Scientific).

2.3. Implantation Procedure

All instruments and lines must be sterile.

1. Hemostatic forceps.
2. Hamilton syringes, 1 and 2 mL.
3. Tefzel tubing (0.03 in. ID × 0.063 in. OD).
4. Tefzel fittings.
5. Tefzel ferrules.
6. Tefzel unions.
7. Towel clamps (four).
8. Bone curettes.
9. Friedman bone rongeurs.
10. Suction tube and tip.

11. Stainless steel basin (small).
12. Periosteal elevators.
13. Scalpel handle with metric rule.

2.4. Other Equipment

1. Carbide burs with excavating tip.
2. Needle holder.
3. Metzenbaum scissors.
4. Stereotaxic frame.
5. Manipulator.
6. Micropositioner (Kopf model 650).
7. Harvard infusion pump (model 44 or 22).
8. Dremel drill.
9. 70% EtOH.
10. Penicillin.
11. Cannola or corn oil.
12. Cold sterilizing agent (Cidex or equivalent).
13. Iodine/povidone scrub (Betadine or equivalent).

3. Methods

3.1. Preparation of SVG Cells for Implantation

1. Transfer cells from liquid nitrogen freezer directly into a beaker of 37°C water.
2. Quickly thaw cells in 37°C water bath.
3. Open vial by wrapping sterile gauze with ethanol around cap.
4. Plate $1 \times 10^6/75$ cm^2 flask or 150,000–200,000 cells/well of a 6-well plate (with or without cover slip) in Eagle's minimum essential medium (EMEM) with 10% FBS, 1% L-glutamine, and 1% gentamycin.
5. Change the medium at 24 h of cell growth.
6. Harvest cells after 24 h.
7. Resuspend aliquots of specific concentrations in 1X PBS, pH 7.5, for implantation.
8. Check cell viability before and after implantation procedure with Trypan Blue stain (0.04%) at 1:20 dilution and count in a Levy-Hausser counting chamber.

3.2. Preparation of Cannulae

1. Get two 26-G, 250 mm long needles from commercial 24-G angiocaths. (Discard the rest.)
2. Holding the needle with a hemostat and the needle hub with a second hemostat over a heat gun, let the plastic warm and then pull back the plastic portion to separate the needle.
3. To prepare the infusion (cannulae) lines, measure 10-cm portions of Teflon tubing with a ruler and cut with a scalpel blade.
4. Apply Super Glue to a 1-cm portion approx 3 mm away from the proximal end of the needle.

5. Insert the proximal end of the needle, approx 1.5 cm into the precut 10-cm Teflon tubing, and allow glue to fix.
6. Test cannulae for leakage (*see* **Subheading 3.3.**).
7. Package two cannulae per autoclave pouch. Autoclave cannulae before using.

3.3. Lines Connections and Testing of Cannulae

1. Attach Tefzel tubing and ferrule to cannulae tubing.
2. Attach union to Tefzel tubing.
3. Attach male Luer-lock to 5-mL syringe filled with saline.
4. Attach male Luer-lock to Tefzel union on tubing.
5. Flush with saline and check for leakage.

3.4. Preparation of the Loading Lines

Loading lines are used to transfer the cells into the infusion line attached to the cannulae and connect the infusion system to the oil lines (**Fig. 1**).

1. Make the loading line with 50-cm sections of Teflon tubing cut with a scalpel blade.
2. Insert Tefzel fittings on both ends of the tubing.
3. Position Tefzel fittings with ferrules on the ends of the line. Ensure that the tip of the flange is flat with the tip of the tubing.
4. Package two lines per autoclave pouch. Autoclave before using.

3.5. Implantation of Cell Suspensions Bilaterally into he Striatum of Primates

3.5.1. Preparation of Cell Suspensions

1. Place the two 1-mL Hamilton syringes on a Harvard infusion pump model 44 (or model 22). This pump will be used for aspiration of the cell suspensions into the infusion lines. Dial in the appropriate syringe settings for the pump corresponding to the description of the Hamilton syringes (1 mL).
2. Attach the two Hamilton syringes to two sterile 2 × 25-cm Tefzel tubing sections (0.03 in. ID × 0.063 in. OD). The tubing will serve as infusion lines for the cell suspensions. Fix the syringes in place on the infusion pump. Set the infusion pump to aspirate at a rate of 100 μL/min. Place the distal end of the tubing in the cell suspension vials. Set the pump to "refill" and withdraw approx 200 μL of cell suspension into each of the two lines; ensure that no air bubbles collect in the lines. Clamp the distal ends of the lines filled with cell suspensions with a sterile hemostat.
3. Using two 1-mL Hamilton syringes, aspirate corn oil into 2 × 35-cm Tefzel tubing until oil is visible in the union. Cap the oil-filled tubing with sterile zero dead volume connectors.
4. Place the syringes attached to the oil infusion lines on the programmable infusion pump.

Cell Loading

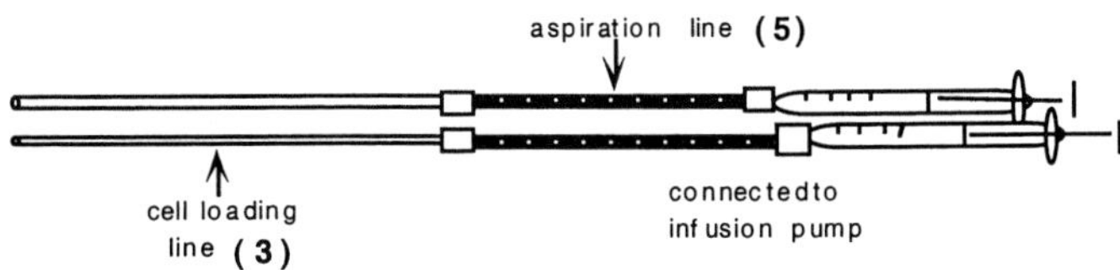

Cell Implantation System

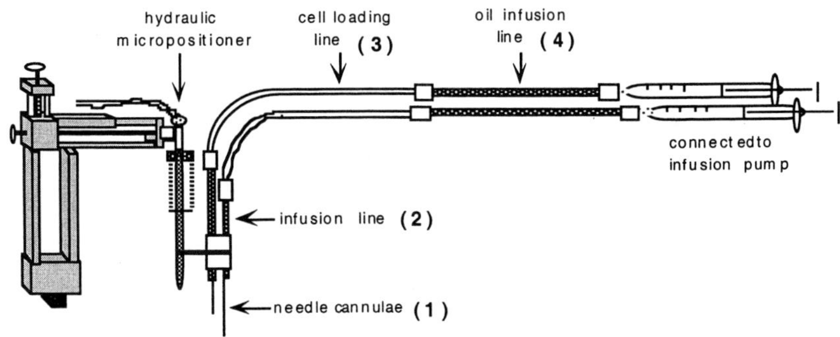

Fig. 1. Implantation system used for cell grafting, consisting of five components: (1) a sterile infusion cannula; (2) a sterile infusion line; (3) a sterile cell loading line; (4) a nonsterile infusion line containing vegetable oil; and (5) a nonsterile aspiration line.

5. Attach each of the loading lines with the cell suspensions to the oil infusion lines using a Tefzel zero dead volume connector. The oil provides an immiscible barrier to the cells (as long as there are no air bubbles) and will not be infused.
6. Remove the hemostats from the opposite end of the cell suspension lines. With a sterile scalpel blade, cut the ends of the lines and prepare to attach them to the cannulae.

3.5.2. Preparing the Cannulae, Pump, and Micropositioner Instrument Settings

1. Attach the double cannulae assembly to the hydraulic arm. The arm is connected to the micropositioner.
2. Check the double cannulae assembly (2 × 25-mm, 26-G needles attached to a 10-cm length of Tefzel tubing, secured in place in a stainless steel clamp). The medial and lateral cannulae should be set 2 mm apart, and the length of the cannula is now adjusted according to dorsoventral coordinates.
3. Check the dimensions with a metric ruler and set at a 90° angle. Then attach the double cannulae assembly to the cell suspension lines using a sterile Tefzel union.
4. Perform a check of the infusion system and concurrently fill the cannulae with cell suspension by setting the pump to "infuse" at a rate of approx 100 µL/min.

Table 1
Recommended Parameters for Cell Infusion

Volume (μL/graft)	Infusion rate (μL/min)	Withdrawal rate (mm/min)
5	0.8	0.8
10	1.6	0.8
20	1.6	0.4

Allow several drops of the cell suspension to come out from the cannulae. Check all infusion lines and connectors during this procedure.

5. Set the Harvard model 44 pump to the determined infusion rate (μL/min) and target volume (μL). (**Table 1**; *see* **Note 2**).

3.5.3. Cell Suspension Infusion

1. Prepare the micropositioner for advancement of the cannulae by setting the cannulae to the anteroposterial and mediolateral baseline coordinates predetermined by MRI. Set the controller to "advance." Press the reset button located on the main unit to "0." Set the run rate on the main unit to "high" (= 64 mm/min). Manually advance the cannulae through the dura. Turn the controller switch to "run." The cannulae will begin to advance toward the target.
2. Monitor the advance of the cannulae tip and stop the hydraulic arm (turn controller to "off") at the specified depth (dorsoventral coordinate). From the micropositioner readout, record the cannulae depth on the surgery record. This will be the implant depth for the target site (corresponding to the dorsoventral coordinate).
3. To set the micropositioner for cannulae withdrawal, select "retract" on the micropositioner controller, select "reset" on the main unit and run rate to "low." Set the main switch unit to the specified withdrawal rate (mm/min).
4. Begin cell suspension infusion and withdrawal of the cannulae simultaneously. Flip the controller switch on the micropositioner to "run" and at the same time turn on the infusion pump (set to "infuse"). Record the start time of implantation (infusion/cannulae withdrawal). Monitor the infusion pump and micropositioner (cannulae withdrawal) during this process.
5. During implantation, periodically check the cannulae position and reduce traction on the dura by occasionally pressing the dura down with a saline-soaked swab.
6. Ensure that the infusion pump and micropositioner are stopped when the calculated infusion volume is achieved per the infusion pump. The time of infusion should be the same for the volume and the distance (e.g., 10 μL at 1.6 μl/min = 6.25 min infusion; 0.8 mm/min × 6.25 min = 5 mm distance). Record the end time of infusion/withdrawal and micropositioner readout depth.
7. Wait 15 min prior to continuing the cannulae withdrawal. Then reset the micropositioner to incrementally faster rates of withdrawal (*see* **Note 3**).

4. Notes

1. The method of cell implantation described has been used safely in a large number of nonhuman primates with only two out of 750 grafts resulting in hemorrhage ***(2)***. This method has also been tested in humans ***(16)***.
2. Cell suspensions are implanted by simultaneous infusion (µl/min) and withdrawal by 2 cannulae to precise medial and lateral locations 2 mm apart in the striatum. The rate of infusion is fixed via a programmable infusion pump. The rate of withdrawal of the two cannulae is fixed (mm/minute) via a micropositioner with hydraulic arm. The controlled rate of infusion and cannulae withdrawal is critical to the correct administration of the implants, both for volume of cells deposited and location of the implant. The implants are placed at six separate successive sites per hemisphere (2× rostral caudate nucleus/2× rostral putamen/2× caudal putamen) in a single surgical session.
3. Repeat the steps described above for the number of implantations to be performed. Ensure that the stereotaxic frame is reset to the next set of coordinates to complete the series of implantations. Prior to each sequential implant, check the patency of infusion lines by turning on the pump and allowing several drops of cell suspension to infuse through the cannulae.

References

1. Kordower, J. H., Palfi, S., Chen, E. Y., Ma, S. Y., Sendera, T., Cochran, E. J., et al. (1999) Clinicopathological findings following intraventricular glial-derived neurotrophic factor treatment in a patient with Parkinson's disease. *Ann. Neurol.* **46,** 419–424.
2. Beck, K. D., Valverde, J., Alexi, T., Poulsen, K., Moffat, B., Vandlen, R. A., et al. (1995) Mesencephalic dopaminergic neurons protected by GDNF from axotomy-induced degeneration in the adult brain. *Nature* **373,** 339–341.
3. Hyman, C., Hofer, M., Barde, Y. A., Juhasz, M., Yancopoulos, G. D., Squinto, S. P., et al. (1991) BDNF is a neurotrophic factor for dopaminergic neurons of the substantia nigra. *Nature* **350,** 230–232.
4. Hoffer, B. J., Hoffman, A., Bowenkamp, K., Huettl, P., Hudson, J., Lin, L. F., et al. (1994) Glial cell line-derived neurotrophic factor reverses toxin-induced injury to midbrain dopaminergic neurons in vivo. *Neurosci. Lett.* **182,** 107–111.
5. Lin, L. F., Doherty, D. H., Lile, J. D., Bektesh, S., and Collins, F. (1993) GDNF: a glial cell line-derived neurotrophic factor for midbrain dopaminergic neurons. *Science* **260,** 1130–1132.
6. Gash, D. M., Zhang, Z., Ovadia, A., Cass, W. A., Yi, A., et al. (1996) Functional recovery in GDNF-treated Parkinsonian monkeys. *Nature* **380,** 252–255.
7. Sauer, H., Rosenblad, C., and Bjorklund, A. (1995) Glial cell line-derived neurotrophic factor but not transforming growth factor beta 3 prevents delayed degeneration of nigral dopaminergic neurons following striatal 6-hydroxydopamine lesion. *Proc. Natl. Acad. Sci. USA* **92,** 8935–8939.
8. Horger, B., Nishimura, M., Armanini, M., Wang, L.-C., Poulsen, K., et al. (1998) Neurturin exerts potent actions on survival and function of midbrain dopaminergic neurons. *J. Neurosci.* **18,** 4929–4937.

9. Milbrandt, J., deSauvage, F. J., Fahrner, T. J., Baloh, R. H., et al. (1998) Persephin, a novel neurotrophic factor related to GDNF and neurturin. *Neuron* **20,** 245–253.
10. Bankiewicz, K. S., Bringas, J., Pivirotto, P., Kutzscher, E., Nagy, D., Emborg, M. E. Technique for bilateral intracranial implantation of cells in monkeys using an automated delivery system. *Cell Transplant* **9,** 595–607.
11. Tuszynski, M. H., Senut, M. C., Ray, J., Roberts, J., Hoi-Sang, U.,and Gage, F. H. (1994) Somatic gene transfer to the adult primate central nervous system: in vitro and in vivo characterization of cells genetically modified to secrete nerve growth factor. *Neurobiol. Dis.* **1,** 67–78.
12. Schinstine, M., Jasodhara, R., and Gage, F. H. (1997) Potential effects of cytokines on transgene expression in primary fibroblasts implanted into rat brain. *Mol. Brain Res.* **47,** 195–201.
13. Major, E. O., Miller, A. E., Mourrain, P., Traub, R. G., de Widt, E., and Sever, J. (1985) Establishment of a line of human fetal glial cells which supports JC virus multiplication. *Proc. Natl. Acad. Sci.* **82,** 1257–1261.
14. Tornatore, C., Bankiewicz, K., Lieberman, D., and Major, E. O. (1993) Implantation and survival of a human fetal brain derived cell line in the basal ganglia of the non-human primate, rhesus monkey. *J. Cell Biochem.* **17E,** 227.
15. Bankiewicz, K. S., Leff, S., Nagy, D., Jungles, S., Rokovich, J, Spratt, K., Cohen, L., et al. (1997) Practical aspects of the development of ex vivo and in vivo gene therapy for Parkinson's disease. *Exp. Neurol.* **144,** 147–156.
16. Quereshi, N. H., Bankiewicz, K. S., Louis, D. N., Hochberg, F., Chiocca, A., and Harsh, G. R. (2000) Multicolumn infusion of gene therapy cells into human brain tumors: technical report. *Neurosurgery* **46,** 633–669.

20

Encapsulated Cell Implants as a Novel Treatment for Parkinson's Disease

Jack L. Tseng and Patrick Aebischer

1. Introduction

Parkinson's disease (PD) is a neurodegenerative disorder characterized by the progressive degeneration of the dopaminergic cells of the substantia nigra pars compacta (SNPc). Systemic levodopa therapy has proved to be an effective initial treatment for this disorder. However, resistance to this therapy inevitably develops with time, necessitating other approaches including surgery. Current experimental surgical treatments for this disorder include pallidal stimulation, pallidal lesion, subthalamic stimulation, and dopaminergic cell transplants. The current limitation of these approaches is that they all treat the symptoms but not the cause, that is, the progressive degeneration of the SNPc goes unabated.

Recently, it has been reported by several groups that neurotrophic factors, specifically two members of the glial cell line-derived neurotrophic factor (GDNF) family, GDNF and neurturin (NTN) are able to prevent degeneration of the dopaminergic cells of the SNPc in nearly all currently available animal models of PD *(1–9)*. Therefore, the administration of these factors may constitute a potential therapy for PD.

1.1. In Vivo and Ex Vivo Gene Therapy

Gene therapy, i.e., the ability to manipulate cells genetically to express a therapeutic protein, is a potentially powerful tool for the treatment of PD. Gene therapy currently involves one of two methods: in vivo and ex vivo. In vivo gene therapy involves the use of viral and chemical agents to transfer genetic

From: *Methods in Molecular Medicine, vol. 62: Parkinson's Disease: Methods and Protocols*
Edited by: M. M. Mouradian © Humana Press Inc., Totowa, NJ

material directly into cells *in situ*. Ex vivo gene therapy consists of the grafting of cells genetically engineered to release a desired protein.

In vivo gene therapy requires the successful transfer of genetic material into the host cell. This transfer can be mediated by viruses or through direct DNA transfer ***(10)***. The most useful of these techniques for gene therapy in neurodegenerative diseases is the employment of viral vectors, since certain viruses can transduce postmitotic neuronal cells ***(11,12)***. The most commonly used viral vectors for in vivo gene therapy in the central nervous system (CNS) are herpes simplex virus-1 (HSV-1) ***(10,13–18)***, adeno-associated virus (AAV) ***(19)***, adenovirus ***(20–24)***, and more recently lentiviruses ***(25)*** .

Ex vivo gene therapy involves the transfer of genetic material to cultured cells that are subsequently implanted into the host organism. The advantage of this method as opposed to in vivo gene therapy is that the efficiency and toxicity of vectors and gene constructs can be tested before transplantation ***(26,27)***. The cultured cells used in ex vivo gene therapy can be either syngeneic, allogeneic, or xenogeneic in nature. The cell types used in ex vivo gene therapy are immortalized cell lines or primary cells. Immortalized cell lines used experimentally for this purpose include fibroblasts ***(28–31)***, neuroblastomas ***(28)***, gliomas ***(32,33)***, and neuroendocrine cells ***(28)***. When allogeneic or xenogeneic immortalized cells are implanted into the host brain without the use of immunosuppression, graft survival is extremely low due to rejection ***(12,26)***. On the other hand, when syngeneic cells are implanted, or when immunosuppression is used with allogeneic or xenogeneic immortalized cells, transgene expression is observed although at much lower levels than that observed in vitro ***(26)***. However, the use of syngeneic cells or immunosuppression often leads to the formation of large tumors, which greatly reduces the window of viable treatment and prevents their use clinically ***(12,28,32)***. To avoid the tumorogenic complications that arise with the use of immortalized cell lines, primary cell cultures have been evaluated ***(12)***. Among these are primary skin fibroblasts ***(29,30,34)***, muscle fibers ***(35)***, and Schwann cells ***(36)***. In animals that have been implanted with these primary cells, transgene expression has been observed up to 6 mo postimplantation ***(35)***. Although transfected primary cells can support long-term in vivo expression, they still have the disadvantage of not being able to be retrieved should the need arises.

1.2. Polymer Encapsulation

Polymer encapsulation of genetically engineered cells is a technique that can bypass several current drawbacks of ex vivo gene therapy including the ability to transplant allogeneic or xenogeneic genetically engineered cells without the necessity for immunosuppression. The continuous release of proteins from the encapsulated cell line and the inflow of nutrients and oxygen into the

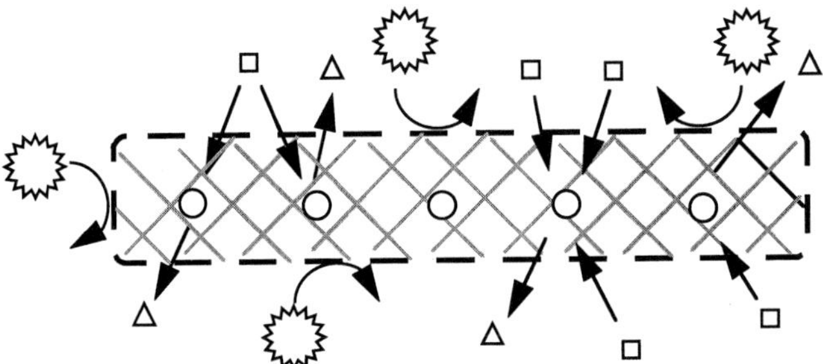

Host's Immunocompetent Cells
Transplanted Cells
Oxygen + Nutrients
Released Protein
Polymer Wall
Matrix

Fig. 1. The principle of polymer encapsulation. The semiporous polymer membrane allows the inflow of oxygen and nutrients and the export of protein while at the same time preventing contact of the implanted cells with the host's immunocompetent cells.

cells are also allowed (**Fig. 1**). At the same time, polymer encapsulation prevents cellular contact with the host's immunocompetent components. In rats, encapsulated cells have been shown to survive for more than 1 yr ***(37)*** whereas nonencapsulated cells either form tumors within days of transplantation or require constant immunosuppression ***(28,32,33)***. Another advantage is that being ensheathed in polymer capsules permits easy and complete retrieval of transplanted cells from the host, if necessary ***(38,39)***. To date, polymer encapsulation of genetically engineered cells is the only ex vivo gene therapy approach that has allowed the delivery of neurotrophic factors from genetically engineered cells in humans ***(40,41)***.

1.3. Delivery Problems

One of the major problems with delivering neurotrophic factors in vivo is the seemingly omnipresent specter of unwanted interactions. Therefore, a more localized delivery of a neurotrophic factor would minimize the risks of unwanted side effects. This problem is highlighted by the results reported by the amyotrophic lateral sclerosis (ALS) ciliary neurotrophic factor (CNTF) treatment study (ACTS) in which adverse effects were encountered with the subcutaneous administration of recombinant human CNTF (rhCNTF) ***(42)***.

High levels of anti-rhCNTF antibodies were detected in the blood of patients who received rhCNTF. On the other hand, a clinical trial utilizing polymer encapsulated cells transfected to release CNTF and implanted in the intrathecal space of ALS patients showed none of the adverse effects reported in the ACTS study ***(40,41)***. The blood-brain barrier (BBB), which effectively hinders the transport of proteins to and from the CNS, forced the ACTS group to administer CNTF systemically at levels that induced peripheral side effects but prevented such untoward effects with intrathecal implants. Thus, encapsulated cells allow the delivery of significantly lower amounts of neurotrophic factor for two reasons. Firstly, the BBB is bypassed with the intrathecal delivery. Second, a continuous delivery device allows steady exposure of target neurons to the therapeutic molecule, which greatly reduces the amount of neurotrophic factor needed for efficacy. Furthermore, the amount of factor that reaches the target neuron through systemic delivery is highly variable depending on several factors such as body temperature, diet, and stress levels ***(43–47)***, whereas CNS implants of polymer encapsulated cells bypass these variables and allow a more consistent delivery of the desired protein.

2. Materials

1. Culture medium
   a. Dulbecco's modified Eagle's medium (DMEM; Life Technologies, Paisley, Scotland),
   b. 10% fetal bovine serum (FBS; Life Technologies).
   c. 1% L-glutamine (Life Technologies).
   d. 1% pencillin/streptomycin (Life Technologies).
2. Sterile saline solution (Hanks' balanced salt solution; Life Technologies).
3. Cells releasing desired protein.
4. Polymer tubing.
5. Silicone tubing.
6. Collagen (Zyderm or Zyplast; Collagen, Palo Alto, CA).
7. Trypsin or cell dissociation medium (Sigma, St. Louis, MO).
8. Needle holder (Roboz, Rockville, MD).
9. Microscissor (Roboz).
10. Forceps (Roboz).
11. Photosensitive acrylate glue (Luxtrak LCM 23; Ablestik, Rancho Dominguez, CA).
12. Polarized blue light (Luxor 3; Ablestik).
13. Glass bead sterilizer (Steri 250; Simon Keller, Burgdorf, Switzerland).
14. Sterilized 80% ethanol or ethylene oxide sterilizer.
15. Dispensing tips (EFD; East Providence, RI).

3. Methods

1. Attach polymer tubing (*see* **Note 1**) of desired length to attachment hub using photosensitive acrylate glue (*see* **Note 2**).

2. Sterilize tubing using either ethylene oxide or sterile 80% ethanol followed by sterile saline solution (*see* **Note 3**).
3. Dissociate cells using either trypsin or cell dissociation medium for 5 min at 37°C and 5% CO_2.
4. Pellet cells by centrifugation (200*g* for 10 min at 4°C).
5. Add appropriate volume of culture medium to obtain twice the desired final concentration (*see* **Note 4**).
6. Make up a 3% matrix (collagen)/sterile saline solution and keep on ice until utilized (*see* **Note 5**).
7. Mix the cell solution with an equal volume of matrix solution in a 1-mL sterile syringe to obtain the final desired concentration.
8. Inject mixture into the polymer tubing through the attached dispensing tip.
9. Heat seal device at both ends using a sterilized needle holder (*see* **Note 6**).
10. Cut off excess tubing and reinforce both ends with photosensitive acrylate glue (LCM 23). Polymerize the glue by exposing to blue light for at least 60 s (*see* **Note 2**).
11. Leave capsules in culture medium at 37°C and 5% CO_2 for 2 d, followed by 3 d at 37°C and 5% CO_2 in differentiating medium (*see* **Note 7**).
12. Implant the capsule into the brain by using a device that is attached to a standard small animal stereotaxic frame (*see* **Fig. 2**).
13. Grab the capsule using forceps where the tips have been coated with silicone tubing (*see* **Note 8**) and leave in sterile saline for 2 min. Place capsule into bottom of outer cannula.
14. Raise outer cannula until the inner obtruder is just touching the top of the capsule.
15. Lower complete device to desired implant location (*see* **Note 9**).
16. Raise outer cannula while keeping inner obtruder in place.
17. Remove device. Capsule is implanted.

4. Notes

1. To be useful in an implant device, the polymer fiber must fulfill several criteria:
   a. Biocompatibility—will the polymer itself induce a response from the host immune system?
   b. Stability—will the polymer degrade with time?
   c. Ease of formation—can the polymer be made into a usable shape?
   d. Relatively controllable ultrastructure—can the polymer's characteristics be altered?
   e. Mechanical resistance—can it withstand the stress of intraparenchymal implantation?

   These questions should be addressed before a polymer is used as an implant device. We find that the polymers polyacrylonitrile-polyvinylchloride (PAN-PVC) and polyether sulfone (PES; AKZO-Fiber Nobel, Wupperthal, Germany) offer a decent combination of these properties. Each of these polymers has advantages and disadvantages. They are both nondegradable. PAN-PVC is typically spun as an asymmetric membrane, whereas PES is typically spun as a sym-

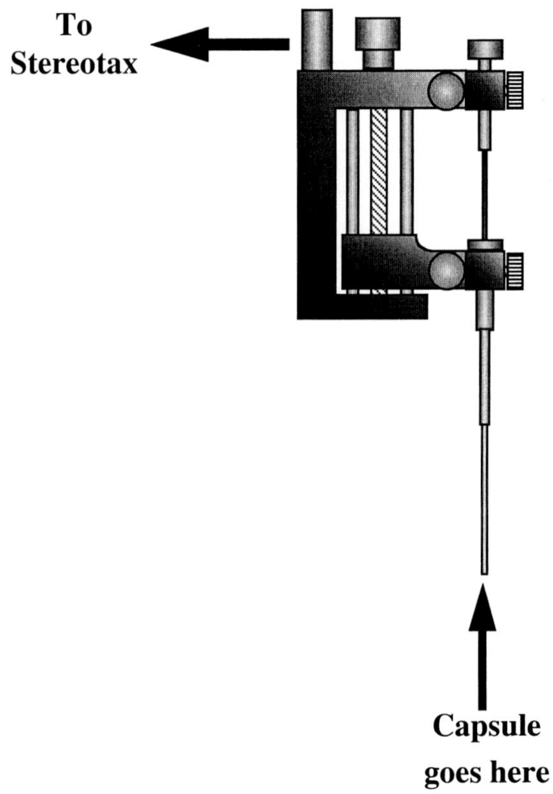

Fig. 2. Diagram of the device used to implant capsules into the brains of rats. The device can be attached to a standard stereotaxic frame to allow precise placement of the capsule in the brain.

metric membrane. Less protein adsorption for PES is compensated for by attainment of a very smooth skin for PAN-PVC, resulting in comparable acceptable biocompatibilities.

2. Make sure that the glue is properly crosslinked (>60 s of exposure to the blue light at a distance of not greater than 0.5 cm). If it is not, the acrylate monomers can be toxic to the cells. When the glue is incompletely polymerized, an oil-like film can be seen emanating from the glue when the capsule is placed into culture medium.
3. If ethylene oxide (ETO) sterilization is used, a minimum of 10 days is needed for evaporation of ETO monomers. For ethanol sterilization, overnight exposure to sterile alcohol followed by several hours of exposure to sterile saline is usually sufficient. Make sure tubes are properly flushed with sterile solution at each step.
4. Double the desired final concentration is chosen when a matrix is required. Otherwise, dilute directly to the desired final concentration.

5. Matrices are used when the cells that one wishes to encapsulate are anchorage dependent. Matrices provide a network of attachment sites for the implanted cells. Because collagen polymerizes at room temperature, it must be kept at 4°C until crosslinking is desired.
6. Preheat the needle holder in a glass bead sterilizer. Remove the needle holder from the sterilizer approx 10–15 s before use to prevent burning of the polymer tubing and evaporation of the culture medium from the capsule.
7. Differentiating medium is utilized when a cell line capable of being made post-mitotic, such as the mouse myoblast line, C_2C_{12}, is encapsulated. For C_2C_{12} cells, low-serum medium (DMEM + 2% FBS + 1% L-glutamine + 1% penicillin/streptomycin) is used to differentiate the cells. Cell lines capable of differentiation are more practical than normal non-postmitotic-capable cell lines (such as baby hamster kidney cells [BHK] or PC12 cells) for the following reasons:
   a. The amount of protein being released can be more precisely controlled.
   b. Cellular debris from dividing and dying cells reaching steady state is reduced, thus reducing the chances of host antibody formation.
8. The silicon tubing prevents damage to the capsule when handling.
9. The device must be lowered slowly (>5 min) into the brain due to the large diameter of the implant cannula. If the device is lowered at a faster rate, damage to brain tissue and excessive immune reaction may occur.

References

1. Hoffer, B. J., Hoffman, A., Bowenkamp, K., Huettl, P., Hudson, J., Martin, D., Lin, L. H., and Gerhardt, G. A. (1994) Glial cell line-derived neurotrophic factor reverses toxin-induced injury to midbrain dopaminergic neurons *in vivo*. *Neurosci. Lett.* **182,** 107–111.
2. Beck, K. D., Valverde, J., Alexi, T., Poulsen, K., Moffat, B., Vandlen, R. A., Rosenthal, A., and Hefti, F. (1995) Mesencephalic dopaminergic neurons protected by GDNF from axotomy-induced degeneration in the adult brain. *Nature.* **373,** 339–341.
3. Bowenkamp, K. E., Hoffman, A. F., Gerhardt, G. A., Henry, M. A., Biddle, P. T., Hoffer, B. J., and Granholm, A. C. (1995) Glial cell line-derived neurotrophic factor supports survival of injured midbrain dopaminergic neurons. *J. Comp. Neurol.* **355,** 479–489.
4. Kearns, C. M., and Gash, D. M. (1995) GDNF protects nigral dopamine neurons against 6-hydroxydopamine *in vivo*. *Brain Res.* **672,** 104–111.
5. Sauer, H., Rosenblad, C., and Björklund, A. (1995) GDNF but not TGF-β3 prevents delayed degeneration of nigral dopaminergic neurons following striatal 6-hydroxydopamine-lesion. *Proc. Natl. Acad. Sci. USA* **92,** 8935–8939.
6. Tomac, A., Lindqvist, E., Lin, L. H., Ögren, S. O., Young, D., Hoffer, B. J., and Olson, L. (1995) Protection and repair of the nigrostriatal dopaminergic system by GDNF *in vivo*. *Nature* **373,** 335–339.
7. Gash, D. M., Zhang, Z., Ovadia, A., Cass, W. A., Yi, A., Simmerman, L., Russell, D., Martin, D., Lapchak, P. A., Collins, F., Hoffer, B. J., and Gerhardt, G. A.

(1996) Functional recovery in parkinsonian monkeys treated with GDNF. *Nature* **380,** 252–255.

8. Tseng, J. L., Baetge, E. E., Zurn, A. D., and Aebischer, P. (1997) GDNF reduces drug-induced rotational behavior following medial forebrain bundle transection by a mechanism *not* involving striatal dopamine. *J. Neurosci.* **17,** 325–333.
9. Tseng, J. L., Bruhn, S. L., Zurn, A. D., and Aebischer, P. (1998) Neurturin protects dopaminergic neurons following medial forebrain bundle axotomy. *Neuroreport* **9,** 1817–1822.
10. Freese, A., Neve, R., and Geller, A. I. (1990) HSV-1 vector mediated neuronal gene delivery: strategies for neuroscience and neurology. *Biochem. Pharm.* **40,** 2189–2199.
11. Ugolini, G., Kuypers, H. G., and Strick, P. L. (1989) Transneuronal transfer of herpes virus from peripheral nerves to cortex and brainstem. *Science* **243,** 89–91.
12. Freese, A. , Stern, M., Kaplitt, M. G., O'Connor, W. M., Abbey, M. V., O'Connor, M. J., and During, M. J. (1996) Prospects for gene therapy in Parkinson's disease. *Movement Disord.* **11,** 469–488.
13. Baringer, J. R. and Sworeland, P. (1973) Recovery of herpes-simplex virus from human trigeminal ganglions. *N. Engl. J. Med.* **228,** 9593–9596.
14. Cook, M. L., Bastone, U. B., and Stevens, J. G. (1974) Evidence that neurons harbor latent herpes simplex virus. *Infect. Immun.* **9,** 946–951.
15. Spaete, R. R. and Frenkel, N. (1982) The herpes simplex virus amplicon: a new eucaryotic defective virus cloning-amplifying vector. *Cell* **30,** 295–304.
16. Palella, T. D., Hidaka, Y., Silverman, L. J., Levine, M., Glorioso, J., and Kelley, W. N. (1989) Expression of human HPRT mRNA in brains of mice infected with a recombinant herpes simplex virus-1 vector. *Gene* **80,** 137–144.
17. Martuza, R. L., Malick, A., Markert, J. M., Ruffner, K. L., and Coen, D. M. (1991) Experimental therapy of human glioma by means of a genetically engineered virus mutant. *Science* **252,** 854–856.
18. During, M. J., Naegele, J. R., O'Malley, K. L., and Geller, A. I. (1994) Long-term behavioral recovery in parkinsonian rats by an HSV vector expressing tyrosine hydroxylase. *Science* **266,** 1399–1403.
19. Kaplitt, M. G., Leone, P., Samulski, R. J., Xiao, X., Pfaff, D. W., O'Malley, K. L., and During, M. J. (1994) Long-term gene expression and phenotypic correction using adeno-associated virus vectors in the mammalian brain. *Nature Genet.* **8,** 148–154.
20. Akli, S., Caillaud, C., Vigne, E., Stratford-Perricaudet, L. D., Poenaru, L., Perricaudet, M., Kahn, A., and Peschanski, M. R. (1993) Transfer of a foreign gene into the brain using adenovirus vectors. *Nature Genet.* **3,** 224–234.
21. Davidson, B. L., Allen, E. D., Kozarsky, K. F., Wilson, J. M., and Roessler, B. J. (1993) A model system for *in vivo* gene transfer into the central nervous system using an adenoviral vector. *Nature Genet.* **3,** 219–223.
22. Le Gal La Salle, G., Robert, J. J., Berrard, S., Ridoux, V., Stratford-Perricaudet, L. D., Perricaudet, M., and Mallet, J. (1993) An adenovirus vector for gene transfer into neurons and glia in the brain. *Science* **259,** 988–990.

23. Neve, R. L. (1993) Adenovirus vectors enter the brain. *Trends Neurosci.* **16,** 251–253.
24. Mallet, J., Le Gal La Salle, G., Robert, J. J., Berrard, S., Ridoux, V., Stratford-Perricaudet, L. D., and Perriaudet, M. (1994) Adenovirus mediated gene transfer to the central nervous system. *Gene Ther.* **1 Suppl 1,** S52.
25. Naldini, L., Blömer, U., Gallay, P., Ory, D., Mulligan, R., Gage, F. H., Verma, I. M., and Trono, D. (1996) *In vivo* gene delivery and stable transduction of nondividing cells by a lentiviral vector. *Science* **272,** 263–267.
26. Suhr, S. T., and Gage, F. H. (1993) Gene therapy for neurologic disease. *Arch. Neurol.* **30,** 1252–1268.
27. Karpati, G., Lochmüller, H., Nalbantoglu, J., and Durham, H. (1996) The principles of gene therapy for the nervous system. *Trends Neurosci.* **19,** 49–54.
28. Horellou, P., Brundin, P., Kalen, P., Mallet, J., and Björklund, A. (1990) *In vivo* release of dopa and dopamine from genetically engineered cells grafted to the denervated rat striatum. *Neuron* **5,** 393–402.
29. Fisher, L. J., Jinnah, H. A., Kale, L. C., Higgins, G. A., and Gage, F. H. (1991) Survival and function of intrastriatally grafted primary fibroblasts genetically modified to produce L-dopa. *Neuron* **6,** 371–380.
30. Kang, U. J., Fisher, L. J., Joh, T. H., O'Malley, K. L., and Gage, F. H. (1993) Regulation of dopamine production by genetically modified primary fibroblasts. *J. Neurosci.* **13,** 5203–5211.
31. Levivier, M., Przedborski, S., Bencsics, C., and Kang, U. J. (1995) Intrastriatal implantation of fibroblasts genetically engineered to produce brain-derived neurotrophic factor prevents degeneration of dopaminergic neurons in a rat model of Parkinson's disease. *J. Neurosci.* **15,** 7810–7820.
32. Uchida, K., Ishii, A., Kaneda, N., Toya, S., Nagatsu, T., and Kohsaka, S. (1990) Tetrahydrobiopterin-dependent production of L-dopa in NRK fibroblasts transfected with tyrosine hydroxylase cDNA: future use for intracerebral grafting. *Neurosci. Lett.* **109,** 282–286.
33. Uchida, K., Tsuzaki, N., Nagatsu, T., and Kohsaka, S. (1992) Tetrahydrobiopterin-dependent functional recovery in 6-hydroxydopamine-treated rats by intracerebral grafting of fibroblasts transfected with tyrosine hydroxylase cDNA. *Dev. Neurosci.* **14,** 173–180.
34. Kawaja, M. D., Fagan, A. M., Firestein, B. L., and Gage, F. H. (1991) Intracerebral grafting of cultured autologous skin fibroblasts into the rat striatum: an assessment of graft size and ultrastructure. *J. Comp. Neurol.* **307,** 695–706.
35. Jiao, S., and Wolff, J. A. (1992) Long-term survival of autologous muscle grafts in rat brain. *Neurosci. Lett.* **137,** 207–210.
36. O'Malley, K., and Geller, A. I. (1992) Gene therapy in neurology: potential application to Parkinson's disease, in *Neurological Disorders: Novel Experimental and Therapeutic Strategies* (Vecsei, L., Freese, A., Swartz, K. J., and Beal, M. F., eds.), Ellis Horwood, West Sussex, England, pp. 223–248.
37. Lindner, M. D., Plone, M. A., Frydel, B., Kaplan, F., Krueger, M., Bell, W. J., et al. (1996) Intraventricular encapsulated CAC cells: viable for at least 500 days *in vivo* without detectable host immune sensitization or adverse effects on behavioral/cognitive function. *Soc. Neurosci. Abstr.* **22,** 306.3.

38. Aebischer, P., Tresco, P. A., Winn, S. R., Greene, L. A., and Jaeger, C. B. (1991) Long-term cross-species brain transplantation of a polymer-encapsulated dopamine-secreting cell line. *Exp. Neurol.* **111,** 269–275.
39. Aebischer, P., Wahlberg, L., Tresco, P. A., and Winn, S. R. (1991) Macroencapsulation of dopamine-secreting cells by coextrusion with an organic polymer solution. *Biomaterials* **12,** 50–56.
40. Aebischer, P., Pochon, N. A.-M., Heyd, B., Déglon, N., Joseph, J.-M., Zurn, A. D., et al. (1996) Gene therapy for amyotrophic lateral sclerosis (ALS) using a polymer encapsulated xenogenic cell line engineered to secrete hCNTF. *Hum. Gene Ther.* **7,** 851–860.
41. Aebischer, P., Schluep, M., Déglon, N., Joseph, J-M., Hirt, L., Heyd, B., Goddard, M. B., Hammang, J. P., Zurn, A. D., Kato, A. C., Regli, F., and Baetge, E. E. (1996) Intrathecal delivery of CNTF using encapsulated genetically modified xenogeneic cells in amyotrophic lateral sclerosis patients. *Nature Med.* **2,** 696–699.
42. ALS CNTF Treatment Study Group (1996) A double-blind placebo-controlled clinical trial of subcutaneous recombinant human ciliary neurotrophic factor (rHCNTF) in amyotrophic lateral sclerosis. *Neurology* **46,** 1244–1249.
43. Oztas, B. and Kaya, M. (1994) The effect of profound hypothermia on blood-brain barrier permeability during pentylenetetrazol-induced seizures. *Epilepsy Res.* **19,** 221–227.
44. Hussain, S. T. and Roots, B. I. (1994) Effect of essential fatty acid deficiency and immunopathological stresses on blood brain barrier (B-BB) in Lewis rats: a biochemical study. *Biochem. Soc. Trans.* **22,** 338S.
45. Ijima, T., Kubota, Y., Kuroiwa, T., and Sankawa, H. (1994) Blood-brain barrier opening following transient reflex sympathetic hypertension. *Acta Neurochir.* **Suppl. 60,** 142–144.
46. Tang, J. P., Xu, Z. Q., Douglas, F. L., Rakhit, A., and Melethil, S. (1993) Increased blood-brain barrier permeability of amino acids in chronic hypertension. *Life Sci.* **53,** 417–420.
47. Wijsman, J. A. and Shivers, R. R. (1993) Heat stress affects blood-brain barrier permeability to horseradish peroxidase in mice. *Acta Neuropathol.* **86,** 49–54.

21

Neural Stem Cell Technology as a Novel Treatment for Parkinson's Disease

Richard J. E. Armstrong, Anne E. Rosser, Stephen B. Dunnett, and Roger A. Barker

1. Introduction

The transplantation of human fetal ventral mesencephalic (VM) tissue for patients with advanced Parkinson's disease (PD) has now proved to be of benefit in early clinical trials *(1–3)*. This has been clearly seen in terms of improved motor function, which has been correlated with increased fluorodopa signal on positron emission tomographic scanning at the site of the implant and the presence of abundant tyrosine hydroxylase (TH)-positive neurons in those patients who have come to postmortem analysis *(4,5)*. However, although the concept of restoration of function through neural transplantation is promising, there are major practical as well as ethical problems with the use of aborted human fetal tissue. In particular, aborted fetal tissue is not available in many countries, and even where it can be obtained, isolation of the VM from the large numbers of fetuses the procedure requires presents major logistical difficulties. For example, in PD the best results have been obtained using an average of six to eight fetuses per patient. Therefore, the search for alternative sources of tissue for transplantation is imperative if the procedure is to be widely adopted in the clinical domain. A number of possibilities are currently being explored experimentally (*see* **Table 1**), although all of them present difficulties that must be overcome before they can be adopted clinically (reviewed in **ref.** ***6***).

1.1. What is a Stem Cell?

The burgeoning field of stem cell biology has attracted considerable interest over the last decade in part due to the unique properties of stem cells that potentially make them an ideal solution to the problems of tissue supply for

From: *Methods in Molecular Medicine, vol. 62: Parkinson's Disease: Methods and Protocols*
Edited by: M. M. Mouradian © Humana Press Inc., Totowa, NJ

Table 1
Alternatives to Primary Human Neuronal Cells for Transplantation in PD

Dopamine-containing polymers that release dopamine slowly over months/years.
Catecholamine-producing cells found naturally within the adult, which may thus be suitable for autotransplantation, e.g., adrenal medulla, carotid body, superior cervical ganglion.
Catecholamine-producing cell lines that may be encapsulated to prevent rejection and spread of the tumour cells out into the host brain, e.g., PC12 cells.
Cells transfected with tyrosine hydroxylase, which potentially allows for the possibility of autotransplantation, e.g., skin fibroblasts.
Xenografts of dopamine-rich tissue, e.g., embryonic porcine ventral mesencephalic tissue.
Neural stem cells.
Embryonic stem (ES) cells.

cell replacement therapies (*see* **Table 2**). A stem cell can be defined as a cell that is capable of self-renewal and multilineage differentiation. In practice this generally means that stem cells undergo asymmetric division to yield another stem cell and a non-self-renewing progenitor cell with a more restricted differentiation potential. The archetypal stem cell, and that which arises earliest in development, is the embryonic stem cell (ES). These totipotent cells can be isolated from the inner cell mass of the blastocyst or from primordial cells of the germ cell lineage. Later in development, tissue-specific stem cells emerge that reside in a specific organ system and under physiological conditions differentiate only into phenotypes appropriate for that tissue. The developmental stages intervening between ES cells and tissue-specific stem cells are uncertain. Techniques for the culture of ES cells are advancing rapidly, and recently human ES cells have been isolated *(7,8)*, although their study and use is strictly regulated and indeed prohibited in some countries. ES cells may ultimately be of use for neural cell replacement therapy *(9)*, but in this chapter we consider the tissue-specific stem cells that are now generally agreed to be present in the brain: neural stem cells.

1.2. Stem Cells in the Central Nervous System

The unambiguous demonstration that stem cells exist in the central nervous system has required analysis at the clonal level. Such experiments require us to follow the fate of individual cells in vitro, which has taken various forms: isolating lone cells in a culture vessel *(10)*; tracking individual cells with time-lapse photomicroscopy *(11)*; identifying cells by virtue of a unique retroviral insertion site *(12)*; and (least satisfactorily) culturing cells at such a low density that they are considered unlikely to aggregate (reviewed in **refs.** *13* and

Table 2
Current Advantages and Disadvantages to Neural Stem Cells as a Treatment for Parkinson's Disease

Advantages	Disadvantages
1. Potential for propagation in culture, increasing number of cells available for clinical transplant programs and thereby reducing the need for large number of fetuses to be available for individual patients.	1. Inability to induce a dopaminergic neuronal phenotype reliably.
2. Potential for producing more homogenous populations of cells for grafting.	2. Inability to alleviate behavioral deficits consistently in animal models of PD.
3. Potential for genetic manipulation of cells prior to grafting, such as transfection with therapeutic genes.	3. Change in characteristics of the cells with long-term expansion in culture may limit their efficacy.
4. Potential to manipulate fate of cells prior to implantation and thus increase their functional efficacy by becoming committed to dopaminergic neurons.	4. Difficulty in maintaining long-term neural stem cells from VM, thus increasing the need for a continual source of embryonic tissue.
5. Possibility of autografting if adult neural stem cells can be harvested efficiently.	5. Still need to use human fetal tissue for clinical allograft programs.
6. Possibly more migratory following implantation into the CNS, which may allow them to effect greater repair.	6. Potential for cells to undergo uncontrolled proliferation and by so doing form tumor masses.
7. Xenogeneic stem cell transplants are potentially less immunogenic than primary xenogeneic tissue.	

14). The use of these techniques has allowed the existence of self-renewing cells that generate neurons and macroglia to be demonstrated in various regions of the developing and adult nervous systems. Such studies have also revealed some of the fundamental properties of these cells (reviewed in **refs. *13–15***):

1. The proliferation of these cells can be elicited by the addition of epigenetic factors. Epidermal growth factor (EGF) and fibroblast growth factor-2 (FGF-2) have been particularly implicated in this regard.
2. Growth factor withdrawal leads to the emergence of variable proportions of neurons, astrocytes, and oligodendrocytes.
3. Cell division is normally asymmetric ***(16)***; hence, even if a culture is established from a single founder cell, it is soon composed of a mixture of stem cells and different progenitors.

Such clonal cultures are of importance in elucidating the basic biology and behavior of these cells, but they are of less use when the aim is to generate large numbers of cells for transplantation experiments; thus, for these purposes population-based approaches are generally used. This approach involves the isolation of a founder population of cells from the region of interest in the developing or adult brain, and the expansion of bulk cultures using growth factors. The mixed founder population further accentuates the heterogeneity of the growing cells promoted by asymmetric division. In recognition of the fact that pure populations of neural stem cells cannot be grown using current methods, we advocate use of the generic term *expanded neural precursor cells* (ENPs) for cell populations grown in this way.

Transplantation experiments using ENPs in animal models of PD are still in their infancy and have yet to reach the levels of success achieved with transplants of primary tissue. At the present time the major limiting factor in the use of these cells in PD is the reliable induction of the dopaminergic phenotype that is necessary if they are ever to be employed in repairing the brain and, thus, curing PD. Although we concentrate here on the potential use of ENPs to replace the lost dopaminergic neurons in PD, it is possible that transplants of these cells can be used as a system to deliver therapeutic molecules such as growth factors ***(17,18)***. Alternatively, it may prove possible to recruit endogenous adult neural precursor cells, which have been shown to be present in the adult human brain, albeit in low numbers ***(19–21)***.

Reliable techniques for growing ENPS have now been well established, although it is clear that great differences exist in ENPs isolated from different regions of different species at different gestational ages. In this chapter we outline the methods that allow differences in the isolation, expansion, and transplantation of these cells to be investigated experimentally.

Unfortunately, there is little consensus on the exact methodologic approach to growing ENP populations, which makes interpretation of the large number of published studies difficult. We describe here the methods used successfully in our laboratory for growing embryonic rat ENP populations, and we attempt to point out the main variations used by others. These basic methods can be simply adapted to allow growth of ENPs from other species, including human, and some of these adaptations are mentioned.

2. Materials

2.1. Cell Culture Reagents

1. Hanks' balanced salt solution (HBSS): The standard solution for dissection and washing of the neural tissue (Life Technologies, Paisley, Scotland).
2. HBSS without calcium/magnesium: Used for making up trypsin inhibitor (Life Technologies).

3. Dulbecco's modified Eagle's medium (DMEM): Used to make up basic culture medium (Life Technologies).
4. Ham's F-12: Used to make up basic culture medium (Life Technologies).
5. Trypsin: Preparation of tissue for culturing and passaging of cells (Worthington Biochemical Corporation, Freehold, NJ).
6. DNase: Preparation of tissue for culturing and passaging of cells (Sigma, Poole, Dorset, UK).
7. Trypsin inhibitor: Preparation of tissue for culturing and passaging of cells (Sigma).
8. Penicillin/streptomycin/amphotericin (PSF): Antimicrobials added to culture medium (Life Technologies).
9. N2: Defined supplement to replace serum in culture medium (Life Technologies).
10. B27: Defined supplement to replace serum in culture medium (Life Technologies).
11. Human recombinant EGF: Mitogen for growing cells (Sigma).
12. Human recombinant FGF-2: Mitogen for growing cells (R&D Systems).
13. T75 tissue culture flasks.
14. Fetal bovine serum (FBS): Standard culture medium (Bio-Whittaker, Wokingham, UK).
15. Heparin: Used in culture with FGF-2 (Sigma).

2.2. Antibodies

TH, γ-aminobutyric acid (GABA), glial fibrillay acidic protein (GFAP), and nestin are polyclonal antibodies; other antibodies are mouse monoclonals in nature. The suggested concentration for use is given in parenthesis (**Table 3**).

1. β-tubulin-III (TuJ1; Sigma) (1:500).
2. Microtubule-associated protein-2ab (MAP-2ab; Sigma) (1:200).
3. Neuronal specific nuclear antigen (NeuN; Chemicon, Tenecula, CA) (1:500).
4. Neurofilament 200 kDa (NF-200; Sigma) (1:200).
5. TH (Institut Jacques-Boy, Bioreme, Reims, France) (1:4000).
6. TH (Chemicon) (1:400).
7. GABA (Sigma) (1:1000).
8. GFAP (Dako, High Wycombe, Bucks, UK) (1:500).
9. Vimentin (Dako) (1:500).
10. Galactocerebroside (Gal-C): ECACC hybridoma clone K07, cell line supernatant (1:30) (Gift of Professor Neil Scolding, Bristol, UK).
11. Nestin (gift of Dr. Ron McKay, Bethesda, MD).
12. MAP2c (Sigma) (1:250).
13. Myelin basic protein (Serotec, Oxford, UK) (1:200).

3. Methods

3.1. Dissection of Embryonic Neural Tissue

1. The initial dissection and preparation of the tissue is identical to that used for primary cultures of embryonic neural cells *(22)* (*see* **Note 1**).
2. The pregnant rats are sacrificed by CO_2 anesthesia and cervical dislocation.

Table 3
Standard Immunocytochemical Markers Used in Cultures[a]

Cell type	Marker
Neuron	General neuronal markers
	β-tubulin III (or TuJ1), MAP-2ab, NeuN, Neurofilament (NF_{200})
	Specific neuronal markers
	TH, GABA, and others
Astrocytes	Glial fibrillary acidic protein, vimentin
Oligodendrocytes	Galactocerebroside-C, myelin basic protein
Precursor/stem cell	Nestin, MAP-2c

[a]*See* **Subheading 2.** for more details on antibodies.

3. The embryos are then removed through an abdominal incision complete with placenta, chorion, and amniotic sacs and placed into a sterile 50 mL universal container in which 20 mL of HBSS has been placed under sterile conditions in a flow hood.
4. The embryos are then transferred to a large Petri dish in a sterile flow hood and the embryos freed from their associated membranes and placed into a second large petri dish containing phosphate-buffered saline (PBS)/0.6% glucose.
5. They are then washed by transferring them across a further two or three Petri dishes containing fresh PBS/0.6% glucose.
6. After washing, the embryos can be dissected. The relevant central nervous system (CNS) region is identified and then dissected out (using a dissecting microscope) with removal of the meninges (*see* **Note 2**).

3.2. Preparation of Embryonic Neural Tissue for Culture

The tissue is prepared in an identical fashion to that used for primary tissue cultures *(22)*.

1. In essence the dissected neural tissue is cut into small pieces and the pieces aspirated with a Pasteur pipet into a 20-mL centrifuge tube along with a few milliliters of PBS/glucose.
2. The tissue is spun at 100*g* for 3 min and then trypsinized.
3. Then 0.5 mL of 0.1% Worthington trypsin is added for 20 min at 37°C.
4. The tissue is spun at 100*g* for 3 min and the trypsin/DNase removed and replaced by Trypsin inhibitor (0.1% in Ca^{2+}/Mg^{2+}– free HBSS, with 0.001% DNase) for 5 min at room temperature.
5. The cells are then washed three or four times in 2–3 mL DMEM, spinning the whole suspension for 3 min, removing the supernatant and repeating.
6. At the end of the washing phase, the tissue is suspended in culture medium (*see* **step 7**) and triturated using 10–15 strokes of a flame-polished Pasteur pipet.

7. The final suspension is now largely in the form of a single cell suspension and is ready for culturing. The viability and density of this suspension is checked using the Trypan Blue exclusion method by mixing equal volumes of the cell suspension and Trypan Blue (5 μL) and placed onto a hemocytometer. The ratio of live to nonlive cells can then be deduced and the percent of viable cells calculated along with a final cell density.

3.3. Propagation of ENPs in Culture

1. The final cell suspension is now ready for growing in culture, assuming the viability of the tissue is >70%.
2. The basic culture medium consists of 70% DMEM, 30% Ham's F-12 with 1% PSF, 1% N2, or 2% B27 along with the mitogens EGF (20 ng/mL) and/or FGF-2 (20 ng/mL) with heparin at a concentration of 5 μg/mL (*see* also **Subheading 2.**).
3. The cells are grown in uncoated T75 flasks containing 20 mL of culture medium. The initial seeding density of the cells can significantly affect the growth characteristics of the cells *(23)*. For bulk cultures the cells are seeded at an initial density of 200,000 cells/mL.
4. Half the culture medium is changed every 4 d and the cultures grown in incubators at 37°C with 5% CO_2.
5. Following an initial phase of death, a robust expansion in cell number can be obtained over time (*see* **Note 3**).

3.4. Passaging and Assessing Expansion of ENPs

As ENPs increase in number, spheres grow in size, meaning that critical diffusable factors are prevented from reaching the center of the sphere. This requires that the spheres be passaged. Similarly, monolayer cultures need passaging to prevent contact-mediated growth arrest. Passaging involves dividing and seeding into new flasks. The variables involved in this process are some of the most critical in achieving successful expansion of ENPs.

3.4.1. When Should the Cultures be Passaged?

1. The two main criteria used are time in culture (e.g., once a week) or a more flexible approach based on the size of the sphere/density of the monolayer culture. The choice of these options depends on the experimental aims, but either may be valid.

3.4.2. How Should the Cultures be Passaged?

1. This depends on the precise growth characteristics of the cultures in question. The standard method involves reducing the ENPs to a single cell suspension through mechanical or enzymatic dissociation.
2. For sphere cultures this involves first harvesting the spheres by centrifugation, and for monolayer cultures cells must be scraped or trypsinized from the culture flask.

3. Following this process, the cells are resuspended in fresh proliferation medium and mechanically dissociated, and the total cell number is determined by the Trypan Blue exclusion technique, as for primary neural tissue (*see* **Subheading 3.2., step 7**).
4. At the end of this passaging procedure, the ENPs are resuspended at a density of 100,000/mL.
5. The expansion ratio can be calculated by dividing the number of cells present at the end of the culture by that which was originally put into culture (*see* **Note 4**).
6. This is the standard method appropriate for rodent cultures; however, for human ENP passaging, an alternative successful approach adopted in our laboratory is an automated sectioning method using the McIiwain tissue chopper *(24)*.

3.5. Assessing the Differentiation of ENPs In Vitro

On withdrawal of the mitogens, ENPs will spontaneously differentiate into terminal phenotypes. These default phenotypes can be assessed using immunocytochemical protocols, akin to those used for primary neuronal cultures (*see* **Subheading 2.** and **Table 3** for details on the standard antibodies used).

In essence an aliquot of cells are removed at the time of passaging and plated onto poly-L-lysine coated 13mm coverslips in the absence of mitogens but the presence of serum (this culture medium consists of DMEM 90%, 1% FBS, and 2% B27).

The cells are grown for the period of interest (often 7 d) and then fixed and their phenotype examined using a range of immunohistochemical markers (for details, *see* **ref.** *25*) (*see* **Notes 5** and **6**).

3.6. Transplantation of ENPs

Transplantation of ENPs into experimental animals (*see* **Fig. 1**) provides a method by which the environment of the cells can be manipulated and their

---

Fig. 1. *(opposite page)* Schematic representation of preparation, differentiation and grafting of ENPs in animal models of Parkinson's disease. 1, A region of the embryonic CNS is dissected and prepared into a cell suspension using a standard method *(22)*. 2, The cell suspension is then grown in the presence of mitogens (EGF, FGF-2, heparin) to form neurospheres (see phase contrast photomicrograph). 3, Differentiation of the ENPs can be achieved through withdrawal of the mitogens and plating the cells on an appropriate substrate. The ENPs then differentiate into neurons (stained with β-tubulin or TuJ1), astrocytes (stained with GFAP), and oligodendrocytes (stained with Gal-C). 4, The standard rat model of PD involves unilateral lesioning of the dopaminergic nigrostriatal pathway. The loss of the dopaminergic input to the striatal complex leads to a rotational bias that can be accentuated by drugs that activate the dopaminergic network such as amphetamine and apomorphine. The loss of this rotational bias after grafting typically reflects restoration of the normal dopaminergic innervation in the lesioned striatum. 5, Grafting of the ENPs to the 6-OHDA-lesioned

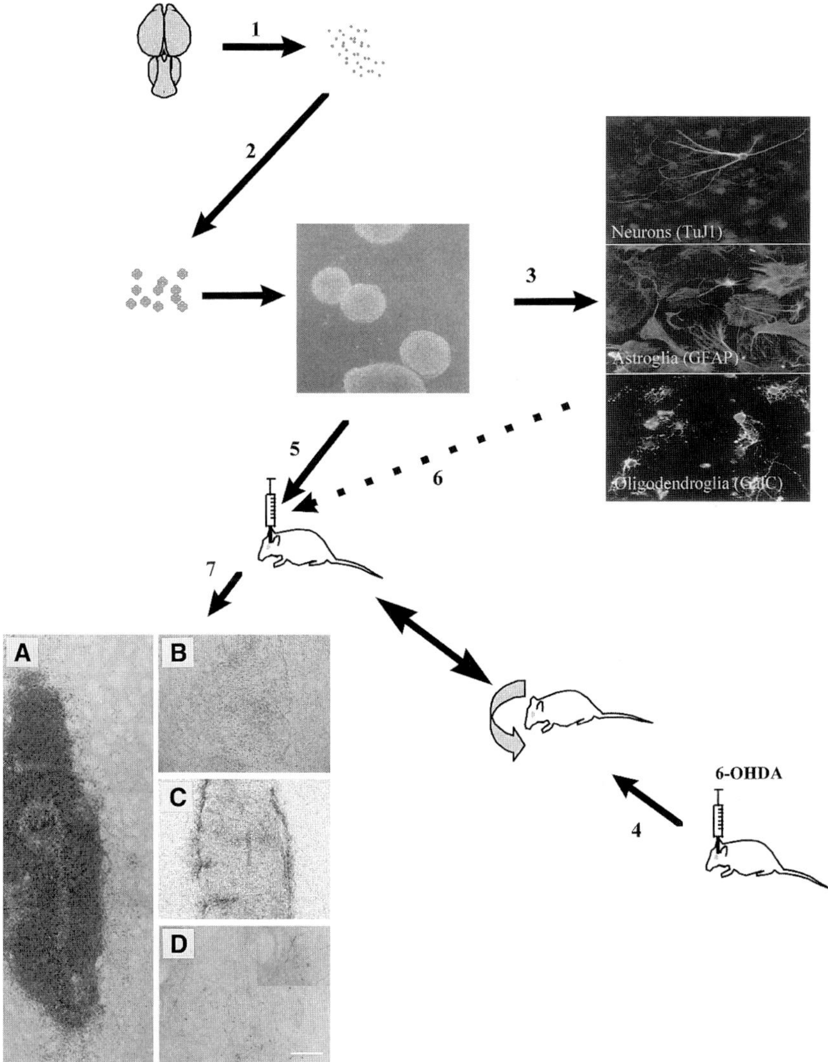

rat model of PD. 6, Grafting of ENPs that have been differentiated in culture prior to implantation (*see* text and **Table 4** for more details). 7, Histologic appearance of ENP grafts several weeks after transplantation. **(A)** Cells can be identified with the use of species-specific markers. In this photomicrograph grafted human ENPs are labeled with human-specific nuclear stain, showing a discrete graft mass with some cells migrating out from graft into host brain. **(B–D)** Characteristic phenotypes can be identified immunohistochemically. **(B)** NeuN-stained neurons in a porcine ENP graft. **(C)** Vimentin-positive astrocytes in adjacent section of same porcine ENP graft. **(D)** TH-positive neurons can occasionally be seen in this porcine ENP graft. Scale bar = 200 µm.

phenotypic potential explored. Transplantation of ENPs into permissive environments such as the developing brain (embryonic or neonatal) and areas of ongoing neurogenesis in the adult brain (such as the hippocampus and subventricular zone) have revealed some plasticity in the neural fates that can be adopted by ENPs (**Table 4**). Perhaps even more surprisingly, experiments in which clonally derived mouse ENPs have been transplanted into the irradiated bone marrow, have revealed that ENPs may adopt nonneural fates, thus suggesting that "tissue-specific" stem cells may retain the potential to generate cells of other organ systems ***(26)***.

The ability of ENPs to adopt appropriate neurochemical phenotypes and mediate functional recovery in animal models of disease remains unclear. In PD models, experiments thus far have shown that TH neurons generally constitute a small proportion of the total differentiated cells and that functional recovery is variable and incomplete ***(27,28)***. The general schema for these experiments is now outlined.

3.6.1. Lesions and Behavioral Assessment

ENPs have been grafted into animal models of PD, in particular the unilateral 6-hyroxydopamine (6-OHDA) lesioned rat (**Table 4**). This model relies on the stereotaxic injection of 6-OHDA into the medial forebrain bundle on one side of the brain, and the resulting dopaminergic imbalance between the two striata causes the animal to rotate spontaneously away from the side of greatest dopaminergic activation (i.e., the animals turn ipsilaterally relative to the lesion; reviewed in **refs.** ***6*** and ***29***). This spontaneous rotational behavior can be exaggerated and quantified using stimulant drugs such as metamphetamine or low-dose apomorphine and automated rotational counters (rotometers). These two drugs work on different parts of the dopaminergic network; metamphetamine stimulates the release of dopamine from the intact side, whereas low-dose apomorphine preferentially activates the supersensitive receptors within the dopamine-deafferented striatum. This understanding of the action of these drugs is important in the interpretation of any grafting experiment as although grafts placed into the dopamine-deafferented striatum are thought to affect drug-induced behavior by a dopaminergic action, they may also have an effect through nonspecific damage of the striatal neurons (*see*, for example, **ref.** ***29***).

3.6.2. Approaches to Transplantation

1. ENPs are grafted into the striatum using standard procedures ***(30)***. The cells may be grafted as undissociated spheres/aggregates ***(27,30)*** or may be dissociated to a coarse single cell suspension at passaging ***(28)*** prior to implantation.
2. When ENPs are grafted as undissociated spheres an estimate of the cell number in the sphere suspension must be obtained; this is most often done by taking

Table 4
Published Studies on the Behavior of Epigenetically Propagated Neural Precursor Cells Following Transplantation[a]

Reference	Tissue source	Pregraft expansion	Host	Time in vivo	Significant findings
Immature host					
Winkler et al., 1998 ***(53)***	E14 mouse striatum, cortex and VM	EGF, 40 d	E15 telencephalic ventricle	5 wk	Only glial differentiation
Brüstle et al., 1998 ***(54)***	7.5–10.5 wk human cortex	EGF + FGF-2, Up to 7 wk	E17–18 telencephalic ventricle	Up to 7 wk	Neurons with regionally appropriate morphology, astrocytes, and oligodendrocytes
Flax et al., 1998 ***(55)***	15-wk human telencephalon	FGF-2, unspecified time	P0 lateral ventricle, cerebellum	24 h to 5 wk	Glial differentiation in cortex; neurons in olfactory bulb and cerebellum; transformation status unclear
Rosser et al., 2000 ***(56)***	22-wk human brain	EGF + FGF-2, 17 d	P1 hippoocampus, striatum	4 wk	Neurons with regionally appropriate morphology; some astroglia
Neurodegenerative disease models					
Minger et al., 1996 ***(51)***	E14 rat basal forebrain	FGF-2, 14 d	Ibotenate-lesioned NBM; frontal cortex[b]	Up to 7 mo	Some ChAT-expressing neurons
Svendsen et al., 1996 ***(35)***	13-wk human VM, E16 rat	EGF, 10–23 d	6-OHDA/ibotenate-lesioned striatum[c]	4 wk	Occasional TH^+ cells seen
Svendsen et al., 1997 ***(28)***	22-wk human brain	EGF + FGF-2, 14–28 d	6-OHDA-lesioned striatum	Up to 20 wk	Functional improvement in two animals with TH^+ cells; predominantly glial differentation

(continued)

Table 4 *(continued)*

Reference	Tissue source	Pregraft expansion	Host	Time in vivo	Significant findings
Stüder et al., 1998 ***(27)***	E12 rat VM	FGF-2, 6–8 d Differentiate, 7 d	6-OHDA-lesioned striatum	11.5–14.5 wk	Significant functional improvement and TH^+ cells reported
Vescovi et al., 1999 ***(44)***	Human 10.5-wk telence-phalon	EGF + FGF-2; 10–11 mo[d] Differentiate 6 d	6-OHDA-lesioned striatum	Up to 1 yr	Neuronal differentiation in graft; TH^+ cells not reported
Corti et al., 1999 ***(57)***	Embryonic human brain	FGF-2, unspecified time	6-OHDA-lesioned striatum	4 wk	Adenovirus-mediated transfection pregraft; regulatable expression of TH transgene
Armstrong et al., 2000 ***(30)***	Human 9-wk striatum	EGF +FGF-2, 10 d	Quinolinic acid-lesioned striatum[c]	12 wk	Significant fiber outgrowth by grafted cells, some DARPP-32 striatal neurons in grafts

[a]Cells used in the above studies were not genetically immortalized. The host species is rat, unless otherwise stated.

[b]Alzheimer's disease model.

[c]Huntington's disease model.

[d]Time in vitro is an estimate calculated on the basis of reported passage number and frequency.

Abbreviations: E, embryonic day; P, postnatal day; VM, ventral mesencephalon; NBM, nucleus basalis magnocellularis; DARPP-32, dopamine and adenosine receptor phosphoprotein (32 kDa).

representative aliquots of the suspension, dissociating them, and determining live cell number as described previously.

3. Cells are loaded into a wide-bore 10 μL Hamilton syringe, to facilitate the delivery of spheres of cells, and ENPs are then grafted into the striatum through a burr hole placed in the skull of the experimental rat.
4. The cells are implanted at a rate of 1 μL/min with a typical deposit being 2 μL in total and containing a total of 500,000 cells.
5. At the end of implantation the cannula is left *in situ* for a further 2 min before removal.
6. The wound is sutured and the animal monitored for behavioral recovery and sacrificed for histology after an appropriate time (**Table 4**) (*see* **Note 7**).

4. Notes

1. Time-mated rats are used so that an accurate gestational age for the litter of embryos can be obtained. The appropriate age for isolation of ENPs from different regions must be determined.
2. Areas from which we and others have reported the successful growth of ENPs include the cerebral cortex *(**11**,**31**)*, striatum *(**23**,**32**)*, hippocampus *(**33**)*, septum *(**34**)*, VM *(**27**,**35**)*, and spinal cord *(**36**)*.
3. The morphologic characteristics of propagating ENPs depend on their region and age of origin. Often cells grow as freely floating, or lightly attached, spheres of cells ("neurospheres;" *see* **Fig. 1**), however, cells may grow as monolayer cultures *(**31**,**33**)*, particularly when derived from young embryos or caudal regions of the neuraxis.
4. The number of times that the cells can be passaged before they enter the phase of decline and growth arrest known as senescence varies according to age and region (A.E. Rosser, unpublished observations).
5. There are no currently available specific markers for neural stem cells within ENP cultures, but nestin is commonly used; it labels immature neuroepithelial precursor cells *(**37**)*. Nestin can also be expressed in developing and adult reactive astrocytes *(**38**)*, but when used in conjunction with bromodeoxyuridine (BrdU) is nonetheless useful for identifying dividing precursor cells.

   It is worth noting that immunocytochemical staining of cells derived from ENPs does not necessarily reveal their full potential, merely their default differentiation pathways, since the absence of a phenotype may simply mean that the necessary signals have not been provided. Questions of fate potential can only be examined by manipulating the environment of the differentiating cells, through transplantation or use of culture supplements (reviewed in **ref. *13***). In the context of this discussion it is also worth noting that TH neurons very rarely emerge spontaneously in culture, although additions to the culture medium may allow small numbers to be obtained *(**27**,**39–41**)*.
6. Parameters that may affect the growth of ENPs:
   a. Gestational age of donor tissue: The gestational age at which the tissue is harvested is important in determining the proliferative potential and may also

be of importance in influencing the phenotypic potential. The greatest expansion is typically seen with cultures derived from the youngest gestational ages, e.g., E12 with the rat VM (AE Rosser, unpublished observations) ***(42,43)***.

b. Regional origin of donor tissue: The extent to which the characteristics of ENPs differ between regions remains to be fully clarified, as does the degree to which ENPs from different regions are plastic in terms of their final phenotype or are fate determined. This may have major implications for transplant studies in that it may be important to select ENPs from specific regions for transplantation into the adult brain, e.g., VM harvested ENPs in PD. Indeed the only studies to date that have shown any functional recovery with ENP grafts in animal models of PD have employed cells derived from the developing VM ***(27,28)***. Cells derived from other regions have not shown any such functional effects, despite good survival of the grafted tissue (R.J.E. Armstrong, et al, unpublished observations) ***(44)***. However, it may be possible (given the putative potential of these cells) that ENPs derived from other brain regions can be induced to develop into TH-positive cells if placed in the appropriate environment or exposed to appropriate developmental signals ***(45)***.

c. Donor species: The basic methods described here are for rat ENPs, but similar approaches have been used to grow ENPs from many species, including mouse, rat, dog, pig, nonhuman primates, and human. Most work to date has concentrated on rat and mouse cells (reviewed in **ref.** ***13***). In studies that addressed species differences explicitly, significant differences have been shown to exist even between species as phylogenetically close as mouse and rat ***(46)***. The underlying mechanisms for this are unknown but will have an impact on their use in transplant paradigms.

d. Mitogen used and other culture supplements: The standard mitogens used in our laboratory, and the majority of others, are EGF and FGF-2 either alone or in combination. The behavior of cells expanded with these growth factors can differ quite significantly, and the relationship between cells responding to EGF and FGF-2 is complex and has been the subject of a number of studies (e.g., **refs.** ***42***, ***43***, and ***47***). The use of heparin in the culture medium in our laboratory has been shown to facilitate the action of FGF-2, possibly through stabilization of this molecule ***(48)***. Other supplements have been shown to affect the behavior of some ENPs in culture, for example, cell surface molecules such as sonic hedgehog ***(49)*** and leukemia-inhibitory factor ***(50)***.

e. Time in culture: It is probable that ENPs alter their characteristics according to the length of time they have spent in culture. For example, rat ENPs grown in culture clearly change over time in terms of the proportion of neurons versus glia they produce ***(12,23)***, although this remains controversial for human ENPs ***(24,44,50)***. In addition, successful grafting in animal models of neurodegenerative disease (including PD), in which a degree of neurochemical differentiation has been observed, has involved ENPs which have been expanded for relatively short periods ***(27,28,30,51)***. Studies that directly address this issue are required.

7. Parameters to consider in transplantation experiments:
   a. Labeling of cells and identification after transplant: The labeling of the grafted cells is especially important in ENP grafts due to their propensity to migrate and not always remain as a discrete graft mass *(28)*. Several markers can be useful in this regard, including the labeling of dividing cells with BrdU prior to implantation, along with species markers in the case of xenografted ENPs (for example, *see* **Fig. 1**). However, there are problems with both of these approaches. BrdU labeling can give false negatives as a result of division of cells postimplantation and dilution of the marker, whereas species-specific markers may show a degree of crossreactivity with the host tissue. Other markers that have been advocated include genetic labels such as *lac*Z or green fluorescent protein and male-to-female grafts identified using a Y-chromosome probe (reviewed in **ref.** ***52***).
   b. Differentiation in vitro prior to grafting: The relatively low numbers of TH-positive cells found after grafting of undifferentiated ENPs has led to the suggestion that this can be improved by predifferentiating the cells prior to transplantation. This has been done using either specific factors known to be important in normal dopaminergic differentiation (e.g., Nurr-1; *see* **ref.** ***45***) or less specific serum factors under specialized culture conditions (roller tube cultures using VM-derived ENPs expanded for short periods) *(27)*.
   c. Immunosuppression in cross-species ENP grafts: The use of different species for isolation and expansion of ENPs has led to a number of studies in which the tissue is xenografted into a rodent host (i.e., across species). To prevent these xenografts from being rejected, immunosuppressive drugs must be given to the host animal. The extent to which immunosuppression affects the behavior of these grafts is not known, but of interest is the observation that xenografted ENP grafts are less immunogenic than primary neural xenografts (R.J.E. Armstrong, unpublished data). The reason for this is not clear at the present time, but it may be important in the future development of any neural xenograft program.

Acknowledgments

R.A.B. and A.E.R. are MRC Clinician Scientists. We would like to thank Pam Tyers for her helpful technical assistance with this paper. Work reported in this chapter has been supported by the Medical Research Council, UK.

References

1. Widner, H. (1998) The Lund programme for Parkinson's disease and patients with MPTP-induced parkinsonism, in *Cell Transplantation in Neurological Disease* (Freeman, T. B. and Widner, H., eds,), Humana Press, Totowa, NJ, pp. 1–17.
2. Rémy, P., Samson, Y., Hantraye, P., Fontaine, A., Defer, G., Mangin, J. F., et al. (1995) Clinical correlates of [^{18}F]fluorodopa uptake in five grafted Parkinsonian patients. *Ann. Neurol.* **38,** 580–588.

3. Fahn, S., Greene, P. E., Tsai, W.-Y., et al. (1999) Double-blind controlled trial of human embryonic dopaminergic tissue transplants in advanced Parkinson's disease: clinical outcomes. *Neurology* **52 (Suppl. 2)**, A405.
4. Kordower, J. H., Freeman, T. B., and Olanow, C. W. (1998) Neuropathology of fetal nigral grafts in patients with Parkinson's disease. *Mov. Disord.* **13,** 88–95.
5. Sawle, G. V. and Myers, R. (1993) The role of positron emission tomography in the assessment of human neurotransplantation. *Trends Neurosci.* **16,** 172–176.
6. Barker, R. A. and Dunnett, S. B. (1999) *Neural repair, Transplantation and Rehabilitation.* Psychology Press, Hove.
7. Shamblott, M. J., Axelman, J., Wang, S., Bugg, E. M., Littlefield, J. W., Donovan, P. J., et al. (1998) Derivation of pluripotent stem cells from cultured human primordial germ cells. *Proc. Natl. Acad. Sci. USA* **95,** 13,726–13,731.
8. Thomson, J. A., Itskovitz-Eldor,J., Shapiro, S. S., Waknitz, M. A., Swiergiel, J. J., Marshall, V. S., et al. (1998) Embryonic stem cell lines derived from human blastocysts. *Science* **282,** 1145–1147.
9. Svendsen, C. N. and Smith, A. G. (1999) New prospects for human stem-cell therapy in the nervous system. *Trends Neurosci.* **22,** 357–364.
10. Reynolds, B. A. and Weiss, S. (1996) Clonal and population analyses demonstrate that an EGF-responsive mammalian embryonic CNS precursor is a stem cell. *Dev. Biol.* **175,** 1–13.
11. Davis, A. A. and Temple, S. (1994) A self-renewing multipotential stem cell in embryonic rat cerebral cortex. *Nature* **372,** 263–266.
12. Palmer, T. D., Takahashi, J., and Gage, F. H. (1997) The adult rat hippocampus contains primordial neural stem cells. *Mol. Cell Neurosci.* **8,** 389–404.
13. Armstrong, R. J. E. and Svendsen, C. N. (2000) Neural stem cells: from cell biology to cell replacement. *Cell Transpl.* **9,** 139–152.
14. Gage, F. H. (2000) Mammalian neural stem cells. *Science* **287,** 1433–1438.
15. Weiss, S., Reynolds, B. A., Vescovi, A. L., Morshead, C., Craig, C. G., and van der Kooy, D. (1996) Is there a neural stem cell in the mammalian forebrain? *Trends Neurosci.* **19,** 387–393.
16. Mayer-Proschel, M., Kalyani, A. J., Mujtaba, T., and Rao, M. S. (1997) Isolation of lineage-restricted neuronal precursors from multipotent neuroepithelial stem cells. *Neuron* **19,** 773–785.
17. Kordower, J. H., Chen, E. Y., Winkler, C., Fricker, R., Charles,V., Messing, A., et al. (1997) Grafts of EGF-responsive neural stem cells derived from GFAP-hNGF transgenic mice: trophic and tropic effects in a rodent model of Huntington's disease. *J. Comp. Neurol.* **387,** 96–113.
18. Dunnett S. B. and Björklund A. (1999) Prospects for new restorative and neuroprotective treatments in Parkinson's disease. *Nature* **399,** A32–A39.
19. Eriksson, P. S. Perfilieva, E., Bjork-Eriksson, T., Alborn, A. M., Nordborg, C., Peterson, D. A., and Gage, F. H. (1998) Neurogenesis in the adult human hippocampus. *Nat. Med.* **4,** 1313–1317.
20. Johansson, C. B., Svensson, M., Wallstedt, L., Janson, A. M., and Frisen, J. (1999) Neural stem cells in the adult human brain *Exp. Cell Res.* **253,** 733–736.

21. Roy, N. S., Wang, S., Jiang, L, Kang, J., Benraiss, A., Harrison-Restelli, C., et al. (2000) In vitro neurogenesis by progenitor cells isolated from the adult human hippocampus. *Nat. Med.* **6,** 271–277
22. Barker, R. A. and Johnson, A. (1995) Nigral and striatal neurons, in *Neural Cell Culture. A Practical Approach* (Cohen, J. and Wilkin, G. P., eds.), IRL Press, Oxford, pp. 25–39.
23. Svendsen, C. N., Fawcett, J. W., Bentlage, C., and Dunnett, S. B. (1995) Increased survival of rat EGF-generated CNS progenitor cells using B27 supplemented medium. *Exp. Brain Res.* **102,** 407–414.
24. Svendsen, C. N., ter Borg, M. G., Armstrong, R. J. E., Rosser, A. E., Chandran, S., Ostenfeld, T., and Caldwell, M. A. (1998) A new method for the rapid and long term growth of human neural precursor cells. *J. Neurosci. Meth.* **85,** 141–153.
25. Rosser, A. E., Tyers, P., ter Borg, M., Dunnett, S. B., and Svendsen, C. N. (1997) Co-expression of MAP-2 and GFAP in cells developing from rat EGF responsive precursor cells. *Dev. Brain Res.* **98,** 291–295.
26. Bjornson, C. R., Rietze, R. L., Reynolds,B. A., Magli, M. C., and Vescovi, A. L. (1999) Turning brain into blood: a hematopoietic fate adopted by adult neural stem cells *in vivo*. *Science* **283,** 534–537.
27. Studer, L., Tabar, V., and McKay, R. D. G. (1998) Transplantation of expanded mesencephalic precursors leads to recovery in parkinsonion rats. *Nat. Neurosci.* **1,** 290–295.
28. Svendsen, C. N., Caldwell, M. A., Shen, J., terBorg, M. G., Rosser, A. E., Tyers, P., Karmiol, S., and Dunnett SB (1997) Long-term survival of human central nervous system progenitor cells transplanted into a rat model of Parkinson's disease. *Exp. Neurol.* **148,** 135–146.
29. Barker, R. A. and Dunnett, S. B. (1994) Ibotenic acid lesions of the striatum reduce apomorphine and amphetamine induced rotation in the 6-hydroxydopamine lesioned rat. *Exp. Brain Res.* **101,** 365–375.
30. Armstrong, R. J. E., Watts, C., Svendsen, C. N., Dunnett, S. B., and Rosser, A. E. (2000) Survival, neuronal differentiation, and fiber outgrowth of propagated human neural precursor grafts in an animal model of Huntington's disease. *Cell Transplant* **9,** 55–64.
31. Johe, K. K., Hazel, T. G., Muller, T., Dugich-Djordjevic, M. M., and McKay, R. D. (1996) Single factors direct the differentiation of stem cells from the fetal and adult central nervous system. *Genes Dev.* **10,** 3129–3140.
32. Reynolds, B. A. and Weiss, S. (1992) Generation of neurons and astrocytes from isolated cells of the adult mammalian central nervous system. *Science* **255,** 1707–1710.
33. Ray, J., Peterson,D. A., Schinstine, M., and Gage, F. H. (1993) Proliferation, differentiation and long-term culture of primary hippocampal neurons. *Proc. Natl. Acad. Sci. USA* **90,** 3602–3606.
34. Temple, S. (1989) Division and differentiation of isolated CNS blast cells in microculture. *Nature* **340,** 471–473.
35. Svendsen, C. N., Clarke, D. J., Rosser, A. E., and Dunnett, S. B. (1996) Survival and differentiation of rat and human epidermal growth factor-responsive precur-

sor cells following grafting into the lesioned adult central nervous system. *Exp. Neurol.* **137,** 376–388.

36. Chandran, S., Svendsen,C., Compston, A., and Scolding, N. (1998) Regional potential for oligodendrocyte generation in the rodent embryonic spinal cord following exposure to EGF and FGF-2. *Glia* **4,** 382–389.
37. Lendahl, U., Zimmerman, L. B., and McKay, R. D. (1990) CNS stem cells express a new class of intermediate filament protein. *Cell* **60,** 585–595.
38. Krum, J. M. and Rosenstein, J. M. (1999) Transient co-expression of nestin, GFAP and vascular endothelial growth factor in mature reactive astroglia following neural grafting or brain wounds. *Exp. Neurol.* **160,** 348–360.
39. Ling, Z. D., Potter, E. D., Lipton, J. W., and Carvey, P. M. (1998) Differentiation of mesencephalic progenitor cells into dopaminergic neurons by cytokines. *Exp. Neurol.* **149,** 411–423.
40. Daadi, M. M. and Weiss, S. (1999) Generation of tyrosine hydroxylase-producing neurons from precursors of the embryonic and adult forebrain. *J. Neurosci.* **19,** 4484–4497.
41. Takahashi, J., Palmer, T. D., and Gage, F. H. (1999) Retinoic acid and neurotrophins collaborate to regulate neurogenesis in adult-derived neural stem cell cultures. *J Neurobiol.* **38,** 65–81.
42. Tropepe, V., Sibilia, M., Ciruna, B. G., Rossant, J., Wagner, E. F., and van der Kooy, D. (1999) Distinct neural stem cells proliferate in response to EGF and FGF in the developing mouse telencephalon. *Dev. Biol.* **208,** 166–188.
43. Kilpatrick, T. J. and Bartlett, P. F. (1995) Cloned multipotential precursors from the mouse cerebrum require FGF-2, whereas glial restricted precursors are stimulated with either FGF-2 or EGF. *J. Neurosci.* **15,** 3653–3661.
44. Vescovi, A. L., Parati, E. A., Gritti, A., Poulin, P., Ferrario, M., Wanke, E., et al. (1999) Isolation and cloning of multipotential stem cells from the embryonic human CNS and establishment of transplantable human neural stem cell lines by epigenetic stimulation. *Exp. Neurol.* **156,** 71–83.
45. Wagner, J., Akerud, P., Castro, D. S., Holme, P. C., Canals, J. M., Snyder, E., Perlman, T., and Arenas, E. (1999) Induction of a midbrain dopaminergic phenotype in Nurr 1-overexpressing neural stem cells by type 1 astrocytes. *Nat. Biotechnol.* **17,** 653–659.
46. Svendsen, C. N., Skepper, J., Rosser ,A. E., ter Borg, M. G., Tyers, P., and Ryken,T. (1997) Restricted growth potential of rat neural precursors as compared to mouse. *Dev. Brain Res.* **99,** 253–258.
47. Ciccolini, F. and Svendsen, C. N. (1998) Fibroblast growth factor 2 (FGF-2) promotes acquisition of epidermal growth factor (EGF) responsiveness in mouse striatal precursor cells: identification of neural precursors responding to both EGF and FGF-2. *J. Neurosci.* **18,** 7869–7880.
48. Caldwell, M. A. and Svendsen, C. N. (1998) Heparin, but not other proteoglycans potentiates the mitogenic effects of FGF-2 on mesencephalic precursor cells. *Exp. Neurol.* **152,** 1–10.

49. Wechsler-Reya, R. J. and Scott, M. P. (1999) Control of neuronal precursor proliferation in the cerebellum by Sonic Hedgehog. *Neuron* **22,** 103–114.
50. Carpenter, M. K., Cui, X., Hu, Z., Jackson, J., Sherman, S., Seiger, A., and Wahlberg, L. U. (1999) *In vitro* expansion of a multipotent population of human neural progenitor cells. *Exp. Neurol.* **158,** 265–278.
51. Minger, S. L., Fisher, L. J., Ray, J., and Gage, F. H. (1996) Long-term survival of transplanted basal forebrain cells following in vitro propagation with fibroblast growth factor-2. *Exp. Neurol.* **141,** 12–24.
52. Harvey, A. (2000) Labeling and identifying grafted cells, in *Neural Transplantation Methods* (Dunnett, S. B., Boulton, A. A., and Baker, G. B., eds.), Humana Press, Totowa, NJ, pp. 133–139.
53. Winkler, C., Fricker, R. A., Gates, M. A., Olsson, M., Hammang, J. P., Carpenter, M. K., and Bjorklund, A. (1998) Incorporation and glial differentiation of mouse EGF-responsive neural progenitor cells after transplantation into the embryonic rat brain. *Mol. Cell Neurosci.* **11,** 99–116.
54. Brüstle, O., Choudhary, K., Karram, K., Huttner, A., Murray, K., Dubois-Dalcq, M., and McKay R. D. (1998) Chimeric brains generated by intraventricular transplantation of fetal human brain cells into embryonic rats. *Nat. Biotechnol.* **16,** 1040–1044.
55. Flax, J. D., Aurora, S., Yang, C., Simonin, C., Wills, A. M., Billinghurst L. L., et al. (1998) Engraftable human neural stem cells respond to developmental cues, replace neurons, and express foreign genes. *Nat. Biotechnol.* **16,** 1033–1039.
56. Rosser, A. E., Tyers, P., and Dunnett, S. B. (2000) Site-specific neuronal integration of EGF and FGF-2-driven human CNS precursors in the neonatal rat brain. *Eur. J. Neurosci.* **12,** 2405–2413.
57. Corti, O., Sanchez-Capello, A., Colin, P., Dumas, S., Bouchet, D., Buc-Caron, M. H., and Mallet, J. (1999) A single adenovirus vector mediates doxycycline-controlled expression of tyrosine hydroxylase in brain grafts of human neural progenitors. *Nat. Biotechnol.* **17,** 349–354.

Index

From: *Methods in Molecular Medicine, vol. 62, Parkinson's Disease: Methods and Protocols*
Edited by: M. M. Mouradian © Humana Press Inc., Totowa, NJ

E

T